Contraception

EDITED BY

Donna Shoupe
Division of Reproductive Endocrinology
Keck School of Medicine
University of Southern California
Los Angeles, CA, USA

WILEY-BLACKWELL

A John Wiley & Sons, Ltd., Publication

This edition first published 2011, © 2011 by Blackwell Publishing Ltd

Blackwell Publishing was acquired by John Wiley & Sons in February 2007. Blackwell's publishing program has been merged with Wiley's global Scientific, Technical and Medical business to form Wiley-Blackwell.

Registered office: John Wiley & Sons Ltd, The Atrium, Southern Gate, Chichester, West Sussex, PO19 8SQ, UK

Editorial offices: 9600 Garsington Road, Oxford, OX4 2DQ, UK
       The Atrium, Southern Gate, Chichester, West Sussex, PO19 8SQ, UK
       111 River Street, Hoboken, NJ 07030-5774, USA

For details of our global editorial offices, for customer services and for information about how to apply for permission to reuse the copyright material in this book please see our website at www.wiley.com/wiley-blackwell

The contents of this work are intended to further general scientific research, understanding, and discussion only and are not intended and should not be relied upon as recommending or promoting a specific method, diagnosis, or treatment by physicians for any particular patient. The publisher and the author make no representations or warranties with respect to the accuracy or completeness of the contents of this work and specifically disclaim all warranties, including without limitation any implied warranties of fitness for a particular purpose. In view of ongoing research, equipment modifications, changes in governmental regulations, and the constant flow of information relating to the use of medicines, equipment, and devices, the reader is urged to review and evaluate the information provided in the package insert or instructions for each medicine, equipment, or device for, among other things, any changes in the instructions or indication of usage and for added warnings and precautions. Readers should consult with a specialist where appropriate. The fact that an organization or Website is referred to in this work as a citation and/or a potential source of further information does not mean that the author or the publisher endorses the information the organization or Website may provide or recommendations it may make. Further, readers should be aware that Internet Websites listed in this work may have changed or disappeared between when this work was written and when it is read. No warranty may be created or extended by any promotional statements for this work. Neither the publisher nor the author shall be liable for any damages arising herefrom.

Library of Congress Cataloging-in-Publication Data

Contraception / edited by Donna Shoupe, Division of Reproductive Endocrinology, Keck School of Medicine, University of Southern California.
     p. ; cm.—(Gynecology in practice)
  Includes bibliographical references and index.
  ISBN 978-1-4443-3351-0 (pbk. : alk. paper)
  1. Contraception. I. Shoupe, Donna, editor. II. Series: Gynecology in practice.
  [DNLM: 1. Contraception–methods. 2. Contraceptive Agents. 3. Contraceptive Devices. 4. Fertilization–drug effects. WP 630]
  RG136.C557 2011
  613.9′43–dc22

                    2010047407

A catalogue record for this book is available from the British Library.

Set in 10/13pt Utopia by Toppan Best-set Premedia Limited, Hong Kong
Printed and bound in Singapore by Fabulous Printers Pte Ltd

1   2011

Contraception

DATE DUE

Contents

Series Foreword

In recent decades, massive advances in medical science and technology have caused an explosion of information available to the practitioner. In the modern information age, it is not unusual for physicians to have a computer in their offices with the capability of accessing medical databases and literature searches. On the other hand, however, there is always a need for concise, readable, and highly practicable written resources. The purpose of this series is to fulfill this need in the field of gynecology.

The *Gynecology in Practice* series aims to present practical clinical guidance on effective patient care for the busy gynecologist. The goal of each volume is to provide an evidence-based approach for specific gynecologic problems. "Evidence at a glance" features in the text provide summaries of key trials or landmark papers that guide practice, and a selected bibliography at the end of each chapter provides a springboard for deeper reading. Even with a practical approach, it is important to review the crucial basic science necessary for effective diagnosis and management. This is reinforced by "Science revisited" boxes that remind readers of crucial anatomic, physiologic or pharmacologic principles for practice.

Each volume is edited by outstanding international experts who have brought together truly gifted clinicians to address many relevant clinical questions in their chapters. The first volumes in the series are on *Chronic Pelvic Pain*, one of the most challenging problems in gynecology, *Disorders of Menstruation*, *Infertility*, and *Contraception*. These will be followed by volumes on *Sexually Transmitted Diseases*, *Menopause*, *Urinary Incontinence*, *Endoscopic Surgeries*, and *Fibroids*, to name a few. I would like to express my gratitude to all the editors and authors, who, despite their other responsibilities, have contributed their time, effort, and expertise to this series.

Finally, I greatly appreciate the support of the staff at Wiley-Blackwell for their outstanding editorial competence. My special thanks go to Martin Sugden, PhD; without his vision and perseverance, this series would not have come to life. My sincere hope is that this novel and exciting series will serve women and their physicians well, and will be part of the diagnostic and therapeutic armamentarium of practicing gynecologists.

Aydin Arici, MD
Professor
Department of Obstetrics, Gynecology, and
Reproductive Sciences
Yale University School of Medicine
New Haven, USA

Preface

When scanning for topics related to world population it is not surprising that family planning is the first entry. This entry, however, is followed by overpopulation, overconsumption, water crisis, sustainable development, food security, green revolution, world energy resources and consumption. An article entitled "The Day of Six Billion" reviews the world population that reached 1 billion in 1804, 2 billion in 1927, 3 billion in 1960, 4 billion in 1974, 5 billion in 1987, and 6 billion in 1999. Some estimates project that the world will reach 7 billion in 2011–12, 8 billion in 2025, 9 billion in 2040, and 10 billion in 2061. These enormous growths in population would place tremendous strains on world energy and food supplies and incite economical and political conflict.

There is evidence, however, that efforts to curb the population explosion have been effective and that another scenario may instead unfold. The global population growth rate, which reached a peak in 1963 (2.2%), has since been steadily slowing and by 2008 was cut by half. While growth rates remain high in Latin America, the Middle East and Sub-Saharan Africa, some countries, especially in central and eastern Europe, have a negative population growth. Within the next 10 years, Japan and some countries in western Europe are expected to have a negative population growth. If these trends continue, the world growth rate may diminish to zero. Addressing these very different possible scenarios, the United Nation's projections for world population in 2050 ranged from 8 billion to 10.5 billion.

Developed countries have traditionally had much lower fertility rates than developing countries, due to a combination of factors relating to greater wealth, education, and urbanization. Although mortality rates are generally lower in developed countries, birth control options are well known and accessible. Many reproductive-aged women in these countries are motivated to use contraceptive methods as they pursue education or job goals or wish to control spacing and number of children. A variety of private and public sector programs help defray the costs of contraceptives for those with limited financial means, and a barrage of mass media advertisements help educate the general public on contraceptive options.

Advances in contraceptive technology, worldwide availability, and effective dissemination of information regarding contraceptive options will continue to play a vital role in the world's economic and political wellbeing. This book is dedicated to those individuals and organizations that have tirelessly advanced these goals around the world. Over the next decade, the impact of their hard work and dedication will continue to show impact and will help to determine which of the scenarios presented above will unfold.

This book is also dedicated to the authors who were willing to take the time to share their expertise. The authors were asked to write a clinically pertinent chapter and include a list of references at the end of the chapter that could be used by interested readers to further expand their knowledge on particular topics. These authors represent a variety of titles, practices, academic backgrounds, and areas of expertise.

The book is divided into three sections. The first section includes chapters on appropriate selection of contraceptive options and cost comparison of contraceptives. Chapter 1 introduces the new Centers for Disease Control and Prevention medical eligibility criteria adaptation for the United States (the US MEC). Chapter 2 presents a comparison of the 1-, 5-, and 10-year present values of the contraceptives available in the United States. These values include the cost of the method, the medical costs of obtaining the method, and the cost of pregnancy as a result of method failure.

The second section of the book includes chapters on the contraceptive options currently available in the United States, with sections on method of action, good candidates, poor candidates, medical eligibility criteria, advantages, noncontraceptive benefits, risks and side effects, patient counseling, available options, new products, supplying the method, and management of problems. Each of the following methods is addressed separately:

- oral contraceptives
- progestin only contraceptives
- contraceptive implants
- contraceptive vaginal ring
- contraceptive patch
- progestin injectables
- intrauterine devices
- spermicides
- vaginal barriers: diaphragm, cervical cap, and female condom
- male condoms
- emergency contraception
- tubal sterilization

The third section of the book includes chapters on various medical conditions and the risks and benefits associated with various contraceptive options:

- postpartum
- adolescents: compliance, ethical and STD issues
- women 35 years and older: safety issues
- perimenopausal contraception—staging of reproductive aging in women
- medical eligibility criteria—WHO MEC and US MEC
- hormonal contraception and mood—depressive disorders, PMDD and PMS, major depressive disorders, postpartum depression, schizophrenia, bipolar, anxiety and panic disorder
- abnormal uterine bleeding—uniform terminology, structural and nonstructural etiologies
- hirsuitism and acne—causes and patient evaluation, diagnosis and treatment
- HIV and other sexually transmitted infections—antiretroviral interactions with hormonal contraceptives, reducing transmission to partners and fetus
- contraception following ectopic pregnancy or spontaneous or induced abortion.

This book is designed to highlight the important issues surrounding contraceptive technology including safety, lifestyle, costs of method, costs of method failure, noncontraceptive benefits, interaction with various medical conditions, and managing side effects. There is an important emphasis on the WHO MEC and CDC modifications as these are the guidelines important to clinicians.

A final tribute is given to those who excel in contraceptive technology and in all areas of human endeavors.

This comprehensive book includes topics on:
- All of the currently available contraceptive methods in the US including those recently introduced
- WHO Medical Eligibility Criteria for contraceptives and CDC modifications
- Selecting contraceptive methods for women with bleeding problems, previous ectopic pregnancy, mood and depressive disorders, hirsutism and acne, perimenopausal women, women with HIV and other STIs.

An important and useful reference for:
- Contraceptive Healthcare Providers
- Gynecologists
- Family Medicine Physicians
- Nurse practitioners
- Internists
- Physician Assistants

Donna Shoupe
Los Angeles

Contributors

Susan A. Ballagh, MD
Department of Obstetrics and Gynecology, Harbor-UCLA Medical Center, Torrance, CA, USA

Paula H. Bednarek, MD, MPH
Department of Obstetrics and Gynecology, Oregon Health & Science University, Portland, OR, USA

Nerys Benfield, MD
Department of Obstetrics Gynecology and Reproductive Sciences, University of California, San Francisco and San Francisco General Hospital, San Francisco, CA, USA

Timothy Campbell, PhD
Economics and Finance, Marshall School of Business, University of Southern California, USA

Catherine Cansino, MD, MPH
Department of Obstetrics and Gynecology, The Ohio State University, Colombus, OH, USA

Mitchell Creinin, MD
Department of Obstetrics, Gynecology and Reproductive Sciences, University of Pittsburgh School of Medicine and Magee Research Institute Hospital, Pittsburgh, PA, USA

Kathryn M. Curtis, PhD
Division of Reproductive Health, Centers for Disease Control and Prevention, Atlanta, GA, USA

Philip D. Darney, MD, MSC
Department of Obstetrics Gynecology and Reproductive Sciences, University of California, San Francisco and San Francisco General Hospital, San Francisco, CA, USA

Alison B. Edelman, MD, MPH
Department of Obstetrics and Gynecology, Oregon Health & Science University, Portland, OR, USA

Ian S. Fraser, AO, MD
Department of Obstetrics, Gynaecology and Neonatology, Queen Elizabeth II Research Institute for Mothers and Infants, University of Sydney, NSW, Australia

Jeffrey T. Jensen, MD, MPH
Department of Obstetrics and Gynecology and Department of Public Health and Preventive Medicine, Oregon Health and Science University, Portland, OR, USA

Ronna Jurow, MD, MS
Department of Obstetrics and Gynecology, Keck School of Medicine, University of Southern California, USA

Andrew M. Kaunitz, MD
Department of Obstetrics and Gynecology, University of Florida College of Medicine, Jacksonville, FL, USA

Charles M. March, MD
Department of Obstetrics and Gynecology, Keck School of Medicine, University of Southern California, USA

Polly A. Marchbanks, PhD
Division of Reproductive Health, Centers for Disease Control and Prevention, Atlanta, GA, USA

Susanna Meredith, MD
Department of Obstetrics and Gynecology, University of Florida College of Medicine, Jacksonville, FL, USA

Daniel R. Mishell Jr, MD
Division of Reproductive Endocrinology and Infertility, Keck School of Medicine, University of Southern California, USA

Anita L. Nelson, MD
Department of Obstetrics and Gynecology, David Geffen School of Medicine at ULCA and Harbor-UCLA Medical Center, Torrance, CA, USA

Melanie Ochalski, MD
Department of Obstetrics and Gynecology and
Reproductive Sciences, Center for Fertility and
Reproductive Endocrinology, University of
Pittsburgh Physicians, Magee-Womens Hospital,
Pittsburgh, PA, USA

Andrea Rapkin, MD
Department of Obstetrics and Gynecology,
David Geffen School of Medicine at UCLA, Los
Angeles, CA, USA

Matthew F. Reeves, MD, MPH
Medical Affairs, WomanCare Global, Chapel
Hill, NC, USA

Regina-Maria Renner, MD, MPH
Department of Obstetrics and Gynecology,
Oregon Health and Science University, Portland,
OR, USA

Frans J.M.E. Roumen, MD, PhD
Department of Obstetrics and Gynaecology,
Atrium Medical Centre Parkstad, Heerlen, The
Netherlands

Jennefer A. Russo, MD
Department of Obstetrics, Gynecology, and
Reproductive Sciences, University of Pittsburgh
Medical Center, Magee-Womens Hospital,
Pittsburgh, PA, USA

Joseph S. Sanfilippo, MD, MBA
Department of Obstetrics and Gynecology and
Reproductive Sciences, Center for Fertility and
Reproductive Endocrinology, University of
Pittsburgh Physicians, Magee-Womens Hospital,
Pittsburgh, PA, USA

Jill L. Schwartz, MD, MPH
Department of Obstetrics and Gynecology,
Eastern Virginia Medical School, Arlington, VA,
USA

Donna Shoupe, MD
Division of Reproductive Endocrinology and
Infertility, Keck School of Medicine, University
of Southern California, CA, USA

Sarita Sonalkar, MD
Department of Obstetrics and Gynecology,
Boston University School of Medicine, Boston,
MA, USA

Stephanie B. Teal, MD, MPH
Department of Obstetrics and Gynecology,
University of Colorado Denver School of
Medicine, Aurora, CO, USA

Naomi K. Tepper, MD, MPH
Division of Reproductive Health, Centers for
Disease Control and Prevention, Atlanta, GA,
USA

Alice Stek, MD
Department of Obstetrics and Gynecology, Keck
School of Medicine, University of Southern
California, Los Angeles, CA, USA

DeShawn L. Taylor, MD, MSc
Department of Obstetrics and Gynecology, Keck
School of Medicine, University of Southern
California, Los Angeles, CA, USA

Section 1

Overview

Contraceptive Use: Guidelines and Effectiveness

Kathryn M. Curtis, Naomi K. Tepper, and Polly A. Marchbanks

Division of Reproductive Health, Centers for Disease Control and Prevention, Atlanta, USA

Introduction

Clinicians are now able to rely on evidence-based guidelines to efficiently incorporate scientific evidence into clinical practice regarding appropriate selection and use of specific contraceptive methods.

Contraceptive effectiveness is also an important factor in contraceptive choice; tools are available to assist providers in communicating contraceptive effectiveness to family planning patients.

Evidence-based guidelines

As the volume of scientific literature rapidly expands, it has become increasingly difficult for individual clinicians to keep up with finding, reading, and interpreting new evidence to put into practice. A PubMed search using the terms "contraception" and "family planning" yielded an average of 130 new articles per month in 2010. Many clinicians rely on evidence-based guidelines to efficiently use the best scientific evidence when making decisions about patient care.

EVIDENCE AT A GLANCE

- The World Health Organization's evidence-based guidance on contraceptive use (WHO Medical Eligibility Criteria for Contraceptive Use (MEC)) is used around the world and has been adapted by several countries, including the United States.
- The Centers for Disease Control and Prevention (CDC) has recently adapted the WHO MEC for use in the United States (US MEC). While the vast majority of the CDC recommendations are identical to the WHO recommendations, some adaptations were made to more accurately focus on methods currently available in the USA, and to better reflect the surgical and medical practices of the USA *(see also Chapter 21).*
- Additional sources of guidance include the National Guidelines Clearinghouse, professional organizations, and international groups.

Clinical practice guidelines have been defined by the Institute of Medicine as "systematically developed statements to assist practitioner and patient decisions about appropriate healthcare for specific clinical circumstances."

EVIDENCE AT A GLANCE

Guidelines that are based on a critical appraisal of the scientific literature, most often through systematic reviews and meta-analyses, are considered "evidence-based guidelines," and have the advantage of

Contraception, First Edition. Edited by Donna Shoupe.

Table 1.1 Elements to consider when choosing an evidence-based clinical practice guideline

1 *Validity*

   a *Scientific evidence:* Were rigorous systematic reviews of the scientific literature conducted and used as the basis of the recommendations, including systematic search of the literature, critical appraisal and grading of the evidence according to some standard grading system, availability of the references and systematic reviews to the users of the guideline?

   b *Decision-making:* Are the methods for translating the evidence to recommendations clearly described?

   c *Benefits and risks:* Are the expected health benefits, potential harms, and alternative interventions described?

2 *Reliability/reproducibility:* Was the guideline sent to external experts for peer review? Has the guideline been piloted or pretested in a clinical setting? Has the process of the guideline development been documented?

3 *Clinical applicability:* Do the goals and rationale of the guideline meet your clinical needs? Is the guideline intended for your patient population and your provider type?

4 *Clinical flexibility:* Does the guideline allow for flexibility in its application? Are patient choices considered?

5 *Clarity:* Is the guideline clearly worded and easy to use?

6 *Scheduled review:* Is the date the guideline was issued included, along with a plan for scheduled review?

7 *Development team:* Did the guideline development team include representatives of all relevant disciplines? Was there consideration of any potential conflicts of interest among the development team, and are the sources of funding clearly documented?

8 *Implementation, dissemination, and evaluation:* Is there a clear plan for implementation, dissemination, and evaluation of the guideline?

Adapted from Vlayen J, Aertgeerts B, Hannes K, Sermeus W, Ramaekers D. A systematic review of appraisal tools for clinical practice guidelines: multiple similarities and one common deficit. Int J Qual Health Care 2005;17:235–42.

linking the recommendation to the scientific evidence.

Evidence-based guidelines are intended to be "assistive rather than directive," and are not meant to replace clinical judgment.

While clinical guidelines can be an efficient way for clinicians to practice evidence-based medicine, these guidelines can be difficult to find; conversely, there may be multiple guidelines on a single topic, perhaps with conflicting recommendations.

Several appraisal systems for clinical guidelines exist, but many of these systems are aimed at organizations that want to undertake a guidelines appraisal process prior to adopting a guideline for their members, rather than at individual clinicians.

Vlayen et al. have proposed 10 dimensions to be considered in any guideline appraisal instrument. We have adapted those 10 dimensions to suggest elements that individual practitioners may want to consider when assessing clinical guidelines for use in their practice (Table 1.1).

Family planning providers frequently face difficult decisions with their patients in the provision of contraceptive methods and management of their use. Because of these challenges, there is a critical need for the use of evidence-based medicine and decision-making in the field of family planning practice.

Development of WHO evidence-based guidance for contraceptive use

In the early 1990s, the Department of Reproductive Health and Research at WHO began addressing the need for evidence-based contraceptive guidance. WHO, the US Agency for International Development (USAID) and others were concerned about unnecessary medical barriers to contraceptive access that were not based on scientific evidence. There was particular concern about medical conditions or other characteristics that were unjustifiably perceived by providers as contraindications to contraceptive use. To address these issues, WHO developed the *Medical Eligibility Criteria for Contraceptive Use* (WHO MEC), first published in 1996, with the intent of improving access to, and quality of, family planning services. This guidance document is currently in its fourth edition and provides recommendations on whether women and men with specific medical conditions and characteristics can safely use various contraceptive methods; for example, whether a woman with hypertension can use combined oral contraceptives or an adolescent can use depot medroxyprogesterone acetate (DMPA).

Currently, the WHO MEC contains recommendations for 18 contraceptive methods and over 160 medical conditions or characteristics. Each medical condition and contraceptive method combination is given a classification from 1 to 4 (Table 1.2), denoting whether or not the contraceptive method is safe to use for women or men with that medical condition or characteristic.

WHO also publishes the *Selected Practice Recommendations for Contraceptive Use* (WHO SPR) that addresses common clinical management questions for contraception. The WHO SPR currently contains 33 evidence-based questions and answers, such as when a woman can start a contraceptive method and when she needs to use a back-up method, what a woman can do if she misses oral contraceptive pills, and what tests or examinations need to be done prior to initiating a method of contraception.

In addition to these two evidence-based guidance documents, WHO also developed two documents that are intended for direct use by family planning providers.

- The *Decision-Making Tool for Family Planning Clients and Providers* is a flip chart meant to assist clients and providers in choosing a method of contraception.

Table 1.2 US Medical Eligibility Criteria for Contraceptive Use Classifications

Classification	Definition
1	No restriction for the use of the contraceptive method
2	The advantages of using the method generally outweigh the theoretical or proven risks
3	The theoretical or proven risks usually outweigh the advantages of using the method
4	An unacceptable health risk if the contraceptive method is used

Source: US Medical Eligibility Criteria for Contraceptive Use, 2010.

- *Family Planning: A Global Handbook for Family Planning Providers* provides a wide range of technical information to assist providers in delivering quality family planning services.

These four documents make up WHO's Four Cornerstones of Family Planning Guidance.

EVIDENCE AT A GLANCE

Both the WHO MEC and the WHO SPR are meant to be used by policy-makers and program managers when developing local clinical guidelines and protocols.

From the beginning, WHO had a vision of guidance based on the best available scientific evidence. The Centers for Disease Control and Prevention (CDC) has worked closely with WHO in identifying the evidence on which the guidance is based. In 2002, WHO, CDC, and the Johns Hopkins Bloomberg School of Public Health developed the Continuous Identification of Research Evidence (CIRE) system to facilitate ongoing identification of scientific evidence relevant to the WHO guidance, conduct of systematic reviews and meta-analyses, and peer review. The CIRE system enables WHO to meet the need of keeping up with the enormous amount of evidence that is produced, but, more importantly, it allows WHO to have an ongoing assessment of whether its recommendations remain consistent with the scientific evidence and facilitates updating the guidance when the evidence warrants.

CDC adaptation of WHO evidence-based guidance for contraceptive use

More recently, CDC has adapted the WHO MEC for use in the United States (US MEC). WHO has always intended for its global guidance to be adapted at the local level for best implementation. Many countries have undertaken various degrees of adaptation, with the United Kingdom as one example of a country having undergone a formal adaptation process.

CDC began its adaptation process by convening a small group of US family planning experts to discuss the need for an adaptation for the United States, the process for such an adaptation, and the scope of the adaptation.

EVIDENCE AT A GLANCE

Because the scientific evidence is the same globally and because CDC had collaborated closely with WHO in the development of the WHO guidance, CDC decided that most of the WHO guidance would be taken directly for use in the United States. Only those recommendations for which there was a compelling reason, either based on new scientific evidence or on the context of family planning provision in the United States, would be considered for adaptation.

The addition of new medical conditions was also considered. Based on a review of existing guidance on medical eligibility criteria from professional and service organizations in the United States, input from key family planning providers, and careful review of the WHO guidance by a small group of experts, six existing WHO recommendations for possible adaptation and six additional medical conditions that could be added were identified. Systematic reviews of the scientific evidence on these 12 topics were conducted and peer reviewed by experts in the United States. CDC then convened a larger meeting of experts, during which the scientific evidence was discussed and draft recommendations were made. Research gaps in the areas addressed were also identified.

The outcome of this meeting was the US *Medical Eligibility Criteria for Contraceptive Use, 2010* (US MEC), published in the series of CDC Morbidity and Mortality Weekly Report (MMWR) Recommendations and Reports.

The vast majority of the CDC recommendations are identical to the WHO recommendations; an example of the guidance is given in Table 1.3. However, some adaptation was made for each of the existing recommendations considered and new recommendations were added for each of the new topics discussed (Table 1.4).

In addition, recommendations for contraceptive methods not currently available in the United States (i.e., levonorgestrel implants, combined injectables, and norethisterone enantate injectables) were removed. Specific recommendations around appropriate settings for female and male sterilization were removed, as many of these do not apply to surgical practice in the United States, although general text about sterilization is included.

Once a clinical guideline is produced, dissemination, implementation, and evaluation of the guideline are essential. A critical component of CDC's dissemination and implementation plan was working closely with partners who provide family planning services or who represent family planning providers in order to effectively disseminate and implement this new guidance.

★ TIPS & TRICKS

The US MEC is available on CDC's website (Table 1.5) in several different formats, along with tools and job aids for providers, speaker presentations, and any updates that are made based on new scientific evidence.

Additional implementation activities include the development of training curricula for different providers and incorporating the guidance into existing clinical standards and guidelines used by various organizations.

Evaluation activities include baseline and follow-up surveys of attitudes and practices among family planning providers, keeping track of where the guidance has been incorporated

Table 1.3 Example of recommendations from US MEC

Condition	COC/P/R	POP	DMPA	Implants	LNG-IUD	Cu-IUD
Smoking						
Age <35	2	1	1	1	1	1
Age ≥35						
<15 cigarettes/day	3	1	1	1	1	1
≥15 cigarettes/day	4	1	1	1	1	1

COC, combined oral contraceptives; P, patch; R, ring: POP, progestin-only pills; DMPA, depot medroxyprogesterone acetate; LNG-IUD, levonorgestrel-releasing intrauterine device; Cu-IUD, copper intrauterine device.
Key:
1 A condition for which there is no restriction for the use of the contraceptive method.
2 A condition where the advantages of using the method generally outweigh the theoretical or proven risks.
3 A condition where the theoretical or proven risks usually outweigh the advantages of using the method.
4 A condition which represents an unacceptable health risk if the contraceptive method is used.

Table 1.4 Topics considered in the US MEC

Existing WHO recommendations adapted for the US MEC	Additional medical conditions added to the US MEC
Breastfeeding and hormonal contraception	Rheumatoid arthritis
Valvular heart disease and IUDs	Endometrial hyperplasia
Postpartum IUD insertion	Inflammatory bowel disease
Ovarian cancer and IUDs	Bariatric surgery
Fibroids and IUDs	Transplantation
DVT/PE and hormonal contraception	Peripartum cardiomyopathy

into clinical practice, and feedback from individual providers and organizations.

A critical component of any evidence-based guidance document is ensuring that guidance is kept up to date through some mechanism of identifying new scientific evidence as it is published, critically appraising that new evidence, and modifying recommendations when the evidence warrants. CDC will continue to use the CIRE system to facilitate this process, and coordinate with WHO on any changes to their guidance, as well as monitoring the evidence and need to refine the US-specific recommendations.

Finally, as with any evidence-based guidance, many of the recommendations could benefit from more or higher-quality evidence. Research gaps pertaining to the WHO and US MEC have been identified and hopefully new research will be conducted to answer these critical questions.

Sources of evidence-based guidelines

There are several additional sources of contraceptive guidance that family planning providers may find useful (Table 1.5).

- The National Guidance Clearinghouse, an initiative of the Agency for Healthcare Research and Quality (AHRQ), is a publicly available and searchable repository for evidence-based guidelines. A recent search using the term "contraception" yielded 114 guidance documents.
- Professional organizations in the United States, such as the American College of Obstetricians and Gynecologists (ACOG), develop guidance for their members and can be a source of guidance for providers.
- In addition, several professional organizations in other countries have evidence-based guidance that may be useful for US providers. For example, the Faculty of Sexual and Reproductive Healthcare in the United Kingdom has several evidence-based guidance documents, in addition to its own adaptations of WHO guidance.

Table 1.5 Websites for sources of evidence-based guidelines

World Health Organization Contraceptive Guidance	www.who.int/reproductivehealth/topics/family_planning/guidelines/en/index.html
United States Medical Eligibility Criteria for Contraceptive Use	www.cdc.gov/reproductivehealth/UnintendedPregnancy/USMEC.htm
National Guidelines Clearinghouse	www.guideline.gov
American College of Obstetricians and Gynecologists	www.acog.org
Faculty of Family Planning and Reproductive Health Care of the Royal College of Obstetricians and Gynecologists, United Kingdom	www.ffprhc.org.uk/
Society of Obstetricians and Gynaecologists of Canada	www.sogc.org/guidelines/#Contraception
Guidelines for the Use of Antiretroviral Agents in HIV-1-Infected Adults and Adolescents	http://aidsinfo.nih.gov/contentfiles/AdultandAdolescentGL.pdf
HIV Drug Interactions, University of Liverpool, United Kingdom	www.hiv-druginteractions.org

- The Society of Obstetricians and Gynaecologists of Canada recently developed guidance for missed hormonal contraceptives.
- Finally, there are other resources that address specific concerns regarding contraceptive use for women with specific medical conditions, such as drug interactions between hormonal contraceptives and antiretroviral therapies among women with HIV/AIDS.

Contraceptive effectiveness

Medical eligibility is only one factor among many that women, couples, and their providers need to consider when choosing a contraceptive method. Cost, risk of sexually transmitted infections, future fertility desires, and patient preference must all be considered as well. One of the most important factors to consider is the effectiveness of the contraceptive method. Any method that is chosen, if not effective for that particular woman, may lead to an unintended pregnancy.

EVIDENCE AT A GLANCE

- Contraceptive effectiveness has been shown to be one of the most important factors considered by women when choosing a method of contraception.

The terms "efficacy" and "effectiveness" are often used interchangeably, but they refer to different concepts. The *efficacy* of a method refers to the reduction in pregnancy caused by use of the method under ideal circumstances and reflects properties of the method itself. The *effectiveness* of a method refers to the reduction in pregnancy caused by use of the method in the real world and reflects properties of the method as well as the user. Both measures need to be considered; however, for the woman facing the contraceptive choice, effectiveness is likely to be the more relevant concern. This does not necessarily imply failure of the method, however.

Almost half of unintended pregnancies result while women are using contraception. The effectiveness of a method is reported as the pregnancy rate during use of that method and is influenced by four factors: (1) capacity to conceive, (2) frequency and timing of intercourse, (3) degree of compliance (i.e., correct and consistent use), and (4) inherent protection of the method. All of these factors should be taken into consideration when discussing method choice for a particular woman.

The distinction between perfect use and typical use is important when assessing the efficacy and effectiveness of contraceptive methods. Perfect use describes the correct and consistent use of the method. Typical use describes how the method is used in the real world. Table 1.6 shows the percentage of women using each method who experienced an unintended pregnancy

Table 1.6 Percentage of women in the United States experiencing an unintended pregnancy during the first year of typical use and the first year of perfect use of contraception and the percentage continuing use at the end of the first year

| Method | % of women experiencing an unintended pregnancy within the first year of use | | % of women continuing use at 1 year[c] |
	Typical use[a]	Perfect use[b]	
No method[d]	85	85	—
Spermicides[e]	29	18	42
Withdrawal	27	4	43
Fertility awareness-based methods[f]	25	—	51
Standard Days method	—	5	—
TwoDay method	—	4	—
Ovulation method	—	3	—
Sponge			
Parous women	32	20	46
Nulliparous women	16	9	57
Diaphragm[g]	16	6	57
Condom[h]			
Female (Reality)	21	5	49
Male	15	2	53
Combined pill and progestin-only pill	8	0.3	68
Evra patch	8	0.3	68
NuvaRing	8	0.3	68
Depo-Provera	3	0.3	56
IUD			
ParaGard (copper T)	0.8	0.6	78
Mirena (LNG-IUS)	0.2	0.2	80
Implanon	0.05	0.05	84
Female sterilization	0.5	0.5	100
Male sterilization	0.15	0.10	100
Emergency contraceptive pills[i]	Treatment initiated within 72 hours after unprotected intercourse reduces the risk of pregnancy by at least 75%		
Lactational amenorrhea method[j]	LAM is a highly effective, *temporary* method of contraception.		

[a] Among *typical* couples who initiate use of a method (not necessarily for the first time), the percentage who experience an accidental pregnancy during the first year if they do not stop use for any other reason. Estimates of the probability of pregnancy during the first year of typical use for spermicides, withdrawal, fertility awareness-based methods, the diaphragm, the male condom, the pill, and Depo-Provera are taken from the 1995 National Survey of Family Growth corrected for under-reporting of abortion; see the text for the derivation of estimates for the other methods.

[b] Among couples who initiate use of a method (not necessarily for the first time) and who use it *perfectly* (both consistently and correctly), the percentage who experience an accidental pregnancy during the first year if they do not stop use for any other reason. See the text for the derivation of the estimate for each method.

(Continued)

Table 1.6 *Footnote continued*

[c]Among couples attempting to avoid pregnancy, the percentage who continue to use a method for 1 year.

[d]The percentages becoming pregnant in columns 2 and 3 are based on data from populations where contraception is not used and from women who cease using contraception in order to become pregnant. Among such populations, about 89% become pregnant within 1 year. This estimate was lowered slightly (to 85%) to represent the percentage who would become pregnant within 1 year among women now relying on reversible methods of contraception if they abandoned contraception altogether.

[e]Foams, creams, gels, vaginal suppositories, and vaginal film.

[f]The Ovulation and TwoDay methods are based on evaluation of cervical mucus. The Standard Days method avoids intercourse on cycle days 8–19.

[g]With spermicidal cream or jelly.

[h]Without spermicides.

[i]The treatment schedule is one dose within 120 hours after unprotected intercourse, and a second dose 12 hours after the first dose. Both doses of Plan B can be taken at the same time. Plan B (1 dose is 1 white pill) is the only dedicated product specifically marketed for emergency contraception. The Food and Drug Administration has in addition declared the following 22 brands of oral contraceptives to be safe and effective for emergency contraception: Ogestrel or Ovral (1 dose is 2 white pills), Levlen or Nordette (1 dose is 4 light-orange pills), Cryselle, Levora, Low-Ogestrel, Lo/Ovral, or Quasence (1 dose is 4 white pills), Tri-Levlen or Triphasil (1 dose is 4 yellow pills), Jolessa, Portia, Seasonale, or Trivora (1 dose is 4 pink pills), Seasonique (1 dose is 4 light-blue-green pills), Empresse (one dose is 4 orange pills), Alesse, Lessina, or Levlite, (1 dose is 5 pink pills), Aviane (one dose is 5 orange pills), and Lutera (one dose is 5 white pills).

[j]However, to maintain effective protection against pregnancy, another method of contraception must be used as soon as menstruation resumes, the frequency or duration of breastfeeds is reduced, bottle feeds are introduced, or the baby reaches 6 months of age.

Source: Trussell J. Contraceptive efficacy. In Hatcher RA, Trussell J, Nelson AL, Cates W, Stewart FH, Kowal D. *Contraceptive Technology: 19th Revised Edition.* New York NY: Ardent Media, 2007.

within the first year of use, separated by perfect use and typical use. Most estimates shown in this table for typical use were derived from the 1995 National Surveys of Family Growth (NSFG) and are therefore nationally representative samples. The estimates reported for perfect use were derived from published studies of those methods. This table highlights the fact that pregnancy rates can vary widely when perfect use and typical use are compared; however, methods that are less user-dependent (such as implants, intrauterine devices, or sterilization) will have typical use rates approaching perfect use rates.

Although effectiveness is an important factor in determining a contraceptive method, many people typically do not have strong background knowledge of effectiveness. Therefore, in order that women, men, and couples truly make an informed choice, healthcare providers must communicate effectiveness in a way that maximizes understanding.

Studies examining the best way to communicate to individuals facing medical decisions have shown that simple aids perform the best. When assessing different ways to communicate contraceptive effectiveness, simple charts comparing one method to another perform better than more complicated charts showing pregnancy rates for each individual method. These charts allow women to focus on understanding the effectiveness of one method relative to another.

Figure 1.1 shows a chart developed by WHO, showing contraceptive methods on a continuum from less effective to more effective. This chart can be helpful in the decision-making process, and can be used as one piece of the larger puzzle, taking into account other factors such as medical conditions, frequency of intercourse, noncontraceptive benefits, and personal preferences. The best method of contraception for a woman is one that she will use correctly and consistently.

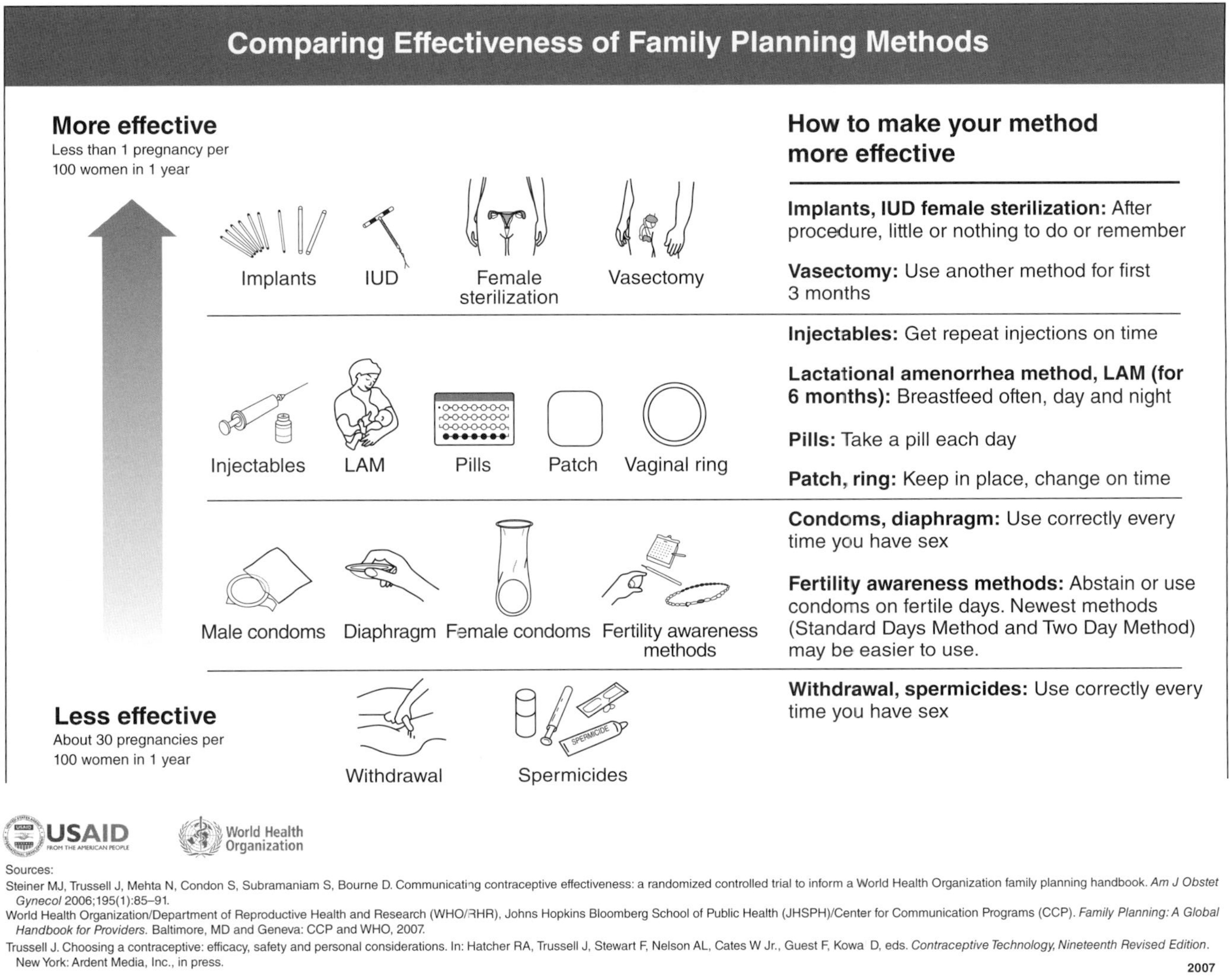

Comparing Effectiveness of Family Planning Methods

More effective
Less than 1 pregnancy per 100 women in 1 year

Implants Injectables IUD Female sterilization Vasectomy

LAM Diaphragm Pills Patch Vaginal ring

Male condoms Female condoms Fertility awareness methods

Withdrawal Spermicides

Less effective
About 30 pregnancies per 100 women in 1 year

How to make your method more effective

Implants, IUD female sterilization: After procedure, little or nothing to do or remember

Vasectomy: Use another method for first 3 months

Injectables: Get repeat injections on time

Lactational amenorrhea method, LAM (for 6 months): Breastfeed often, day and night

Pills: Take a pill each day

Patch, ring: Keep in place, change on time

Condoms, diaphragm: Use correctly every time you have sex

Fertility awareness methods: Abstain or use condoms on fertile days. Newest methods (Standard Days Method and Two Day Method) may be easier to use.

Withdrawal, spermicides: Use correctly every time you have sex

USAID World Health Organization

Sources:
Steiner MJ, Trussell J, Mehta N, Condon S, Subramaniam S, Bourne D. Communicating contraceptive effectiveness: a randomized controlled trial to inform a World Health Organization family planning handbook. *Am J Obstet Gynecol* 2006;195(1):85–91.
World Health Organization/Department of Reproductive Health and Research (WHO/RHR), Johns Hopkins Bloomberg School of Public Health (JHSPH)/Center for Communication Programs (CCP). *Family Planning: A Global Handbook for Providers.* Baltimore, MD and Geneva: CCP and WHO, 2007.
Trussell J. Choosing a contraceptive: efficacy, safety and personal considerations. In: Hatcher RA, Trussell J, Stewart F, Nelson AL, Cates W Jr., Guest F, Kowa D, eds. *Contraceptive Technology, Nineteenth Revised Edition.* New York: Ardent Media, Inc., in press.

2007

Figure 1.1 Comparing effectiveness of family planning methods. Source: World Health Organization Department of Reproductive Health and Research (WHO/RHR) and Johns Hopkins Bloomberg School of Public Health/Center for Communication Programs (CCP) IP. Family Planning: A Global Handbook for Providers. Baltimore and Geneva: CCP and WHO; 2007.

Disclaimer

The findings and conclusions in this report are those of the authors and do not necessarily represent the official position of the Centers for Disease Control and Prevention.

Selected references

Centers for Disease Control and Prevention. United States Medical Eligibility Criteria for Contraceptive Use, 2010. MMWR 2010;59 (No. RR-4):1–85.

Feder G, Eccles M, Grol R, Griffiths C, Grimshaw J. Clinical guidelines: using clinical guidelines. BMJ 1999;318:728–30.

Finer LB, Henshaw SK. Disparities in rates of unintended pregnancy in the United States, 1994 and 2001. Perspect Sex Reprod Health 2006;38:90–6.

Fu H, Darroch JE, Haas T, Ranjit N. Contraceptive failure rates: new estimates from the 1995 National Survey of Family Growth. Fam Plann Perspect 1999;31:56–63.

Grimes DA. Evidence-based family planning: the paradigm for the third millennium. Eur J Contracept Reprod Health Care 2000;5:287–94.

Mohllajee AP, Curtis KM, Flanagan RG, Rinehart W, Gaffield ML, Peterson HB. Keeping up with evidence a new system for WHO's evidence-based family planning guidance. Am J Prev Med 2005;28:483–90.

Sackett DL, Rosenberg WM, Gray JA, Haynes RB, Richardson WS. Evidence based medicine: what it is and what it isn't. BMJ 1996;312:71–2.

Shaneyfelt TM, Centor RM. Reassessment of clinical practice guidelines: go gently into that good night. JAMA 2009;301:868–9.

Shelton JD, Angle MA, Jacobstein RA. Medical barriers to access to family planning. Lancet 1992;340:1334–5.

Steiner M, Dominik R, Trussell J, Hertz-Picciott I. Measuring contraceptive effectiveness: a conceptual framework. Obstet Gynecol 1996;88:24S-30S.

Steiner MJ, Trussell J, Mehta N, Condon S, Subramaniam S, Bourne D. Communicating contraceptive effectiveness: A randomized controlled trial to inform a World Health Organization family planning handbook. Am J Obstet Gynecol 2006;195:85–91.

Stephen G, Brechin S, Glasier A. Using formal consensus methods to adapt World Health Organization Medical Eligibility Criteria for contraceptive use. Contraception 2008;78: 300–8.

Trussell J. Choosing a contraceptive: efficacy, safety, and personal considerations. In: Hatcher RA, Trussell J, Nelson A, Cates W Jr, Stewart FH, Kowal D, eds. Contraceptive technology, 19th ed. New York: Ardent Media, Inc.; 2007. pp. 19–47.

Vlayen J, Aertgeerts B, Hannes K, Sermeus W, Ramaekers D. A systematic review of appraisal tools for clinical practice guidelines: multiple similarities and one common deficit. Int J Qual Health Care 2005;17:235–42.

Woolf SH, Grol R, Hutchinson A, Eccles M, Grimshaw J. Clinical guidelines: potential benefits, limitations, and harms of clinical guidelines. BMJ 1999;318:527–30.

WHO. Selected practice recommendations for contraceptive use: 2008 update. Available from: http://www.who.int/reproductive-health/publications/spr/spr_2008_update.pdf.

WHO. Medical eligibility criteria for contraceptive use, 4th ed. Geneva: World Health Organization; 2009.

WHO and Johns Hopkins Bloomberg School of Public Health Center for Communication Programs (CCP). Decision-making tool for family planning clients and providers. Baltimore, Maryland: CCP and Geneva: World Health Organization; 2005.

WHO/RHR and Johns Hopkins Bloomberg School of Public Health/Center for Communication Programs. Family planning: a global handbook for providers. Baltimore, Maryland: CCP and Geneva: WHO; 2007.

Cost and Availability of Contraceptive Methods

Donna Shoupe[1] and Timothy Campbell[2]

[1]Division of Reproductive Endocrinology and Infertility, Keck School of Medicine, University of Southern California, USA
[2]Economics and Finance, Marshall School of Business, University of Southern California, USA

Selecting the right contraceptive method

This chapter presents a comparison of the effectiveness and the costs of a broad selection of contraceptive methods currently available to U.S. women. Of course cost is not the only consideration in the choice of contraceptives. A typical U.S. woman spends about 40 years of her life managing her fertility. For most of these years, women are choosing a contraceptive method that fits their lifestyle, income, and age. Other considerations in this selection process may include an ever increasing list of factors including efficacy, noncontraceptive benefits, ease of use, side effects, reversibility, cooperation of a partner, religious beliefs, risk of acquiring a sexually transmitted disease (STD), availability of medical coverage, and personal medical problems. But increasingly, cost is an important consideration (Table 2.1).

EVIDENCE AT A GLANCE

The costs considered in this chapter include the initial and ongoing cost of the device and the medical services to install or prescribe as well as the expected cost of pregnancy, taking into account the probability the chosen method will not be effective. The primary conclusions, documented below, are:

- All contraceptives are cost-effective when used in a typical fashion.
- Effective methods of contraception are highly cost-effective over time.
- The consistent and proper use of any user-dependent method profoundly affects the cost-effectiveness of the method.
- For sexually active women at risk of pregnancy, using no method of contraception is the highest-cost option.

The most popular contraceptive choice for U.S. women is the oral contraceptive pill (OCP) (Table 2.2). The OCP has a high efficacy if taken properly, a well-known daily schedule of intake, and a constant monthly cost. Permanent sterilization is the second most common contraceptive method, but is limited to those women who have completed their family. The male condom is the third most widely used method of contraception: it is inexpensive to purchase and easy to find.

In a typical population, the high failure rates of the male condom and other barrier methods result in a relatively low cost-effectiveness. Even though injectable, intrauterine device (IUD), and implant methods have high efficacy, low maintenance demands, and low long-term cost, they attract a small (but growing) percentage of users.

Contraception, First Edition. Edited by Donna Shoupe.
© 2011 Blackwell Publishing Ltd. Published 2011 by Blackwell Publishing Ltd.

Table 2.1 Factors that may be factors to consider when selecting the best contraceptive method

Efficacy	Importance of using method with "near zero" failure
Costs	Income/access to medical insurance or public assistance
Costs relating to method	Upfront cost of method and required medical visits to get method
	Insertion or surgical cost/removal cost
	Ongoing monthly costs
	Method cost/required ongoing medical exams/visits
	Costs of method failure
	High cost of continuing pregnancy
	Lower costs of emergency contraception or termination
	Costs due to side effects
	Extra medical visits for complication, medications, or sanitary supplies
	Complications of insertion/surgery
	Savings due to contraceptive and noncontraceptive benefits
	Fewer medical visits, medications, or sanitary supplies
	Fewer hospitalizations, surgery
Personal lifestyle issues	Cooperation of partner to use method or avoid contact at specific times
	Option for male sterilization
	Personal ability and willingness to plan for sex
	Risk of STIs and need for protection/monogamous relationship
	Whether or when pregnancy is desired
	Useful life of product
	Reversibility of method/speed of reversibility of method
	Regularity of menstrual cycles
	Ability to accurately tract cycles and avoid contact
	Choice on what would happen with a method failure: maintained or terminated
	Opinion on using emergency contraception and ability to keep it available
	Religious constraints
	Fertility potential
	Frequency of sex
	Age/years until perimenopause/menopause
	Known infertility factors
Ease of use	Comfort level with using/inserting a contraceptive device
	Ability to follow directions and comply with treatment requirements
	Ability and willingness to keep ongoing healthcare visits
Side effects	Attitude toward altering natural bleeding patterns
	Attitude towards a method that alters sexual experience
	Method side effects
	Hormonal side effects
	Device related problems/vaginal irritation, discharge, infection or presence of device/string
Noncontraceptive benefits of method	Presence of acne
	Problems with PMS, PMDD, cyclic mood swings
	Problems with irregular or heavy bleeding /Benefit of lighter or less frequent menses
	Presence of pelvic pain associated with endometriosis
	Problems with ovarian cyst formation
	Need of STI protection
	Catamenial problems

Table 2.1 *Continued*

Safety/health status	Cardiovascular risk factors
	Smoking, hypertension, longstanding diabetes, known vascular disease
	Migraines with or without aura or localizing signs
	Age over 35 with other factors
	Obesity
	Other medical problems
	Allergies
	Side effects from previous use of method

PMS, premenstrual syndrome; PMDD premenstrual dysphoric disorder; STI, sexually transmitted infection.

Table 2.2 Contraceptive choices in the United States

Contraceptive method	% of market
Pill	30.6
Tubal ligation	27.0
Male condom	18.0
Vasectomy	9.2
Injectable	5.3
Withdrawal	4.0
IUD	2.0
Natural family planning	1.6
Implant	1.2
Diaphragm	0.3
Other methods	0.9

Adapted from Mosher WD et al., Use of contraception and use of family planning services in the United States: 1982–2002. National Center for Health Statistics. Vital Health Stat Series No. 350. 2004.

Condoms and other barrier methods

Barrier methods are the oldest and most widely used contraceptives in the world. They include male and female condoms, spermicides (gel/jelly/foams/films/suppository/cream), cervical caps/shields, diaphragms, and contraceptive sponges.

Male condoms are inexpensive and generally cost less than $1 per condom. They are available in a variety of styles and are sold without prescription in drugstores and some bathroom vending machines. The cost of spermicides is around $1–2 per use. The cost per year of using a male condom with spermicide averages $166–249, assuming 83 acts of intercourse per woman per year. Female condoms are also available over the counter in drugstores and some supermarkets for $2.50–5.00 each. Diaphragms require a medical visit and fitting ($100–200) and generally cost from $15–75. Cervical caps also require a medical visit but do not require a fitting and are slightly more expensive than diaphragms ($60–70) plus the cost of spermicide ($1–2 per use). Only one contraceptive sponge ($2–3) is made in the United States but other foreign-made sponges are available online.

Natural family planning

Natural family planning may be an effective method for highly motivated and disciplined couples, but in typical populations there is a 25% failure rate during the first year of use. These methods are basically cost free, although potential costs include a thermometer ($10), cycle beads ($15), or classes that teach the various methods.

Examples of methods based on fertility awareness are basal body temperature, calendar, cervical mucus, standard days, symptothermal, and lactational amenorrhea.

Contraceptive pills and other hormonal methods

Hormonal methods of contraception include the combined oral contraceptive pill, minipill, vaginal ring, skin patch, injection, and implant (all discussed in later chapters).

Combined OCPs were introduced in the 1960s and quickly became the most popular contraceptive method in the United States. The market now offers a variety of hormonal methods containing "selective" progestins, lower-dose estrogens and progestins, new regimens, and new delivery methods. All of the hormonal methods require an initial healthcare visit, costing $100–300.

For injectables, although a self-injectable (subcutaneous) form is available, most women use the intramuscular form of the medication and many pay for an additional three clinic visits per year in addition to the cost of the injectable ($100–300/year).

The costs of combination oral contraceptives vary widely, depending on the availability of insurance coverage or public assistance, and are also affected by whether the prescribed product is generic or proprietary. Oral contraceptives cost $100–600 a year and the minipill varies between $30 and $60/month. Skin patches and the vaginal ring do not have a generic form and tend to be at the higher end of the price range. The cost of the implant plus cost of insertion is $400–627 and the cost of removal of the implant plus office visit is $200–346.

Intrauterine devices/systems

Recently, intrauterine devices (IUDs) have been gaining popularity as a very effective, easy to use, and a safe method of birth control. There are two types: hormonal (Mirena) and copper-containing (Paragard). The upfront costs, including the purchase price of the IUD ($300–806) plus the examination and insertion fee ($150–300) are relatively high compared to other methods. However, since the effectiveness is so high for the life of the IUDs (5–10 years or more), the method is one of the cheapest when one considers more than the first year. There is also a cost of visit and removal ($170–300). The copper IUD costs less and lasts longer than the levonorgestrel-releasing IUD.

Female and male sterilization

Female and male sterilization have become very popular forms of contraception for couples that have finished their families. Today, female or male sterilization is the contraceptive choice of 45% of couples, greater than any other single method. Sterilization methods for women include: tubal ligation; postpartum, during cesarian section or interval tubal ligation; and hysterocopic insertion (Essure coils). For men, the procedure is vasectomy.

- The cost of laparoscopic tubal ligation is typically $1,500–6,000, although in some hospitals costs can reach $13,000 or more for an outpatient procedure.
- Hysteroscopic coils (Essure) are a permanent birth control method that does not require an incision or general anesthesia. Tiny metal coils are inserted into the fallopian tubes using a hysterscope. The procedure can be done in a physician's office but requires radiologic confirmation of tubal blockage 3 months after the procedure. The cost of the procedure can range from $2,300 to $4,000.
- Adiana, approved by the Food and Drug Authority (FDA) in July 2009, also uses a hysteroscope but is different as a catheter is placed in the intramural portion of the tube where low-level radiofrequency radiation causes tubal destruction.
- Vasectomy is the cheapest method in this group, costing $350–1,000. It is highly effective. There is also the cost of a repeat semen analysis 3 months after the procedure. Considering the moderate upfront costs, this method offers one of the lowest-cost methods for contraceptive protection.

Birth control methods in development

That one half of all pregnancies in the United States are not intended reflects a dissatisfaction with, and underuse of, the currently available methods. New methods are being designed and tested with the aim of finding a better fit between the user and the method, finding more effective, cheaper, safer, and easier-to-use methods, and designing methods for particular populations such as older women, teenagers, breastfeeding women, women with medical problems, and men. Attention is also directed to increasing protection from STDs. Examples of many of the new birth control methods currently under development are listed in Table 2.3.

> **⚙ SCIENCE REVISITED**
>
> Many of the recently developed methods offer a secondary indication that provides a noncontraceptive benefit such as bleeding control, avoidance of bleeding, or protection from sexually transmitted diseases (STDs).

Table 2.3 New contraceptives in development

Advances in female contraceptives	
OCPs with new progestins, regimens, and/or estrogens	Estradiol valerate in combination pill
	Dinogest, chlormadinone acetate in combination pills
	Progestin-only pills (desogestrel only)
Contraceptive microbicides offering protection from HIV and STIs	
New IUDs	Frameless with copper, frameless with levonorgestrel
New combination rings	EE and nestorone, EE and ST-1435/nestorone; progestin-only rings (nestorone, progesterone)
New patches	EE and levonorgestrel, EE and gestodene
Second-generation implants	Jadelle-2 implants with levonorgestrel, nestorone implants
New injectables	Norethisterone and estradiol valerate; Uniject single-use syringe for self-injecting
Spray-on contraceptives	Nestorone for breast-feeding women
New methods for transcervical sterilization	Quinacrine (sclerosing agent)
	Radiofrequency energy to scar fallopian tube
	Plastic implants—same idea as Essure
New cheaper female condoms	Synthetic latex (FC2), VA or Reddy, or V-Amour female condom with soft sponge to hold it in place; PATH woman's condom with dissolving capsule and urethane foam
Vaccine against HCG (immunocontraceptives)	
Minicomputers designed to interpret urinary hormone levels and predict fertile days	
Advances in male contraceptives	
Vas deferens	Sperm-blocking polymer gel (styrene maleic anhydride and DMSO)
	Silicone plugs
	Soft hollow plug ("shug")
	Battery-powered capsule emitting low-dose electrical impulse
Pills, patches, injections, and implants to deliver various formulations of testosterone or MENT (potent substitute for testosterone)	Monthly or bimonthly injections of: undecanoate, testosterone undecanoate, testosterone, and enanthate nortestosterone alone or with a progestin, etonogestrel, or GnRH implants with depot testosterone
New nonlatex condoms	Polyurethane, SEBS, Tactylon

EE, ethinyl estradiol; GnRH, gonadotropin releasing hormone; HCG, human chorionic gonadotropin; IUD, intrauterine device; OCP, oral contracptive pill; SEBS, styrene ethylene butylene styrene; STI, sexually transmitted infection.

Cost saving of contraceptive methods

The upfront and ongoing costs of all of the various contraceptives are more than offset by the medical costs saved by preventing pregnancy. Consistent and proper use of any method makes the method more cost-effective.

It is estimated that use of contraceptives saves around $19 billion in direct medical costs each year in the United States. These are costs that would otherwise be paid by sexually active reproductive-aged women and their families, medical insurance companies, or public assistance programs. The high-efficacy methods prevent pregnancy more often than less effective methods; even though they have substantial upfront costs, the more effective methods over time often result in the most cost savings in a typical population. The economic savings from contraceptives are particularly high in the adolescent population (ages 15–19), where 85% of the pregnancies are unintended and where there are higher than average rates of STDs and terminations.

An economic analysis comparing actual private and public sector costs reported that use of any of the 11 available contraceptive methods substantially saved healthcare dollars. In the private sector, savings ranged from $308 for the implant at 1 year of use to over $4,000 for the male condom at 5 years of use. In the public sector, the savings were smaller and ranged from $60 for the implant at 1 year to over $2,000 for the male condom at 5 years of use. This analysis included the medical costs associated with unintended pregnancy, method cost, and cost of treatment for STDs. Combining male condoms with other methods further reduced medical care costs.

In a study comparing the cost of publicly funded family planning services through Family PACT program in 2002 to the public sector expenditures that would have occurred in the absence of unintended pregnancy, the provision of effective methods of contraception to low-income individuals resulted in substantial cost savings to local, state, and federal government. The total public sector cost savings of the pregnancies prevented was over $1.1–2.2 billion. Every dollar spent saved the public sector $2.76–5.33.

Cost comparisons of current contraceptive methods

- A recent study comparing 16 contraceptive methods over a 5-year period used a sensitivity analysis incorporating failure rates, adverse event rates, and resource utilization. The costs of method failures included costs from the anticipated number of ectopic pregnancy, spontaneous or induced abortion, or term pregnancy. The probability of each outcome as well as the probability of method failure was obtained from the literature. In order to estimate costs for barrier methods, each woman was assumed to have 83 sexual acts per year. After 5 years, any contraceptive method was more cost-effective than "no method" and the least expensive methods were the copper-T IUD, vasectomy, and levonorgestrel IUD. (The Essure method was not included in this analysis.)

- In another study comparing hysteroscopic tubal occlusion (Essure), performed in the office setting, with laparoscopic bilateral tubal ligation over a 5-year time period, the authors reported a substantial cost saving of 33% over 5 years for hysterscopic tubal occlusion.

- A case–control study within a UK community health service compared the cost-effectiveness of the implant (Implanon) and oral contraceptives over 36 months. Cost-effectiveness was calculated using actual costs of provision of the methods plus cost of pregnancies in both cohorts. At 12 months the cost of the implant was half the cost of the oral contraceptives. The conclusion of the authors was that although long-acting reversible contraception is perceived to be expensive, it is actually highly cost-effective compared to methods that have lower upfront costs but higher failure rates.

Present value comparison of US contraceptive methods

In order to compare all currently available methods of contraception, the present value of identifiable costs, including expected costs of pregnancy due to method failures are calculated (Table 2.4). Assumptions underlying these calculations are shown below

Table 2.4 Percentage of U.S. women with an unintended pregnancy during the first year of typical or perfect use of a contraceptive method; percentage continuing method after 1 year of use

Method	Women with unintended pregnancy in 1st year		Women continuing use at 1 year (%)
	Typical use (%)	Perfect use (%)	
No method	85	85	
Spermicides	29	18	42
Withdrawal	27	4	43
Fertility awareness-based methods	25		51
Standard days method	25	5	
TwoDay method	25	4	
Ovulation method	25	3	
Sponge (parous)	32	20	46
Sponge (nulliparous)	16	9	57
Diaphragm	16	6	57
Female condom (Reality)	21	5	49
Male condom	15	2	53
Combined pill and progestin-only pill	8	0.3	68
Patch (Evra patch)	8	0.3	68
Ring (NuvaRing)	8	0.3	68
Injectable (DPMA)	3	0.3	56
Cu-IUD (ParaGard)	0.8	0.6	78
LNG-IUS (Mirena)	0.2	0.2	80
Implant (Implanon)	0.05	0.05	84
Female sterilization	0.5	0.5	100
Male sterilization	0.15	0.10	100

Adapted from Trussell J. Contraceptive efficacy. In Hatcher RA, Trussell J, Nelson AL, Cates W, Stewart FH, Kowal D. Contraceptive technology. 19th revised ed. New York, NY: Ardent Media; 2007.

EVIDENCE AT A GLANCE

Net present value (NPV) takes the stream of future costs over 1, 3 or 5 years into the future and summarizes this stream in a single number. It is the sum of each of these future costs, adjusted for how far in the future they are expected to be incurred. The adjustment incorporates the financial cost of delayed access to cash, or the opportunity cost of financing these costs. NPV is a widely accepted methodology used across all industries for combining revenues and costs distributed over time.

Total present value (TPV) represents the discounted sum of three distinct costs:
- Initial cost, such as the cost of inserting an IUD.
- Ongoing or annual cost, such as the annual cost of birth control pills.
- Expected cost of pregnancy (probability of pregnancy times cost of dealing with pregnancy), given an assumed probability that pregnancy will occur for each method of birth control.

The cost of removal of a device is prorated per year of life expectancy of the device.

The assumed **annual discount rate** is 10%.

These calculations assume that, should pregnancy occur, the patient will, once again continue the same method of birth control and incur the same probability of pregnancy in all subsequent years. The probability of pregnancy is assumed to remain constant over time. This means that for birth control methods where the probability of pregnancy is relatively high, the expected costs of pregnancy can overwhelm the other costs of that method of birth control.

Upper and lower costs of methods and method failure were obtained from the literature. Method failure factors in anticipated rates and costs of term pregnancy, induced or spontaneous termination, ectopic pregnancy, caesarian section, and complications.

Termination only as an option cost $350–650. Emergency contraception was not included in this analysis.

Failure rates for typical and perfect use of various methods are taken from the literature. Induced termination rates for unintended pregnancies, spontaneous abortion rates, and term pregnancy rates from unintended and intended pregnancies are also obtained from the literature.

Potential savings from noncontraceptive benefits was not included. Potential extra costs resulting from side effects and/or complications of the methods were not included.

The results of this analysis are similar to the findings of the studies mentioned above and confirm that, in a typical population, methods that do not rely on proper use by the user are the most cost-effective.

Comparison of the cost estimates shown in Tables 2.5–2.7 demonstrate the heavy impact of method effectiveness on method cost. Factors that impact on method costs are listed under the cost section in Table 2.4 and are reflected as minimum and maximum cost ranges.

⚠ CAUTION

Over time, the present values of less effective methods in a typical population are high because of their higher failure rate and high cost of pregnancy.

As the last row of Table 2.6 demonstrates, in a typical population lack of use of any contraceptive is prohibitively expensive, and therefore has the highest present values. This is simply because the probability of pregnancy is very high and its costs are very high as well.

EVIDENCE AT A GLANCE

- Generally, compared to other reversible contraceptive methods, **tubal ligation** becomes very cost-effective after 10 years of use. If out-of-pocket costs are low, it can be a very cost-effective method within a shorter time period.
- Perfect use of **OCPs** for 4 years is cost equivalent to 1 year of typical use, because of the higher failure rate of typical use.
- The third-tier group includes most of the **barrier methods** plus **periodic abstinence** and **withdrawal**. The costs of these methods are competitive with the second-tier group for about 3 years, but thereafter the costs of these methods become quite high as a result of method failure.

In a *theoretical population with perfect use* (Table 2.7), the barrier methods and natural family planning methods are among the least expensive. This confirms the dominant impact on the cost of each method of the cost of dealing with unintended pregnancy. But even in this "perfect" population IUDs (especially the 380) and vasectomy are still cost-effective: they are more or less equivalent to the barrier methods and, after 5–10 years, are the least expensive methods.

Table 2.5 Present value (PV) of various contraceptive methods in a general population with **typical** use of method

Method	3-year PV ($)		5-year PV ($)		10-year PV ($)		Breakeven years of 380 IUD use	
	Min	Max	Min	Max	Min	Max	Min	Max
IUD 380	480	990	550	1,085	680	1,260		
IUD levo	760	1,280	810	1,370	920	1,540		
Vasectomy	417	1,220	430	1,230	440	1,250		
Implant	730	1,290	820	1,470	980	1,790		
OCPs	1,440	3,915	2,120	5,550	3,340	8,490	<1	<1
Injectable	1,130	2,410	1,625	3,420	2,515	5,230	<1	<1
Essure	2,380	3,950	2,402	3,970	2,440	4,010	>10	>10
Male condom with spermicide	2,590	3,560	3,820	5,200	6,033	8,180	<1	<1
Cervical cap (nulip)	2,290	3,200	3,360	4,600	5,290	7,120	<1	<1
Diaphragm	2,240	3,104	3,310	4,500	5,245	7,020	<1	<1
Periodic abstinence	2,870	3,520	4,370	5,360	7,090	8,690	<1	<1
Sponge (nulip)	2,410	3,120	3,590	4,620	5,720	7,340	<1	<1
Withdrawal	3,100	3,800	4,720	5,790	7,660	9,380	<1	<1
Female condom	3,130	4,400	4,670	6,490	7,430	10,260	<1	<1
Spermicides	3,620	4,080	5,470	6,220	8,820	10,080	<1	<1
Tubal ligation	1,610	6,270	1,640	6,307	1,690	6,370	>10	>10
Cervical cap (parous)	4,120	5,450	6,160	8,030	9,830	12,680	<1	<1
Sponge (parous)	4,250	5,370	6,390	8,050	10,260	12,900	<1	<1
None	9,750	11,950	14,870	18,220	24,100	29,530	<1	<1

Method failures were based on typical use, and resulted in one of four outcomes: birth, spontaneous abortion, induced abortion, or ectopic pregnancy. Maximum and minimum estimates of method and pregnancy costs in a typical population are shown. The breakeven column shows the number of years of a particular method when the cost equals the (primarily upfront) cost of the IUD 380. Numbers are rounded.

Table 2.6 Present value (PV) of various contraceptive methods in a general population with **perfect** use of method

Method	3-yr PV $		5-yr PV $		10-yr PV $		Breakeven years of 380 IUD use	
	Min	Max	Min	Max	Min	Max	Min	Max
Withdrawal	**460**	**563**	**700**	**860**	**1,130**	**1,390**	2	5
Periodic Abstinence	**574**	**580**	870	875	1,420	1,420	2	3.5
Male condom	**1,100**	**1,730**	1,540	2,420	2,350	3,660	<1	<1
IUD 380	460	960	520	1,040	630	1,190		
IUS levo	760	1,280	810	1,370	920	1,540		
Vasectomy	**410**	1,210	**420**	1,220	**430**	**1,230**	<1	<1
OCPs	560	2,830	770	3,900	1,160	5,820	1	<1
Diaphragm	1,090	1,700	1,560	2,360	2,410	3,550	<1	<1
Injectable	820	2,030	1,150	2,840	1,750	4,290	<1	<1
Female condom	1,300	2,150	1,870	3,060	2,900	4,700	<1	<1
Implant	750	1,290	840	1,470	1,000	1,790		
Cervical cap (nulip)	1,480	2,220	2,130	3,100	3,300	4,690	<1	<1
Sponge (nulip)	1,610	2,130	2,370	3,120	3,740	4,910	<1	<1
Spermicides	2,350	3,100	3,550	4,650	5,700	7,440	<1	<1
Essure	2,370	3,911	2,380	3,913	2,410	3,920	>10	>10
Sponge (parous)	2,870	3,680	4,290	5,480	6,860	8,730	<1	<1
Cervical cap (parous)	3,430	4,610	5,110	6,740	8,130	10,600	<1	<1
Tubal ligation	**1,610**	6,270	1,640	6,310	1,690	6,370	>10	>10
None	**9,760**	**4,370**	**14,870**	**18,220**	**24,100**	**29,530**	<1	<1

Method failures resulted in one of four outcomes: birth, spontaneous abortion, induced abortion, or ectopic pregnancy. Minimum and maximum costs are shown for each method.

Table 2.7 Present value (PV) with outcomes in a selected population with typical failure rates and all selecting pregnancy termination

Method	3-yr PV $		5-yr PV $		10-yr PV $		Breakeven years of 380 IUD use	
	Min	Max	Min	Max	Min	Max	Min	Max
Periodic abstinence	**218**	**400**	**330**	**620**	540	1,000	5	7
Withdrawal	240	440	360	660	580	1,080	5	6
Vasectomy	400	1,200	400	1,200	**400**	1,200		
Male condom	542	1,690	782	2,360	1,220	3,560	<1	<1
Injectable	810	2,040	1,140	2,850	1,730	4,310	<1	<1
Cervical cap (nulip)	590	1,210	770	1,570	1,100	2,200	<1	1
Spermicides	540	1,050	780	1,510	1,220	2,350	2	6
Diaphragm	544	1,110	730	1,460	1,050	2,100	<1	1–2
None	**740**	**1,370**	**1,130**	**2,090**	**1,830**	**3,400**	1	2
380 Cu-IUD	400	890	430	930	470	1,020		
OCP	600	2,920	800	4,030	1,250	6,040	1	
Levo IUS	740	1,250		780	1,330	860	1,480	
Cervical cap (parous)	730	1,470	980	1,960	1,440	2,840	<1	<1
Sponge (nulip)	720	1,130	1,010	1,590	1,530	2,420	<1	1
Sponge (parous)	860	1,380	1,220	1,980	1,870	3,060	<1	<1
Female condom	900	1,790	1,270	2,510	1,930	3,800	<1	<1
Tubal ligation	1,550	6,210	1,560	6,210	1,560	6,220	>10	>10
Implant	730	1,280	810	1,460	970	1,771		
Essure	2,350	3,910	2,350	3,910	2,360	3,920	>10	>10

When considering cost of a method, this table compares present value costs for women who plan on termination of pregnancy only. The minimum and maximum costs of method and medical costs are listed separately.

Selected references

Andrade A, Wildemeersch D. Menstrual blood loss in women using the frameless FibroPlant LNG-IUD. Contraception 2009;79(2):134–8.

Family PACT. Cost-benefit analysis of the California Family PACT program for calendar year 2007. Available from: http://bixbycenter.ucsf.edu/publications/files/FamilyPACTCost-BenefitAnalysis2007_2010Apr.pdf

INFO Project Population Report. New contraceptive choices. Center for Communications Programs, the John Hopkins Bloomberg School of Public Health Series M, Number 19, April 2005. Available from: http://info.k4health.org/pr/m19/

Kost K, Forrest JD, Harlap S. Comparing the health risks and benefits of contraceptive choices. Fam Plann Perspect 1991;23:54–61.

Kraemer DF, Yen PY, Nicols M. An economic comparison of female sterilization of hysterscopic tubal occlusion with laparoscopic bilateral tubal ligation. Contraception 2009;80(3):256–60.

Lipetz C, Phillips CJ, Charlotte F. the cost-effectiveness of a long-acting reversible contraceptive (Implanon) relative to oral contraception in a community setting. Contraception 2009;79(4): 304–9.

Mayo Clinic staff. Brith control basics. Available from: http://mayoclinic.com/health/birth-control/BI99999/PAGE=BI00005

Trussell J. Contraceptive efficacy. In: Hatcher RA, Trussell J, Nelson AL, Cates W, Stewart FH, Kowal D. Contraceptive technology, 19th revised ed. New York, NY: Ardent Media; 2007.

Trussell J, Koenig J, Stewart F, Darroch JE. Medical care cost savings from adolescent contraceptive use. Fam Plann Perspect 1997;29:6. Available from: http://www.guttmacher.org/pubs/journals/2924897.html

Trussell J, Lalla AM, Doan QV, Reyes E, Pinto L, Gricar J. Cost-effectiveness of contraceptives in the United States. Contraception 2009;79: 5–14.

Varney SJ, Guest JF. Relative cost-effectiveness of Depo-Provera, Implanon, and Mirena in reversible long-term hormonal contraception in the UK. Pharmacoeconomics 2004;22(17): 1141–51.

Section 2

Individual Contraceptive Methods

3

Combination Oral Contraceptives

Daniel R. Mishell Jr

Division of Reproductive Endocrinology and Infertility, Keck School of Medicine, University of Southern California, USA

Mechanism of action and effectiveness

Combination oral contraceptives (OCs) primarily work by inhibiting the midcycle luteinizing hormone (LH) surge and preventing ovulation. All OCs also act on other areas of the reproductive tract in the following ways:

- Making the cervical mucus thick, viscid, and scanty, thus preventing sperm penetration and inhibiting sperm capacitation
- Decreasing uterine and oviduct motility, thus inhibiting ova and sperm transport
- Decreasing endometrial glandular production of glycogen thus decreasing sperm survival.

The typical-use pregnancy rate varies depending on the population being tested but ranges from 2% to 8% per year. The perfect-use pregnancy rate of combination OCs is 0.3% per year. OCs are in the second tier of contraceptive effectiveness, as they are subject to user error.

Combination OCs provide effective contraception if they are started within 5 days or the first day of menstruation and taken daily.

- If started any other time, back-up method is needed for 7 days
- If more than 2 pills missed, back-up method is needed for 7 days
- Higher failure rates are seen in women weighing over 160 pounds (73 kg).

No significant differences in efficacy have been demonstrated between various OCs on the market today.

Good candidates

- Healthy reproductive-aged women with no contraindications
- Sexually active girls are eligible to start OCs after having at least three regular, presumably ovulatory, cycles
- Reproductive-aged women with heavy monthly bleeding, catamenial problems such as premenstrual dysphoric disease, or acne
- Healthy perimenopausal women who are normotensive nonsmokers, with no migraines, no known vascular disease, and no diabetes (see Chapters 17 and 18).

OCs can be used following pregnancy in non-breast-feeding women:

- Immediately after a first or second trimester spontaneous or induced abortion (ovulation usually occurs between 2 and 4 weeks after a spontaneous or induced abortion).
- OCs are initiated 3–4 weeks after delivery in women delivering after 28 weeks.
- Ovulation is usually delayed beyond 6 weeks after a term delivery but may occur as earlier in a non-breast-feeding woman.
- The delay in starting OCs is due to the normally increased risk of thromboembolism

occurring postpartum, which may be further enhanced by the hypercoagulable state associated with estrogen-containing contraceptive.

> ⚠ CAUTION
>
> When combination OCs are **not** used for contraceptive protection:
> * Candidates must meet the WHO MEC and US MEC guidelines
> * Health care providers should use good clinical judgment when counseling about contraceptive options.

OCs can be used in women with premature ovarian failure, and in anovulatory women with oligomenorrhea, polycystic ovarian syndrome (PCOS) with androgen excess, or dysfunctional bleeding:

* OCs inhibit ovarian testosterone secretion and increase sex hormone-binding globulins (SHBG), thus reducing levels of biologically active testosterone and lessening the manifestations of hyperandrogenism.
* OCs, the patch, and ring will control and usually reduce uterine bleeding and protect the user from endometrial hyperplasia due to unopposed estrogen.

Poor candidates

> ⚠ CAUTION
>
> Cigarette smoking increases the risk of serious adverse effects on the heart and blood vessels from oral contraceptive use. This risk increases with age and with the amount of smoking (15 or more cigarettes/day has been associated with a significantly increased risk) and is quite marked in women over 35 years of age. Women who use oral contraceptives should not smoke.

Contraindications to combination OC use include the following:

* History of heart attack or stroke, current chest pain
* Thrombophlebitis or thromboembolic disorders
* Cerebrovascular or coronary artery disease
* Hereditary or acquired blood clotting disorders: If a woman has known thrombophilic mutation she should not take a combination OC. It is not cost-effective to screen for thrombophilic mutation before use of OCs unless there is a family or individual history of venous thromboembolism (VTE)
* Known or suspected breast, endometrial, cervical, vaginal, or certain hormonally sensitive cancers
* Unexplained (undiagnosed) vaginal bleeding
* Hepatic adenomas or carcinoma, liver failure, active liver disease
* Cholestatic jaundice of pregnancy or during previous OC use
* Known or suspected pregnancy
* Uncontrolled hypertension; hypertension in women over 35 years of age
* Diabetes mellitus with vascular disease
* Smoking in women over 35 years of age
* Migraine with aura, localizing symptoms, or peripheral neurologic symptoms; migraines that worsen in frequency or severity with use of OCs, or migraines in women over 35 years of age
* Functional heart disease
* Nursing:
  * Using an estrogen-containing contraceptive may diminish the amount of milk produced (estrogen inhibits prolactin's action on the breast.)
  * Women who are exclusively breast-feeding every 4 hours, including night-time, and not having menstruation, will not ovulate until 6 months after delivery and do not need contraception before that time.
  * If supplemental feeding is introduced, ovulation can resume. Use of progestin-only methods of contraception does not diminish the amount of breast milk and is recommended.

Other risk factors to consider when prescribing oral contraceptives

* Heavy cigarette smoking under the age of 35
* The presence of migraine headaches without aura in women under 35 years of age (if they worsen with on OC use, OCs should be discontinued)

- Undiagnosed causes of amenorrhea:
  - Combination OCs can be given to women with hypothalamic amenorrhea, or pituitary microadenoma (with follow-up) but not when amenorrhea is due to a prolactin-secreting pituitary macroadenoma.
  - Work-up for galactorrhea while taking these agents can include measurement of serum prolactin 2 weeks after stopping OCs. If the prolactin level is elevated, a further diagnostic evaluation is indicated.
- Obesity is a risk factor for VTE and extreme obesity (BMI > 40) is a strong risk consideration when counseling on OC use. WHO MEC lists ≥30 BMI as a category 2 for OCs (the absolute risk remains small). Long-standing obesity, especially with the presence of other risk, may warrant a higher category.
- Women with a history of gestational diabetes may take low-dose OC formulations, as data indicates that OCs do not clinically affect glucose tolerance or accelerate the development of diabetes mellitus.
- Insulin-dependent diabetes without vascular disease in women under 35 is no longer considered to be a risk. Use of low-dose OCs in women with insulin dependency does not accelerate the disease process and these women are at high risk for pregnancy complications.
- The presence of varicose veins is not a contraindication to combination OC use.

Medical eligibility criteria

> ☆ **TIPS & TRICKS**
>
> The World Health Organization has established medical eligibility criteria (WHO MEC) for use of OCs with estrogen plus progestin, progestin-only OCs, and the nonhormonal contraceptives. These recommendations are summarized in Table 3.1. The Centers for Disease Control and Prevention (CDC) has recently published some modifications to these recommendations (US MEC) (see Chapters 1 and 19).

Advantages of low-dose oral contraceptives

Low-dose OCs are:

- Highly effective if taken properly
- Rapidly reversible within a few months of discontinuing
- Relatively easy to use
- Safe: healthy, normotensive, nonsmoking, women without migraines can safely use OCs during their reproductive years.

OCs are associated with noncontraceptive benefits including bleeding control, less dysmenorrhea, reduced premenstrual dysphoric disorder (PMDD), lowered risk of ovarian and endometrial cancer. In addition, their cost in some settings may be low.

Noncontraceptive health benefits

In addition to providing effective contraception, OCs also promote many health benefits. The following noncontraceptive benefits are listed in the package insert:

OCs are associated with decreased risk of:

- Blood loss and iron deficiency
- Pain or other cycle-related symptoms
- Ovarian cysts
- Ectopic pregnancy
- Noncancerous cysts or lumps in the breast
- Acute pelvic inflammatory disease (PID)
- Ovarian and endometrial cancer

Benefits from antiestrogenic action of progestins

As a result of the antiestrogenic action of the progestins in OCs, there is less endometrial proliferation and the thickness of the endometrium is less than in an ovulatory cycle. This results in a reduction in the amount of blood loss from 35 mL in a normal menstrual cycle to around 20 mL. Women on OCs, compared to those not on OCs, are about half as likely to have iron deficiency anemia, and are significantly less likely to have heavy bleeding episodes, irregular bleeding, intermenstrual bleeding, or the surgical procedures used to treat these conditions. After 1 year of OC use, the chance of developing endometrial

Table 3.1 Summary of medical eligibility criteria for contraception from WHO guidelines

	COCs	Progestin-only OCs	Cu-IUD
Venous cardiovascular disease			
History of DVT or PE	4	2	1
Family history of VTE	2	1	1
Thrombophilia	4	2	1
Varicose veins	1	1	1
Superficial VT	2	1	1
Obesity: BMI > 30	2	1	1
Arterial cardiovascular disease			
Ischemic heart disease	4	3	1
Stroke history	4	2	1
Hypertension			
Uncontrolled	4	2	1
Controlled	3	2	1
Smoking			
Age < 35	2	1	1
Age > 35 (<15/day)	3	1	1
Age > 35 (>15/day)	4	1	1
Hyperlipidemia	2	2	1
Headache			
No migraine	1	1	1
Migraine w/out aura (age < 35)	2	2	1
Migraine w/out aura (age > 35)	3	2	1
Migraine with aura	4	2	1
Valvular heart disease			
Uncomplicated	2	1	1
Complicated (AF)	4	1	2
Diabetes			
History of gestational diabetes	1	1	1
Non-insulin-dependent	2	2	1
Insulin-dependent	2	2	1
Vascular disease or duration > 20 yrs	4	2	1
Epilepsy			
No drugs	1	1	1
Anticonvulsants	3	3	1
Depression	1	1	1
Thyroid disease	1	1	1
Breast diseases			
Benign	1	1	1
Family history of cancer	1	1	1
Personal history of breast cancer	4	4	1
Anemias			
Thalassemia	1	1	2
Sickle cell disease	2	1	2
Iron deficiency	1	1	2
SLE			
No vascular disease	2	1	1
Vascular disease	4	2	1

Table 3.1 *Continued*

	COCs	Progestin-only OCs	Cu-IUD
Antibiotics			
Rifampicin	3	3	1
Broad spectrum	2	2	1
ARV	1	1	2
Antifungals	1–2–3	1–2	1
HIV/AIDS			
HIV	1	1	2
AIDS no ARV	1	1	3
AIDS with ARV	2	2	2

AF, atrial fibrillation; ARV, antiretroviral; BMI, body mass index; COC, combined oral contraceptive; Cu-IUD, copper-containing intrauterine device; DVT, deep venous thrombosis; OC, oral contraceptive; PE, pulmonary embolism; SLE, systemic lupus erythematosus; VTE, venous thromboembolism.

Key:

Category	Description	Interpretation when clinical judgment is available	Interpretation when clinical judgment is limited
1	No restriction for the contraceptive method	Use the method in any circumstance	Use the method
2	The advantages of using the method generally outweigh the theoretical or proven risks	Generally use the method	Use the method
3	The theoretical or proven risks usually outweigh the advantages of using the method. Safe use requires careful clinical judgment and access to clinical services	Use of method not usually recommended unless other more appropriate methods are not available or not acceptable	Do not use the method
4	A condition which represents an unacceptable health risk if the contraceptive method is used	Method not to be used	Do not use the method

Adapted from http://whqlibdoc.who.int/publications/2004/9241562668.pdf and www.infoforhealth.org.

cancer is reduced by 50%. There is further reduction in risk with longer duration of use and the reduced risk persists for at least 15 years after stopping OCs.

OC use is associated with a reduced incidence of benign breast disease. Current OC users have an 85% reduction in the incidence of fibroadenomas and a 50% reduction in chronic cystic changes and nonbiopsied breast lumps.

Benefits from inhibition of ovulation

Other noncontraceptive medical benefits of OCs result from their action of inhibition of ovulation.

OC users have 63% less dysmenorrhea and 29% less premenstrual syndrome than nonusers. Additionally, OC users have a significant reduction in the development of ovarian cysts although the magnitude of the reduction in risk is greatest with combination formulations containing 30–35 μg of estrogen. Development of ovarian cancer is significantly reduced in OC users. After 1 year of use the risk is reduced by 50% and after 10 years of use it is reduced by 80%. Protection lasts for at least 15 years after OCs are stopped. Reduction of the risk of developing ovarian cancer extends to women with the *BRCA* mutations.

Other benefits

- Combination OCs decrease the severity of acne. Several formulations are approved for the treatment of acne, after successful randomized trials demonstrated a significant benefit.
- Several studies show a 50% lowered risk of developing rheumatoid arthritis in OC users.
- The risk of developing PID from gonorrhea or chlamydia in OC users in most studies is reduced by 50%. Even though the incidence of cervical infection with *Chlamydia trachomatis* is increased in OC users compared with controls, the incidence of chlamydial PID in users is only half that of control subjects. OCs reduce the risk of ectopic pregnancy by more than 90% in current users and may reduce the incidence in former users by decreasing their chance of developing PID.
- OC use in perimenopausal women (Chapter 18) has been shown in some studies to increase bone mineral density and decrease the risk of postmenopausal osteoporosis fractures.
- OC use is associated with a 20% reduction in the development of colon and rectal cancer. In an analysis of a large British General Practitioners study (1968–1992), OC users had reduced risk of developing all cancer compared to nonusers. The risk of endometrial and ovarian cancer in users was reduced about 50%. Breast cancer risk with current and past use of OCs was not increased compared with nonusers in women 35–65. Combined OC (COC) use in women with a family history of breast cancer or with a *BRCA* mutation was not increased.

Because OCs have many noncontraceptive health benefits and because they can be used safely in normotensive, nonsmoking women, in 1991 the class labeling for OCs was updated to read:

⚠ CAUTION

The benefits of oral contraceptive use by healthy nonsmoking women over 40 may outweigh the possible risks. Of course, older women, as all women who take oral contraceptives, should take the lowest possible dose formulation that is effective.

Risks associated with the use of oral contraceptives

Neoplastic effects

Breast cancer

Because estrogen stimulates the growth of breast tissue, there are concerns that the high dose of estrogen in OCs can either promote or initiate breast cancer. For over 40 years, extensive study has been done to determine the relationship between OCs and the development of breast cancer. It is reassuring that the vast number of studies show small or no increased risk in breast cancer in OC users. By age 65, the risk of having had breast cancer diagnosis is the same in ever users as in never users. The dose or type of either steroid, or years of use, are not related to risk. Women with a family history of breast cancer or those with the *BRCA* mutation do not have an added increased risk of diagnosis of breast cancer with COC use.

- In 1996, a reanalysis was done on the entire worldwide epidemiologic data. The analysis indicated that women on OCs compared to nonusers had a slightly increased risk of having breast cancer (relative risk (RR) 1.24, confidence interval (CI) 1.15–1.30). The risk declined steadily after stopping COCs, and was not significantly increased after 10 or more years after stopping (RR 1.01, CI 0.96–1.05).
- While taking combination OCs, there is a 0.5 excess cancers per 10,000 women aged 16–19 and 5 excess cancers in women aged 25–29.
- The cancer in OC users was less advanced clinically and the risk of having breast cancer spread beyond the breast was significantly reduced (RR 0.88, CI 0.81–0.95) compared with nonusers.
- By age 50, the cumulative risk of breast cancer was equal in COC users and never users.
- In a large case control study by the Centers for Disease Control, the relative risk of diagnosis of breast cancer in women aged 35 to 65 was 1.0 for current users and 0.9 for former OC users. The Royal College of General Practitioners (RCGP) study of 744,000 women–years of users and 339,000 women–years of never

users, the relative risk of breast cancer diagnosis was 0.98.

Cervical cancer

Evidence indicates that use of OCs for 5 or more years may increase the risk of cervical cancer. There are 14 types of human papillomavirus (HPV) that are recognized to be the major cause of the disease. Women taking OCs should have routine cervical cytologic screenings for HPV. It appears that HPV-positive women on OCs are a high risk group and require appropriate screening and follow-up.

Endometrial cancer

All but 2 of 12 case–control studies and 3 cohort studies have found that OC use has a protective effect against endometrial cancer, the third most common cancer among U.S. women.

The RCGP study reported a relative risk of uterine cancer of 0.58 (CI 0.42–0.79) that persisted after OC discontinuation. After at least 1 year of OC use, women have an age-adjusted relative risk of 0.5 for diagnosis of endometrial cancer between ages 40 and 55 as compared with nonusers. The risk is reduced to 60% after 4 years of use.

Ovarian cancer

OCs reduce the risk of the four main histologic types of epithelial ovarian cancer (serous, mucinous, endometrioid, and clear cell), the risk of invasive ovarian cancers, and those with low malignant potential. The decrease in risk increases from about a 40% reduction with 4 years of use, to a 53% reduction with 8 years of use, and to a 60% reduction with 12 years of use. The reduced risk continues for at least 20 years after stopping OC use.

- All but 2 of the 22 case control and 2 cohort studies report a reduced risk of epithelial ovarian cancers in OC users. The summary relative risk among ever users of COCs was 0.6, a 40% reduction. In the RCGP study the risk of ovarian cancer with COC use was 0.58. The protective effect occurs in women of low parity who are at greatest risk for this type of cancer.

- Studies report a 50% risk of developing ovarian cancer with OC use in women with *BRCA1* and *BRCA2* mutations.
- OCs reduce the risk of developing cystadenomas, cystic teratomas and endometriomas.

Liver adenoma and cancer

- There does not appear to be an increased risk of developing benign hepatic tumors in users of OCs containing ethinyl estradiol formulations.
- WHO's large multicenter epidemiologic study showed no increase in liver cancer with OC use, regardless of duration of use.
- The development of benign hepatocellular adenoma was reported to be increased in long-term users of high-dose OCs, particularly those containing mestranol.

Pituitary adenoma

Although OCs may mask the predominant symptoms produced by prolactinoma–amenorrhea and galactorrhea, data from three studies indicate that OC users do not have an increased incidence of prolactin-secreting pituitary adenomas.

Malignant melanoma

The result of several large studies of long duration of OC use indicates no increased risk of malignant melanoma.

Colon and rectal cancer

A meta-analysis reported that OC use decreased the risk of developing colon and rectal cancer by 20%. The RCGP study reported that OC use was associated with a significant decreased relative risk (0.72) of developing colorectal cancer.

Reproductive effects

Discontinuation of the use of low-dose formulations causes a reduction in conception rates for at least the first six cycles after discontinuation. The delay to return of conception after discontinuing OCs is greater among older, premenopausal women. By 2–3 years after the discontinuation of OCs or barrier methods, fertility rates are equal.

The rate of spontaneous abortion or the incidence of chromosomal abnormalities in abortuses or infants is not increased in women who conceive after stopping OC use, even if conception occurred in the first month after the OC was discontinued.

A review of prospective epidemiologic studies found there is no increased risk of congenital malformations overall among the offspring of OC users. There is no increased risk of congenital heart defects or limb reduction defects in users of OCs if OC is ingested during the first few months of pregnancy.

Metabolic effects

The magnitude of the metabolic effects of the synthetic steroids in OC formulations is directly related to the dosage and potency of the steroids in the formulations. Fortunately, the more common adverse effects are relatively mild.

The incidence of all estrogenic side effects, including the serious side effects, is much less with use of lower estrogen dose formulations than that which occurred with use of high estrogen dose formulations.

Thromboembolic risks

> ✋ CAUTION
>
> Combination OCs may impact coagulation factors and increase the risk of deep venous thrombosis, pulmonary embolism, stroke and myocardial infarction. It is generally accepted that the risks associated with OCs in most women are lower than those from pregnancy and birth.

Ethinyl estradiol, the synthetic estrogen in combination OCs, causes increases in hepatic production of several globulins, including factors V, VIII, X, and fibrinogen. These factors enhance thrombosis, while another globulin, angiotensinogen, can increase blood pressure. The impact of ethinyl estradiol on these globulins is directly correlated with the amount of estrogen in the formulation. Epidemiologic studies report that the incidence of both arterial and venous thrombosis is directly related to the dose of estrogen.

The effect of OCs on parameters that inhibit coagulation, such as protein S, protein C, and antithrombin III, is not as well understood, although an inherited deficiency in these globulins substantially increases a user's risk of devel-

oping thrombosis. Users of OCs who have an activated protein C resistance have a 30-fold increased risk of deep venous thrombosis (DVT) compared to normal nonusers. Women with a personal or family history of thrombotic events should be screened for coagulation deficiencies.

Monitoring blood pressure is recommended for women on OCs, as about 1 in 200 women on a ≤35-μg estrogen OC will develop clinical hypertension.

Progesterone and androgenic progestins do not significantly affect the synthesis of globulins except that androgenic progestins decrease synthesis of SHBG.

Venous thromboembolism

The risk of VTE is related to the dose of estrogen and progestin in the formulation. A large observational study reported that the incidence of venous thromboembolic events among users of OCs containing 20–50 μg ethinyl estradiol was 15 per 100,000 woman–years, higher than the 5 per 100,000 rate of women of reproductive age, but much less than the rate of 60 per 100,000 woman–years associated with pregnancy.

There is some evidence that the risk of VTE in women taking OCs containing desogestrel or gestodene is increased about 1.5–2.5 times compared to women on OCs with levonorgestrel. The incidence in third-generation OCs (gestodene and desogestrel) users is reported to be approximately 25 per 100,000 women. The risk is increased in women over 35 who smoke, or in subgroups with additional risk factors.

A large observational study reported that the risk of VTE with an OC containing drosperinone and 30 μg of ethinyl estradiol was the same as an OC containing levonorgestrel and the same dose of estrogen.

Myocardial infarction

> ✋ CAUTION
>
> A WHO report stated that women who do not smoke, who have their blood pressure checked, and do not have hypertension or diabetes are at no increased risk of myocardial infarction if they use combined OCs regardless of their age.

Epidemiologic studies of humans and studies with primates have not observed an acceleration of atherosclerosis with the ingestion of OCs. Epidemiologic studies also report no increased risk of myocardial infarction (MI) in former OCs users, and two recent U.S. case–control studies reported no significantly increased risk of MI in OC users.

There is a significantly increased incidence of MI in older OC users who have risk factors that cause arterial narrowing, such as pre-existing hypercholesterolemia, hypertension, diabetes mellitus, or smoking more than 15 cigarettes a day.

A case–control study of women admitted to a group of New England hospitals between 1985 and 1988 reported that the relative risk of MI among current OC users was not significantly increased (RR 1.1, CI 0.4–3.1). Women who smoked at least 25 cigarettes a day and used OC had a threefold increased risk of MI. Smoking alone increased the risk of MI by about ninefold. These data, along with other, indicate that smoking and OCs act synergistically.

Studies by the Royal College and WHO reported that the risk of MI in OC users with hypertension was several-fold greater than in normotensive users.

Stroke

As with findings of OCs and MI as mentioned above, studies show that the significant increased risk of stroke in OC users was mainly limited to older women who also smoked and/or were hypertensive.

It is strongly recommended that OCs not be prescribed to women with uncontrolled hypertension or migraine headaches with aura, or those over 35 who smoke or have hypertension.

Diabetes risk

The effect on glucose metabolism is primarily related to the dose, potency, and chemical structure of the progestin. The estrogen component appears to act synergistically with the progestin to impair glucose tolerance.

The large RCGP cohort study reported no increased risk of diabetes mellitus in current OC users (RR 0.80) or former COC users (RR 0.82), even in women who had used OCs for ≥10 years.

The Nurses Health Study reported on more than 1 million person–years of follow-up of OC users. Although type 2 diabetes mellitus was diagnosed in >2000 women, the risk was not increased in current OC users (RR 0.71). It was slightly increased in past high-dose OC users (RR 1.11) but not in low-dose users.

Cardiovascular disease risk

The estrogen in OCs increases levels of high-density lipoprotein (HDL) cholesterol, total cholesterol, and triglycerides, and decreases levels of low-density lipoprotein (LDL). The progestin component decreases HDL, total cholesterol, and triglycerides, and increases LDL.

Current studies of several OC formulations containing levonorgestrel, norethindrone, and the newer nonandrogenic progestins report a significant increase in triglyceride levels but little change in HDL, LDL, and total cholesterol levels, signifying that the effects of the estrogen component are offset by the progestin component.

Patient counseling

First visit

At the initial visit a history, vital signs (*particularly blood pressure*), weight, and physical examination including pelvic and Pap smear are done to determine that there are no medical contraindications for OCs. For medicolegal reasons it is best to use either a written informed consent signed by the woman or note on the woman's medical record that the benefits and risks have been explained to her and that she has been encouraged to read the patient package insert.

- The patient should be counseled to take a pill every day, preferably at the same time each day.
- The patient should be counseled as to whether she will be taking placebo pills or skipping a certain number of days each cycle.
- The patient should understand that not starting a new pack on time or missing pills can result in increased pregnancy risk. Skipping two or more pills or not starting on time should be followed up by using a back-up method of contraception for 7 days.

- If the woman has no contraindications to estrogen/progestin use, no routine laboratory tests are needed prior to initiation.
- Cervical cytology with HPV screening should be obtained on the first visit.
- Lab tests can include: A liver panel is indicated for those with a significant past history of liver disease, a lipid panel in women with a family history of early (<50 years of age) cardiovascular disease, and HgA_{1c} in women with strong family history of diabetes.

Follow-up visits

Scheduling a 3 month follow-up visit should be considered and is recommended. During this and all subsequent visits, a history of bleeding and side effects (headaches, acne, breast tenderness) is obtained, and blood pressure is measured. After this visit the user should be seen annually, at which time a history is taken, blood pressure and body weight measured, and a physical examination (including breast, abdominal, and pelvic examination with appropriate cervical cytology as needed) performed.

Annual cervical cytology is indicated in HPV-positive users of OCs as they are a relatively high-risk group for development of cervical neoplasia.

- Periodic measurement of a lipid panel is advisable in women with a family history of early vascular disease or early MI (in family members under the age of 50).
- Low-dose OCs can be used in women with dysplidemia, other than hypertriglyceridemia (>300 mg/dL), as they have a beneficial effect upon the lipid profile, raising HDL cholesterol and lowering LDL. However, they do increase trigylcerides.
- For woman with a family history of diabetes or personal history of gestational diabetes, a HgA_{1c} or 2-hour postprandial blood glucose

test should be tested periodically. If abnormal, a glucose tolerance test is indicated.
- If the woman has a past history of liver disease, a normal liver panel should be documented as needed.

There is no need for a rest period after a few years of OC use as it does not serve any value.

Selecting the right oral contraceptive: type of formulation

In determining which formulation to use, it is best to prescribe a OC with less than 30 µg of ethinyl estradiol, since these pills are associated with less cardiovascular risk, as well as less estrogenic side effects than the higher doses. The Food and Drug Administration (FDA) recommends that the product prescribed should be one that contains the least amount of estrogen and progestin that is compatible with a low failure rate and the needs of the individual woman.

There are few randomized studies comparing the different marketed formulations, and until large-scale comparative studies are performed, clinicians may be heavily influenced by OC performance among women in their practice.

- Many OC formulations, including many with 20 µg ethinyl estradiol, are available as generics.
- For women with androgen excess, consider the most recently developed progestins desogestrel, norgestimate, and drosperinone, and dienogest (antiandrogenic activity) as these have less androgenic activity than the older progestins and some of the formulations containing these new progestins are approved to treat acne.
- The progestin drosperinone has antiandrogenic as well as antimineralocorticoid properties, and OCs containing it are approved to treat acne and premenstrual dysphoria disorder in women desiring contraception. The 20 ug and 30 ug OC formulation are available with the supplement folic acid [levomefolate].
- A novel contraceptive pill containing estradiol valerate and dienogest (gonane progestin) is available in Europe and has just been approved

by the FDA. Natazia (Qlaira in Europe) will be the first four-phase oral contraceptive to be marketed in the United States. Bleeding control is considered to be a strength.

- A three-month version of the pill was introduced in 2003 (Seasonale) designed to give the benefit of less frequent periods at the potential drawback of breakthrough spotting or bleeding. Seasonique is a similar formulation containing low-dose estrogen pills instead of placebo pills.
- A continuous daily OC formulation is designed to completely eliminate withdrawal bleeding (Anya or Lybrel).
- OCs with the new 24–4 regimens are associated with good bleeding control and less bleeding each month. There are two available branded products (Lo-Estrin 24 Fe and Yaz). Generic regimens of extended cycles are used by some healthcare providers.

The pill packets with placebo are designed to allow the user to take a pill every day. Placebo pills may contain an iron supplement or low-dose estrogen.

Drug interactions

- Although synthetic sex steroids can inhibit the biotransformation of certain drugs such as phenazone and meperidine (by substrate competition), such interference has not been shown to be clinically important.
- Some drugs will induce hepatic enzymes that increase the metabolism of steroids and significantly interfere with the action of OCs.
- Failure rates with barbiturates, sulfonamides, cyclophosphamide, and particularly rifampin are relatively high.
- Failure rates are also reported to be increased in women on antiretroviral medications used to treat HIV (OCs with antiretrovirals is category 2—see Table 3.1).
- There are some limited clinical data concerning OC failure in users of antibiotics (penicillin, ampicillin, and sulfonamides), analgesics, and barbiturates.
- Consideration of higher-dose OCs in women with epilepsy requiring medication may be considered. Second-generation antiepileptic

medication increases the metabolism of the estrogenic but not progestogenic portion of the formulation, and data suggests that it does not affect the OC failure rate.

Supplying the method

Because the orally administered estrogen in OCs is thrombogenic and increases the risk of venous and arterial thrombosis in a dose-dependent fashion, researchers have directed their efforts in reducing the dose. The dose of the progestin has also been reduced along with introduction of new progestins that, while still are derivatives of testosterone, are more selective and have less androgenic activity. More recent OC developments have been directed toward modifying the traditional 21–7 treatment regimen. The first extended regimen OC was approved by the FDA in 2003. Several recently introduced OCs have shortened the 7-day interval to a 4-day interval to improve bleeding profiles and decrease the incidence of ovulation (pill failure) when there is a delay in starting a new pack.

The generic OC package insert contains a long list of noncontraceptive benefits (see above). Additionally, several pills now include specific secondary benefits such as decreased acne, treatment for PMDD, or bleeding control.

New products

A new four-phase OC, Natazia, was been is approved by the FDA in May, 2010. It is the first OC to contain estradiol valerate and dienogest and is packaged in a 28-day cycle pack.

Management of problems

It is generally the progestin component that linked to a failure of withdrawal bleeding or amenorrhea. Progestins decrease synthesis of endometrial estrogen receptors and decrease endometrial growth.

A high progestin to estrogen ratio may cause a failure of withdrawal bleeding. Although not important medically, bleeding serves as a signal that the woman is not pregnant and switching to an OC with a higher estrogen to progestin ratio is often recommended. Alternatively, switching to an OC formulation with estrogen in the placebo pills may be a good choice.

For women with complaints of breakthrough bleeding, switching to an extended regimen or to an OC with a higher estrogen to progestin ratio is recommended. Oral formulations with 20 µg of estrogen of progestin may allow more unscheduled bleeding and if persistent, switching to a higher dose pill or switching to one with a shortened placebo period (24/4), may solve the problem.

The most frequent symptoms produced by the estrogen component include nausea (a central nervous system effect), breast tenderness, and fluid retention due to decreased sodium excretion. Estrogen can also cause development of melasma (pigmentation of the malar eminences). Melasma is accentuated by sunlight and may take a long time to fade after discontinuation of OCs.

If estrogenic or progestogenic side effects occur with one oral formulation, a different agent with less estrogenic or progestogenic activity can be selected. All but one of the progestins currently used in OCs are structurally related to testosterone and may produce androgenic side effects including weight gain, acne, and nervousness.

- Estrogens decrease sebum production and progestins increase it: formulations with high progestin dominance are poor choices for women with acne. Several OC formulations with low-androgenic progestins are now approved to treat acne (Yaz, Ortho-Tricylen; see Chapter 22).
- Fear of weight gain may be associated with poor compliance, especially in adolescents. A 2000 U.K. review article reported that there is no evidence that modern low-dose OCs cause weight gain; however, switching to another low-dose OC may improve further compliance in a concerned user.
- OCs may increase vaginal discharge (*leukorrhea*), and more frequent candida vaginitis is reported. Switching to an OC with a lower estrogen dose for women with frequent vaginal problems is recommended.
- Some research links OCs with decreased libido. There are several mechanisms that may play a role including increases in SHBG and suppression of ovarian androgens that leads to decreases in biologically active testosterone. However, a 2007 study in 1700 users found that OC users had no change in sexual satisfaction. Exogenous supplementation of androgens is under study to see if it may play a role in younger and older women.
- Current evidence indicates that COCs do not increase the incidence of depression (see Chapter 20).

Selected references

Abdollahi MC. Obesity: risk of venous thrombosis and the interaction with coagularion factor levels and oral contraceptive use. Thromb Haemost 2003;89:493–8.

Beral V, Hermon C, Kay C, et al. Mortality associated with oral contraceptive use: 25 year follow up of cohort of 46000 women from Royal College of General Practitioners' Oral Contraception Study. BMJ 1999;318:96.

Burkman R, Schlesselman J, Zieman M: Safety concerns and health benefits associated with oral contraception. Am J Obstet Gyn 2004; 190;S5.

Collaborative Group on Hormonal Factors in Breast Cancer. Breast cancer and hormonal contraceptives: Collaborative reanalysis of individual data on 53,297 women with breast cancer and 100,239 women without breast cancer from 54 epidemiological studies. Lancet 1996;347:1713.

Croft P, Hannaford PC. Risk factors for acute myocardial infarction in women. BMJ 1989; 298:165.

Dinger JC, Heinemann LAJ, Kühl-Habich D. The safety of a drospirenone-containing oral contraceptive: final results from the European Active Surveillance study on Oral Contraceptives based on 142,475 women-years of observation. Contraception 2007;75:344.

Donaghy M, Chang CL, Poulter N. Duration, frequency, recency, and type of migraine and the risk of ischaemic stroke in women of childbearing age. J Neurol Neurosurg Psychiatry 2002;73:747–50.

ESHRE Capri Workshop Group. Noncontraceptive health benefits of combined oral contraception. Hum Reprod Update 2005;11:513–525.

Gerstman BB, Piper JM, Tomita DK, et al. Oral contraceptive estrogen dose and the risk of deep venous thromboembolic disease. Am J Epidemiol 1991; 133:32.

Gillum LA, Mamidipudi SK, Johnston SC. Ischemic stroke risk with oral contraceptives: a metanalysis. JAMA, 2000, 284:72–8.

Hankinson SE, Colditz GA, Hunter DJ, et al: A quantitative assessment of oral contraceptive use and risk of ovarian cancer. Obstet Gynecol 1992; 80:708.

Khader YS et al. Oral contraceptives use and the risk of myocardial infarction: a meta-analysis. Contraception, 2003, 68:11–7.

Hannaford PC, Kay CR. Oral contraceptives and diabetes mellitus. BMJ 1989; 299:315.

Hannaford PC, Selvaraj S, Elliot AM, Angus V, Iversen L, Lee AJ. Cancer risk among users of oral contraceptives: cohort data from Royal College of General Practitioner's oral contraception study. BMJ 2007;335:651.

Holt VL, Cushing-Haugen KL, Daling JR. Body weight and risk of oral contraceptive failure. Obstet Gynecol 2002;99:820–7.

Heinemann LAJ, Dinger JC. Range of published estimates of venous thromboembolism incidence in young women. Contraception 2007; 75:328.

Heit JA, Kobbervig CE, James AH, Petterson TM, Bailey KR, Melton LJ III: Trends in the incidence of venous thromboembolism during pregnancy or postpartum: a 30-year population-based study. Ann Int Med 2005; 143:697.

Marchbanks PA, McDonald JA, Wilson HG, et al. Oral contraceptives and the risk of breast cancer. N Engl J Med 2002;346:2025.

Martinelli I, Sacchi E, Landi G, Taioli E, Duna F, Mannucci PM. High risk of cerebral-vein thrombosis in carriers of a prothrombin-gene mutation and in users of oral contraceptives. N Engl J Med 1998;338:1793–7.

Narod SA, Dube MP, Klijn J, et al. Oral contraceptive and the risk of breast cancer in BRCA1 and BRCA2 mutation carriers. J Natl Cancer Inst 2002;94:1773–9.

Nightingale AL, Lawrenson RA, Simpson EL, Williams TJ, MacRae KD, Farmer RD. The effects of age, body mass index, smoking and general health on the risk of venous thromboembolism in users of combined oral contraceptives. Eur J Contracept Reprod Health Care 2000;5:265–74.

Poulter NR for the World Health Organization Collaborative Study of Cardiovascular Disease and Steroid Hormone Contraception. Venous thromboembolic disease and combined oral contraceptives: Results of international multi-centre case-control study. Lancet 1995;346:1571.

Rosenberg L, Palmer FJ, Rao RS, Shapiro S. Low-dose oral contraceptive use and the risk of myocardial infarction. Arch Int Med 2001:161; 1065–70.

Roumen FJME, Apter D, Mulders TMT, et al: Efficacy, tolerability and acceptability of a novel contraceptive vaginal ring releasing etonogestrel and ethinyl oestradiol. Hum Reprod 2001;16:469.

Schwartz SM, Petitti DB, Siscovick DS, et al. Stroke and use of low-dose oral contraceptives in young women: A pooled analysis of two US studies. Stroke 1998;29:2277.

Sidney S, Siscovick DS, Petitti DB, et al. Myocardial infarction and use of low-dose oral contraceptives: A pooled analysis of two US studies. Circulation 1998;98:1.

Tanis BC et al. Oral contraceptives and the risk of myocardial infarction. N Engl J Med 2001:345; 1787–93.

Van den Bosch MA, Kemmeren JM, Tanis BC, et al. The RATIO study: oral contraceptives and the risk of peripheral arterial disease in young women. J Thromb Haemost 2003;1: 439–44.

WHO. Venous thromboembolic disease and combined oral contraceptives: results of international muticentre case-control study. World Health Organization Collaborative Study of Cardiovascular Disease and Steroid Hormone Contraception. Lancet 1995;346:1575–82.

4

Progestin-only Oral Contraceptive Pills

Regina-Maria Renner[1] and Jeffrey T. Jensen[1,2]

[1]Departments of Obstetrics and Gynecology and
[2]Department of Public Health and Preventive Medicine, Oregon Health & Science University, Portland, OR, USA

Method of action

The progestogen-only pill (POP), also referred to as the "minipill," contains a synthetic progestogen hormone, but no estrogen. Although POPs have been available since the 1960s, they only contribute a small percentage to the oral contraceptive market share. Progestogens are also called progestins or gestagens, and are synthetic agonists of the progesterone receptors.

They prevent pregnancy via the following mechanisms:

- Ovulation suppression: The POP disrupts ovulation by suppressing mid-cycle peaks of luteinizing hormone (LH) and follicle stimulating hormone (FSH). Detailed studies of ovulation with different POPs demonstrate that this occurs in approximately 50–60% of cycles in users of formulations containing norethindrone (NET), 72% in levonorgestrel (LNG) users, and 97.3% among desogestrel users.
- Cervical mucus effects: The characteristics of cervical mucus change throughout the normal menstrual cycle. At the time of ovulation the mucus is abundant and more fluid, allowing sperm penetration. Progestogens reduce the amount and increase the viscosity of cervical mucus. This thick, tenacious mucus decreases sperm penetration and is the most immediate and protective contraceptive mechanism of the POP.

> ✋ CAUTION
>
> Since this effect on cervical mucus only persists for approximately 24 hours after taking the pill, regular dosing is required for the highest efficacy.

- Tubal effects: Fertilization normally occurs in the tube. Progestogens decrease tubal motility and cilia activity, decreasing the likelihood of adequate sperm and ova transport and fertilization.
- Endometrial effects: Progestogens decrease endometrial proliferation, and over time this lead to an inactive endometrium as shown on endometrial biopsies of women taking POPs. These changes include a reduction in number and size of endometrial glands. Progestogens down-regulate both estrogen and progesterone receptor synthesis in the endometrium. It is unknown whether these endometrial changes affect sperm transport or implantation.

One or more of these mechanisms prevent fertility, and the importance of the various effects may differ between cycles and with the different POP formulations.

Effectiveness

The failure rate for the POP (0.6%) is slightly higher than that of combined oral contraceptive pills (COC) (0.2%), with published failure estimates for the POP ranging from 0.5% to 13%. One randomized controlled trial compared two COCs (ethinyl estradiol [EE]/levonorgestrel [LNG] and mestranol [MES]/norethindrone [NET]) and two POPs (NET and LNG) and reported no statistically significant difference in 2-year pregnancy rates between the EE/LNG (4.5%) and LNG alone group (9.5%). However, the magnitude of the point estimates of failure suggest a twofold increase risk of failure with the POP, and the study had limited statistical power to exclude a difference due to poor enrollment and high loss rate for reasons other than pregnancy. A cohort study of 6779 woman-years using POPs found a Pearl index of 0.56 per 100 women–years, compared to 0.20 per 100 in 48,692 woman–years of combination pill use.

Contraceptive failure that occurs while a method is used as directed is called *method, or perfect-use failure*. When pregnancy results from inconsistent or incorrect use of a method, this is considered a *user, or typical-use failure*.

Data from the 2002 National Survey of Family Growth has been used to provide estimates of the *first-year failure rate* associated with use of a contraceptive method. For all users of oral contraceptives (both combined and POP), perfect-use failure is estimated at 0.3%, while typical use first year failure is 8%. This wide variation between perfect and typical-use failure indicates that patterns of use influence efficacy more than the type of pill. In other words, correct and consistent use of the POP would be expected to result in a lower failure rate than typical or inconsistent use of a combined pill.

One can imagine many scenarios where this could occur. For example, a breast-feeding mother may feel reassured about the absence of a deleterious effect on nursing with use of the POP, and become an extremely dedicated pill-taker after counseling on the importance of consistent dosing at the same time each day. Another new mother, encouraged by her provider to use a "more effective" combined pill, may worry about effects on nursing, or perceive a reduction in milk volume, and become an inconsistent pill-taker.

The efficacy of *different POP formulations* has been studied. Rice and colleagues found that a POP with desogestrel 75 µg inhibited ovulation more consistently than the POP with LNG 30 µg. Korver and coworkers found that this effect was maintained for desogestrel even with a delay in ingestion of up to 12 hours. In a large open-label noncomparator multicenter trial, the crude Pearl Index (PI) of this formulation was 0.41 and the adjusted (perfect-use) PI was 0.14.

Since the POP may be prescribed to women with absolute or relative contraindications to estrogen, it is important to know if *medical comorbidities* affect efficacy. One such potential factor is obesity. Recent reports have suggested an interaction between obesity and an increase risk of OC failure, but not all studies demonstrate this effect. Since both volume of distribution and metabolism are influenced by obesity, the risk of failure may be increased with very low dose pills such as the POP. However, data from the large prospective Oxford Family Planning Association contraceptive study did not demonstrate any influence of body weight on the risk of accidental pregnancy with either POP or combined oral contraceptives. Data from the 2002 National Survey of Family Growth (NSFG) also failed to demonstrate an interaction between obesity and OC failure, but did not separately evaluate combined and progestogen-only pills.

As is true for COCs, the typical use failure rate is strongly influenced by a variety of factors, including user compliance, age (Pearl index of 3.1 in young women vs 1 in women over age 40) and frequency of coitus. A back-up method (i.e., condoms) is recommended in case of delayed or forgotten POPs, when taking medications that may interfere with POPs, or when suffering from diarrhea or vomiting. The highest efficacy will be seen in women who are highly motivated to be perfect users, and in women with lower fertility (e.g. advanced maternal age, concurrent breast-feeding).

Pharmacokinetics and its implications

The amount of the synthetic progestin in POPs is 75% lower than the amount used in a COC. The serum progestin level peaks about 2 hours after oral administration and rapidly declines to undetectable levels after 24 hours. This is especially true for NET with a half-life of approximately 7 hours compared to 16 hours for LNG. The progestogen effect on the cervical mucus is rapidly reversed; several studies have demonstrated that cervical mucus permeability to sperm returns to baseline about 24 hours after the last pill. Therefore, to optimize efficacy, POPs should be taken at about the same time (±3 hours) each day, and continuously, without any placebo days. While this general recommendation makes sense for routine practice, there is considerable variation in the pharmacokinetics between individuals and studies, and no clinical data has correlated pregnancy rates with timeliness in taking POPs.

Pharmacodynamics

The synthetic progestogens used in the POP are derivatives of 19-nortestosterone, and bind not only to progesterone receptors but also to estrogen, testosterone, and corticoid receptors with variable affinity. Thus, depending on the type of progestin and route of administration, they not only have progestational effects on various target organs, but also may have estrogenic, androgenic, and gluco- or mineralocorticoid effects. NET and LNG have similar biological effects; they both display progestational, androgenic, and antiestrogenic effects; they both lack glucocorticoid effects; and most studies demonstrate no estrogenic effects. POPs have androgenic activity which decreases the circulating levels of sex hormone binding globulin (SHBG). This leads to an increase in free steroid levels such as levonorgestrel and testosterone. Desogestrel seems to have less androgenic effects than LNG and NET.

Good candidates

There are relatively few contraindications to the use of the POP. They are particularly well suited for women who desire oral contraception and are:

- motivated and compliant pill takers at any age
- are 40 years or older
- are breast-feeding (see the sections on "Advantages" and "Medical eligibility criteria" for details)
- have contraindications to estrogen (see World Health Organization Medical Eligibility Criteria)
- report side effects with combined pills that may be related to the estrogen component of

the pill: these include decreased libido, gastrointestinal upset, breast tenderness or headaches
- are obese (as POPS do not increase the risk of venous thromboembolism (VTE)).

Poor candidates

Women who

- have a history of prior oral contraceptive failure or who report difficulty remembering to take the pill.
- will have difficult taking the pill at the same time each day (±3 hours), since this will increase the risk for method failure (see details on efficacy above); this may include many adolescents.
- cannot tolerate an irregular bleeding pattern or amenorrhea.
- have contraindication based on the medical eligibility criteria of the World Health Organization [see below].
- have abnormal vaginal bleeding of unknown origin. POPS should not be prescribed until an explanation has been determined.
- have polycystic ovarian syndrome. These patients have symptoms of androgen excess. A combined pill is preferred, as these will suppress gonadotropins and reduce ovarian production of androgens, as well as increase SHBG to lower free testosterone levels. The unopposed androgenic activity of POPs could aggravate the hyperandrogenicity.
- are breast-feeding Latina women with a history of gestational diabetes. These women should be told about a possible increase in the risk of diabetes. Please see below for details.

Medical eligibility criteria

> ☆ TIPS & TRICKS
>
> The World Health Organization (WHO) has published medical eligibility criteria (WHO MEC) available in a number of printed forms as well as on the WHO website (http://www.who.int/reproductivehealth/publications/family_planning/9789241563888/en)

in which the risk level for use of a contraceptive method in the setting of a variety of medical conditions is assessed.

For each condition, eligibility to use the method is assigned using a numeric scale: Category 1 indicates that the method can be used without restrictions; Category 2 indicates that advantages generally outweigh theoretical or proven risk; Category 3 indicates that the method is not usually recommended unless other, more appropriate methods are not available or not acceptable; and Category 4 indicates that the method is not to be used.

Since the POP does not contain estrogen, there is no increase in the risk of thrombosis, and most women with medical comorbidities can safely take POPs (MEC category 1 or 2). The only contraindication with a *category 4* is current breast cancer.

A *category 3* has been assigned for the following conditions:

- past history of breast cancer
- certain anticonvulsants and rifampin, both due to drug interactions that may increase metabolism
- liver disease with severe cirrhosis
- liver tumors or active viral hepatitis, since POPs are metabolized in the liver
- postpartum and breastfeeding less than 6 weeks postpartum
- current deep vein thrombosis (DVT)

Since the POP does not contain estrogen, these common *contraindications for COCs* **do not restrict** *the use of POPs*, including:

- diabetes mellitus with end-organ damage or >20 years duration
- symptomatic gallstones without cholecystectomy
- hormone-related cholestasis in the past
- migraine headache in women older than 35 years or with aura
- hypertension
- ischemic heart disease

- smoking of more than 15 cigarettes daily in women older than 35 years
- stroke
- major surgery with prolonged immobilization
- complicated valvular hear disease
- history of deep vein thrombosis

However, if a woman develops migraines with aura, ischemic heart disease or a stroke while using the POP, they should be stopped according to the WHO criteria.

Postpartum/breastfeeding

POPs are considered category 3 (method not usually recommended unless other, more appropriate methods are not available or not acceptable) in the first six weeks postpartum when breastfeeding. After six weeks, a risk category one is assigned. In contrast, combined pills are considered category 4 until 6 weeks and remain category 3 for the first six months post partum while nursing. Use of the POP in breastfeeding women is discussed in further detail in the next section.

Obesity

In the Multiple Environmental and Genetic Assessment of risk factors for venous thrombosis (MEGA) study, the joint effects of obesity, OC use, and prothrombotic mutations on the risk of VTE venous thrombosis were analyzed. Obese women who used combined oral contraceptives had a 24-fold higher thrombotic risk than women with a normal BMI who did not use OCs. Therefore, obese women have a relative contraindication to combined OC use, and the estrogen free POP presents an attractive oral contraceptive alternative. However, obesity may also affect OC efficacy.

While the results of database and prospective studies do not demonstrate a consistent association between obesity and OC failure, the mechanisms that might explain failure in obese women have not been fully evaluated. Therefore, obese women should receive particular counseling regarding the need for compliance with the dose schedule during use of the POP.

Advantages

POPs have a *simple* and *fixed pill-taking regimen*. The simple regimen of a daily pill without placebo pills or a pill-free interval facilitates compliance.

The available data suggests a rapid *return of fertility* after stopping POPs, independent of the length of time POPs have been taken. In one study, the first ovulation after discontinuing the desogestrel POP occurred after 7 days. Since NET and LNG pills are less likely to suppress ovulation, a return to fertility would be expected to occur as soon as cervical mucus changes reverse.

Safety profile

POPs are safe for almost all women, and are an alternative for women with contraindications to estrogen. In general, the principal risks associated with combined pills are due to estrogen-induced effects on the liver that result in a net prothrombotic effect. These altered *effects on coagulation* are not observed with POPs. However, since only a few studies have directly compared POPs with combined pills, drawing conclusions about the actual differences in *safety profile* is difficult. POPs have not been found to be associated with hypertension, cardiovascular disease, stroke, acute myocardial infarction, venous thromboembolism, coagulation factors or birth defects in children of women who took the medications in pregnancy.

A large multicenter, international study sponsored by WHO investigated the risks of cardiovascular disease (CVD) associated with the use of oral and injectable progestogen-only and combined injectable contraceptives (see Table 4.1). The adjusted odds ratio (OR) for all CVDs combined was not significantly elevated, at 1.14 (95% CI: 0.79–1.63) for current use of POPs compared to nonusers of any type of steroid hormone contraceptive (SHC). Furthermore, no significant change in risk was noted for stroke, venous thromboembolism, or acute myocardial infarction.

A large Danish cohort study found no association between use of POPs containing LNG 30 µg, norethisterone 350 µg, or desogestrel 75 µg, and the risk of venous thromboembolism when compared with nonusers of oral contraceptives. COCs, in contrast, were associated with an increased risk for venous thrombosis. For the same dose of estrogen and the same length of use, oral contraceptives with desogestrel (RR 1.82 [1.49–2.22]), gestodene (RR 1.86 [1.59–2.18]), drospirenone

(RR 1.64 [1.27–2.10]) or cyproterone (RR 1.88 [1.47–2.42] were associated with a significantly higher risk of venous thrombosis than oral contraceptives with LNG. The risk of venous thrombosis in current users of COCs decreases with duration of use and decreasing estrogen dose.

The lack of association with thrombosis represents a major benefit of POPs. They represent a highly effective and safe option for women at high risk, as they offer excellent protection against pregnancy, a condition associated with a greatly increased risk of thrombosis. Compared to COCs, the POPs have relatively few category 3 or 4 exclusions listed in the WHO Medical Eligibility Criteria (WHO MEC) for contraception users. It is important to understand that much of the precautions and warnings sections for labeling in the United States reflect required statements for the use of synthetic estrogens or progestins alone or in combination. The principal risk of combined OCs is thrombosis (an estrogen effect). For POPs, however, labeling statements regarding thrombosis risk are not appropriate in view of the absence of estrogen and the lower dose of progestin. The WHO MEC provides better guidance.

Breast-feeding

A recent systematic review of five randomized controlled trials (RCTs) assessing hormonal contraceptives while breast-feeding found no clinically important impact of POP use on milk volume, milk composition or infant growth when taken in the first 14 days postpartum. The timing of initiation (6 weeks versus 6 months postpartum or resumption of menses) did not affect contraceptive continuation or pregnancy rates. The WHO trial included in the systematic review showed a significant decline in milk volume with COCs compared to POPs. Of note, the overall quality of the reviewed studies was considered to be poor.

A more recent study documented that use of desogestrel 75 µg/day did not change the amount and composition of breast milk, nor did it affect growth and development of the breast-fed children. Only very small amounts of the progestogen are passed into the breast milk. Some data suggests that women who use POPs breast-feed longer and add supplementary feeding at a later time.

Table 4.1 Odds ratios (95% CI) for all CVD combined (stroke, venous thromboembolism, or acute myocardial infarction) in relation to current use of progestogen-only and injectable steroid hormone contraceptives

	Cases	Control subjects	Odds ratio (95% CI) Crude		Adjusted	
CVD Combined (Stroke, VTE, and AMI)						
Nonusers	2,668	8,266	1.00	(ref)	1.00	(ref)†
Oral progestogens (all)	53	141	1.22	(0.86–1.72)	1.14	(0.79–1.63)
Continuous POP only	51	129	1.30	(0.91–1.86)	1.19	(0.82–1.74)
Progestogen-only injectable	37	122	0.99	(0.68–1.46)	1.02	(0.68–1.54)
Combined injectable**	13	43	0.97	(0.52–1.82)	0.95	(0.49–1.86)
All stroke*						
Nonusers	1,774	5,183	1.00	(ref)	1.00	(ref)‡
Oral progestogens (all)	29	70	1.26	(0.78–2.03)	1.01	(0.60–1.69)
Continuous POP only	27	60	1.33	(0.80–2.21)	1.07	(0.62–1.86)
Progestogen-only injectable	25	81	0.93	(0.58–1.48)	0.89	(0.53–1.49)
Combined injectable**	9	26	0.97	(0.45–2.10)	0.88	(0.38–2.06)‡‡
VTE						
Nonusers	635	2,288	1.00	(ref)	1.00	(ref)§
Oral progestogens (all)	21	64	1.30	(0.75–2.25)	1.74	(0.76–3.99)
Continuous POP only	21	63	1.33	(0.77–2.31)	1.82	(0.79–4.22)
Progestogen-only injectable	11	34	1.27	(0.63–2.57)	2.19	(0.66–7.26)
Combined injectable**	3	10	1.21	(0.33–4.48)	1.30	(0.35–4.81)‡‡
AMI						
Nonusers	259	795	1.00	(ref)	1.00	(ref)#
Oral progestogens (all)	3	7	1.27	(0.31–5.10)	0.87	(0.15–5.01)
Continuous POP only	3	6	1.40	(0.34–5.83)	0.98	(0.16–5.97)
Progestogen-only injectable	1	7	0.52	(0.06–4.38)	0.66	(0.07–6.00)
Combined injectable**	1	7	0.50	(0.06–4.21)	0.25	(0.01–8.09)§§

*Hemorrhagic, ischemic, and unspecified stroke.
†Adjusted for HBP and smoking categories. Excluding 13 cases (11 nonusers, two users) and five control subjects (nonusers) with unknown HBP or smoking categories.
‡Adjusted for HBP, marital status and smoking categories. Excluding 12 cases (10 nonusers, two users) and four control subjects (nonusers) with unknown HBP or smoking categories.
§Adjusted for BMI categories. Excluding 24 cases (22 nonusers, two users) and 85 control subjects (78 nonusers, seven users) with unknown BMI.
#Adjusted for HBP, diabetes and smoking categories.
**Latin America only.
††Adjusted for HBP, RHD, HIP, and smoking categories.
‡‡Adjusted for HBP and family history of premature heart attack.
§§Adjusted for HBP, number of live births, family history of premature stroke, family history of premature heart attack and smoking categories.
CVD, cardiovascular disease; VTE, venous thromboembolism; AMI, acute myocardial infarction; SHC, steroid hormone contraceptives; POP, progestogen-only pills; HBP, high blood pressure; BMI, body mass index; RHD, rheumatic heart disease; HIP, hypertension in pregnancy.
Reproduced from WHO, *Contraception* 1998; 57: 315–324 with permission from Elsevier.

Correct and consistent use of the method should always be stressed, but counseling should also emphasize that the method is highly effective. Overly pessimistic counseling regarding the efficacy of the POP may encourage some breast-feeding women to discontinuing nursing in order to initiate combined pills. Available data does not support the category 3 recommendation to avoid the POP in the puerperium. Although WHO recommend that breast-feeding women wait until 6 weeks postpartum to initiate POPs, they can be started earlier.

Metabolic effects

No significant metabolic effects have been observed during or following use of the POP. Specifically, lipid levels, carbohydrate metabolism, and coagulation factors remain unchanged.

The effect of steroidal contraceptives on *carbohydrate metabolism* in women without diabetes was examined in a recent Cochrane review that included two trials with POPs. In a double-blind, randomized, multicenter study in Finland, Kivela and colleagues measured glucose, insulin and glycosylated hemoglobin (HbA_{1C}) levels in 84 women using either the desogestrel ($75\,\mu g$) or LNG ($30\,\mu g$) POP and found no clinically significant difference in any of these measures from baseline values in either group after three or seven cycles of use. In the second, smaller trial, fasting plasma glucose stayed within the normal range for women using norethisterone $350\,\mu g$ versus LNG $30\,\mu g$ at 6 months. In women with diabetes mellitus use of POP has not been associated with changes in blood glucose levels, required insulin dose, retinopathy or weight.

In general, progesterone opposes the activity of estrogen. The progestogen component of a combined OCPs has been found to increase LDL cholesterol and decrease HDLs and triglycerides; thereby modulating the opposite estrogen effects.

Studies of POPs have shown a negligible effect on *lipids*, with slight decrease in HDL and triglycerides. No difference in lipid profiles were observed in the previously mentioned trial comparing NET $350\,\mu g$ and LNG $30\,\mu g$. These studies evaluating lipids, a surrogate marker for cardiovascular disease risk, are consistent with the findings from the WHO study that showed no association of POPs and cardiovascular disease.

POPs have little or no effect on the synthesis of hepatic globulins, and do not directly influence the *coagulation system*. There is no effect on the development of liver adenomas or liver cancer, although these are listed as contraindications in the product labeling.

Epidemiologic and prospective studies have not detected any effect on the development of prolactinomas, gallbladder disease or irritable bowel syndrome. No clinically significant thyroid function changes have been observed.

A recent systematic review on safety of contraceptive methods for women with systemic lupus erythematosus (SLE) included four studies. None of these demonstrated any increase in disease activity with use of POPs.

Bone mineral density

A systematic review on bone mineral density (BMD) and progestogen-only contraception confirmed a reversible decrease in bone density in users of injectable depot medroxyprogesterone acetate (DMPA), but this effect was not observed in users of the POP.

In the only study that specifically investigated POPs, a beneficial effect on BMD was observed. Lactating women using the POP experienced a significantly smaller percentage loss of bone mineral density after 6 months compared to women using barrier methods, and after 12 months their bone mineral density was almost 3% higher than postpartum.

Noncontraceptive benefits

Combined pills offer a number of noncontraceptive benefits including menstrual cycle regularity, treatment of menorrhagia, reduced dysmenorrhea, decreased pelvic pain related to endometriosis, improvement in premenstrual syndrome, decreased acne, decreased hirsutism, improved BMD, prevention of menstrual migraines, and decreased risk of endometrial, ovarian and colorectal cancer. Many of these benefits are estrogen related and driven by reliable ovulation suppression, stabilization of the endometrium and decrease in free serum androgens. Beneficial effects on acne and hirsutism are due to estrogen-induced increase in sex hormone binding globulin (SHBG) which binds androgens and due to suppressed luteinizing hormone(LH)-driven ovarian androgen production.

EVIDENCE AT A GLANCE

- Data is sparse as to whether POPs have the same noncontraceptive benefits as COCs.
- Specifically, estrogen-mediated benefits are not achieved with POPs; such as reliable stabilization of the endometrium or improvement of acne.
- However, women that experience estrogen-related side effects with combined pills should experience beneficial effects with the POP.

Dysmenorrhea

Two German prospective, noncomparative multicenter observational studies evaluated the effects of the POP Cerazette, a 75 µg/day desogestrel pill, in 403 women with estrogen-related symptoms during previous COC use and in 406 women with dysmenorrhea. Symptom-related assessments were made at baseline and after 3–4 months, along with bleeding pattern and treatment satisfaction. Estrogen-related symptoms resolved or improved in over 70% of women. Nausea improved/resolved most (92% of women), followed by breast tenderness (90%), estrogen-related headache (84%) and edema (74%).

In the dysmenorrhea study, symptoms resolved or considerably improved in 93% of the study subjects and analgesic use dropped from 70% of women at baseline to 8% at study end. Adverse events, mainly bleeding irregularities, were reported by 7–8% of both study populations. Approximately 90% of women in both studies were satisfied with treatment and 85% wished to continue treatment after study completion.

Heavy bleeding

Studies finding efficacy for progestogen treatment of heavy bleeding have used higher dose POPs not approved for contraception (see next section).

Dermatitis

Other noncontraceptive benefits include a case report in which estrogen dermatitis related to the menstrual cycle responded to a POP.

Risks and side effects

Change in menstrual cycle bleeding

Change in menstrual cycle bleeding is frequently observed on POPs. The most common change is short irregular cycles (up to 40% of cycles) with prolonged bleeding occurring less frequently (up to 10%). In an observational study of 358 women on POPs for at least 6 months, the unpredictable pattern manifested as irregular bleeding in 23%, amenorrhea in 8%, and mixture of regular and irregular bleeding or amenorrhea in 29%. About 40% of women in this study reported regular cycles.

Two RCTs that compared POPs and COCs in the same study demonstrated that abnormal bleeding occurs more frequently in women taking the progestogen-only pill. In an RCT with 66 women, 72% of POP users and significantly fewer (30%) of COC users reported intercyclic bleeding.

Further evidence comes from a large study that analyzed menstrual diary records obtained from 5257 women admitted to 6 clinical trials using 9 different methods of contraception (one natural fertility awareness and eight hormonal—COC, POP, vaginal ring or DMPA). Women using the nonhormonal fertility awareness method reliably experienced regular cycles and averaged 3 bleeding/spotting episodes of length 5 days in each 90-day reference period. Combined pill users had more regular patterns than any other hormonally-treated group, with short (4-day) episodes and 23–24 day bleeding-free intervals.

EVIDENCE AT A GLANCE

In contrast, POP users experienced menstrual disturbance in 25–48% of cycles, and had more frequent, longer bleeding episodes and shorter, less predictable bleed-free intervals than COC users The two POPs (LNG 0.03 µg and norethindrone 0.35 µg) produced higher numbers of bleeding/spotting days (15–18 days) in the first 90-day reference period and more episodes (3–4 episodes) than any of the COCs (Figure 4.1).

In the second 90-day reference period, however, POP users recorded less spotting than COC users: more than 50% of women using the POP had no spotting days at all, and spotting episodes occurred only rarely. Users of the norethindrone 0.35 µg pill had bleeding episodes with a mean length (4.7–5.0 days) almost identical to that of untreated women. The bleeding-free interval (mean 23 days) was approximately 2 days shorter than normally cycling women. Bleeding-free intervals among LNG 0.03 µg users were only 20–21 days, and 25% of subjects had intervals whose average length was 18 days or less. Although bleeding patterns became less irregular as the year progressed, 50% of all subjects using the POPs still had intramenstrual intervals which differed by at least 10 and 8 days, in the norethindrone and LNG group respectively, in the fourth reference period. Infrequent bleeding was reported in between 11% and 33%. None of the women using either POP experienced amenorrhea, and frequent or prolonged bleeding was rarely recorded after the first 90 days of method use.

In clinical trials with POPs, bleeding changes represent the most common complaint (40–60%) and reason for discontinuation (up to 25%). The detailed calendar study revealed marked differences between individuals in terms of their acceptance of bleeding disturbances, suggesting the importance of counseling. Women using DMPA tolerated far greater menstrual disruption than subjects using any other method. One explanation was that DMPA users were counseled to expect irregular patterns and possibly amenorrhea, while OC users were not warned of potential bleeding problems, so when problems occurred they were more likely to discontinue the method.

Functional cysts or persistent follicles

Since the POPs do not contain estrogen, they do not inhibit FSH-induced follicle growth. Furthermore, the levels of progestogen are below the minimal dose to reliably inhibit ovulation Therefore, women on POPs have a higher proportion of functional cysts or persistent follicles than COC users. The cysts typically undergo spontaneous regression and are usually uncomplicated.

In an observational study, 8 of the 21 POP users were noted to have an ovarian cyst after the first month. Three cysts regressed during the next cycle. Of the 13 women with normal ovaries initially, 4 developed a new functional cyst of which 2 were associated with pain. Of the 12 women with cysts, 7 complained of pain at some time during the monitored cycle. Among 21 control women only one symptom-free cyst was shown on the initial postmenstrual ultrasound scan and this resolved painlessly during the scanned cycle with ovulation from the opposite ovary.

Ectopic pregnancy

Data are inconclusive as to whether women using POPs are at increased risk of ectopic pregnancy compared to women using combined pills or nonhormonal methods. The absolute risk is not increased compared to woman not using OCs. However, up to 10% of pregnancies that occur in women using a POP are ectopic. Most data regarding ectopic risk stems from retrospective and cohort studies assessing POPs.

One RCT comparing COC with POP reported 2 ectopic pregnancies in the POP arm of 22 women and none in the COC arm. Decreased tubal motility (a contraceptive mechanism of action) possibly contributes to the risk of ectopic pregnancy when fertilization occurs. A history of ectopic pregnancy is not considered a contraindication to POP use in product labeling, or in the WHO MEC. However, clinicians and patients should always be alert to symptoms of ectopic pregnancy.

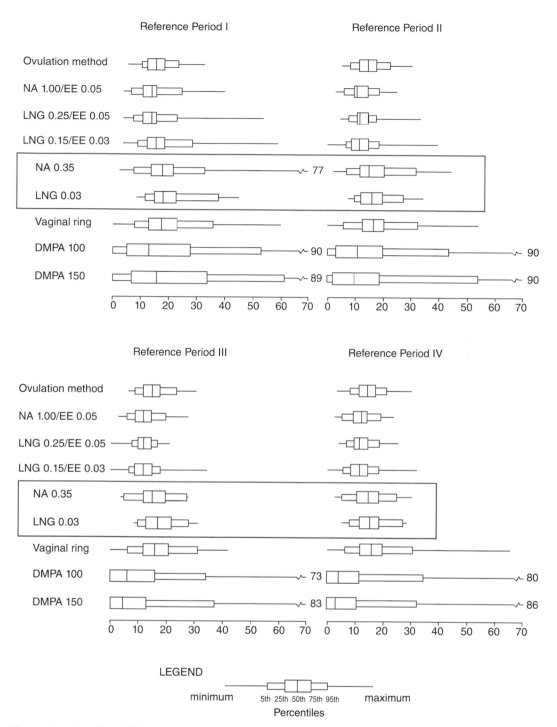

Figure 4.1 Number of bleeding/spotting days with different contraceptives. DMPA 100, depot medroxyprogesterone acetate 100 μg intramuscular; DMPA 150, depot medroxyprogesterone acetate 150 μg intramuscular; ING 0.15/EE 0.03, levonorgestrel 0.15 μg + ethinyl estradiol 0.03 μg; LNG 0.03, levonorgestrel 0.03 μg; LNG 0.25/EE 0.05, levonorgestrel 0.25 μg + ethinyl estradiol 0.05 μg; NA 0.35, norethisterone acetate 0.35 μg; NA 1.0/EE 0.05, norethisterone acetate 1.0 μg + ethinyl estradiol 0.05 μg; vaginal ring, levonorgestrel 20 μg. Reproduced from Belsey EM, *Contraception* 1988; 38:181–206 with permission from Elsevier.

Type 2 diabetes mellitus

A threefold increased long-term *risk of type 2 diabetes mellitus* has been described in one study of Latina women with gestational diabetes who took POPs postpartum, while a cohort using combined OCs in the same study did not demonstrate an increased risk. However, no significant metabolic effects in women with diabetes mellitus have been noted.

A 2008 retrospective chart review by Nelson and colleagues found no increase in the risk of developing diabetes in either COC or POP users compared to those women using a nonhormonal method. While 36% of POP users experienced a deterioration of glucose tolerance, this occurred in 34% of users of combined pills and in 23% of women using a nonhormonal method. Only among users of DMPA (42%) was the risk of impaired glucose tolerance statistically significantly increased. These findings were independent of breastfeeding status. While women with a history of gestational diabetes are at high risk for developing type 2 diabetes, there is still insufficient evidence to suggest that hormonal contraception greatly influences the long-term risk.

★ TIPS & TRICKS

Use of the POP in women with a history of gestational diabetes has been assigned risk category 1 in the WHO MEC.

Sexually transmitted infections

COCs decrease the risk of pelvic inflammatory disease (PID). Although cervical mucus effects are a primary mechanism of action for the POP, a case-control study did not show a decrease in the risk of any sexually transmitted infections (STIs) or PID with POP use.

Acne

As explained above, a number of effects that are estrogen-induced combine to improve acne in most users of combined pills. Therefore, switching to a POP may worsen acne, or return the skin condition to baseline. The LNG POP has been associated with acne due to its androgenic effects. POPs decrease SHBG, which results in an increase in free androgens.

Breast disease

The Oxford Family Planning Association long-term prospective study reported outcomes from women using oral contraception followed up until 1994. These reports included information on women using the POP. Both high dose ($\geq 50\,\mu g$ EE) and low dose ($<50\,\mu g$ EE) combined pills reduced the risk of *benign breast disease* (fibroadenoma and chronic cystic disease), but this protection was not observed among women using POPs.

The association of OCs with *breast cancer* has been evaluated in a number of studies. Compared to COCs, the epidemiological evidence on POPs and breast cancer risk is based on much smaller populations of users.

- In a large reanalysis of previous studies of hormonal contraceptives and breast cancer risk published in 1996, less than 1% of women were POP users. The relative risk (RR) for current or recent (past 5 years) users was 1.17, similar to that found in COC users. For both COCs and POPs, the elevation in risk decreased after discontinuing the OCP and vanished after 10 years.

- The International Agency for Research on Cancer (IARC) performed an evaluation of cancer risk with progestogen-only hormonal contraceptives that included the 1996 reanalysis as well as 4 additional case-control studies of POP users not included in the reanalysis. They concluded that "Overall, there was no evidence of an increased risk of breast cancer" with progestogen-only contraceptives, but that the evidence was inadequate to exclude a carcinogenic effect of progestogens.

- The percentage of women taking POPs was higher (approximately 8%) in a national population-based case-control study in New Zealand. The relative risk (RR) of breast cancer was increased in current young (25–34 years) and recent (within 10 years) users, but not in "ever users" and past users of POPs.

- More recent data provides additional reassurance. The Women's CARE study, a large population-based case-control study conducted by the U.S. National Institutes of Health, found no increased risk of breast cancer with current or past use of POPs compared to never users.

- A prospective cohort study conducted in Norway and Sweden found that women who had ever exclusively used POPs were not at an increased breast cancer risk. In this study, only the subgroup of current/recent users of POPs had an increased risk of breast cancer (RR 1.6, CI 1.1–2.5) (similar to COCs) as compared with never use.
- A systematic review suggested that the use of OCs does not significantly modify the risk of breast cancer among women with a *familial history of breast cancer*; however, evidence from four of the studies showed that some women may be at a greater risk; particularly women who took OCs prior to 1975.
- Population-based and case-control studies of the role of oral contraceptives, particularly the low-dose oral contraceptive preparations, on breast cancer risk among *BRCA1/2 mutation carriers* have also generated mixed results. No data specifically for POPs exists.

EVIDENCE AT A GLANCE

Taken together, all of these studies point to the fact that synthetic steroids may be growth factors for existing breast cancers leading to earlier diagnosis, but do not initiate new breast cancers. This would explain the small increase in risk observed with current, but not past users, and the absence of an overall increase in risk in ever users compared to never users.

Ovarian cancer

COCs reduce the risk of ovarian cancer. There are no studies that separate the effects of POPs. The large Royal College of General Practitioners update included POP users in the general population of low-dose pill users. Although the biologic mechanisms that protect OC users against ovarian cancer are incompletely understood, one hypothesis is that ovarian cancer is related to ovulation. Since inhibition of ovulation is not a regular mechanism of the POP, extension of the health benefit of reduced ovarian cancer cannot be assumed.

Endometrial cancer

Progestogens suppress endometrial mitotic activity. While data on the specific effect of POPs on endometrial cancer risk is limited, a reduction in risk with exposure to combined pills is a well-established benefit. A population-based case-control study in Sweden showed a 30% decreased risk of endometrial cancer in ever users of any kind of OCPs. Use of POPs was associated with a trend toward decreased risk in this study, but this did not reach statistical significance, likely due to low numbers.

Other cancers

There are no data on POPs in relation to liver, colorectal, kidney or gallbladder cancers, pituitary tumors, or malignant melanoma.

Other reported side effects

The progestogens used in POPs are derivatives of 19-nortestosterone, and therefore are considered to have androgenic effects. These have been implicated in the following complaints: increased appetite and weight gain; depression, fatigue and tiredness; decreased libido; acne and oily skin; and hirsutism. Other infrequently reported side effects include headache, nausea and breast tenderness. However, available data does not provide proof of a causal relationship between POP use and any of these symptoms, and the dose of progestogen in a POP is lower than in a COC. A recent Cochrane review on progestogen-only contraceptive use in obese women did not identify a relationship between POP use and weight gain.

Interactions with other drugs

Though not well studied, the low progestogen dose may increase the risk for insufficient hormone levels and decreased efficacy due to *interacting with other drugs*. Decreased absorption, increased serum protein binding and liver metabolism are mechanisms of interaction that decrease the serum free steroid levels. Drugs that may interfere with the metabolism of COCs and possibly POPs include those listed in Table 4.2.

Combined use with barrier methods such as condoms is advisable if temporary concomitant use of one of the medications listed in Table 4.2

Table 4.2 Drugs that may interfere with metabolism of COCs

Anticonvulsants	Barbiturates: phenobarbital, primidone Carbamazepine Felbamate Oxacarbazepine Phenytoin Topiramate Vigabatrin
Anti-infective agents	Rifabutin Rifampicin
Antiretrovirals	Protease inhibitors: nelfinavir, ritonavir, lopinavir/ritonavir Nevirapine
Herbal	Saint John's wort
Possibly	Ethosuximide Griseofulvin Troglitazone

is required. If long-term use of one of these medications is required, an alternative contraceptive method (e.g. DMPA, implant, IUD) should be used. For women whose bleeding patterns have stabilized, unexpected bleeding when taking other medications could indicate that serum steroid levels have been reduced. Particular care should be given to women who are taking several other drugs.

Key history and physical elements

Breast-feeding patients, or patients with contraindications to the use of estrogen, such as migraine with aura or diabetes with vascular changes, who are otherwise good candidates for oral contraception, are the appropriate target group for POPs. See the WHO MEC for more details. Pregnancy should be excluded before starting POPs, and in case of irregular vaginal bleeding, a diagnosis should be identified.

Patient counseling

Directions on how to take POPs

- Take POP at the same time every day.
- After taking the last pill of a pack, start the first pill of the next pack on the next day without taking a break.

- Have the next pack available before finishing the current pack.

Efficacy and specific concerns

The patient should be counseled as to the advantages of the medication as well as the risks and side effects (as described above). In particular, she should be advised about the likelihood of bleeding pattern changes, to ensure that she accepts the possibility of these changes and is mentally prepared. This can increase tolerance to bleeding changes and continuation rate. The patient should be counseled to contact the provider if she desires to discontinue the method (so that an alternative can be discussed) or in case of prolonged or heavy bleeding.

Timing of initiation and backup method

No backup method is needed if POPs are started:

- during the first 5 days of the menstrual period
- between 6 weeks and 6 months postpartum if a woman is fully or nearly fully breast-feeding and amenorrheic
- within the first 21 days postpartum if not breast-feeding
- immediately after an abortion
- the day after stopping another hormonal method. If switching off COCs, skip the inactive/placebo pills.

A woman can start POPs at any time if it is reasonably certain that she is not pregnant ("quick start" method). In this case, and in all other cases when the woman could be at risk of early ovulation, a backup method (i.e., male condom, abstinence) is recommended for the first 7 days taking the POP. Additional reasons for using at least 48 hours of a backup method are:

- any time the daily POP has been taken more than 3 hours late.
- episodes of vomiting or diarrhea until 48 hours after the symptoms have subsided.

Switching

- Switching to a *new brand of POPs* can be done at any time during the cycle or at the end of the last pack.

- Switching *to POPs from COCs* should occur at the end of the 21 active COC pills (discarding the placebos).
- Switching to *COCs from POPs* should take place on the first day of menses, or at any point during the POP package.

Unprotected intercourse

In case of unprotected intercourse (missed, or late for a pill), patients should use emergency contraception (EC; see Chapter 13). Having a prescription for EC available at home facilitates access and timely use. Since EC is safe, and most effective when used as soon as possible after unprotected intercourse, patients should be encouraged to use it without delay. Contacting a clinician is not necessary before using the method. Use of the regular POP can resume the next day. Bleeding may be disrupted.

A pregnancy test is recommended if:

- the menstrual period is late and pills have been taken later or missed during the most recent cycle
- two periods in a row were missed despite taking all pills correctly
- there are concerns about a pregnancy for other reasons.

The patient should be told not to not stop taking the pill while waiting to take a pregnancy test. There is no harm to a pregnancy if the pills are continued. She should stop the pills only after a positive test is confirmed.

Drug interactions

The patient should be advised to consult a pharmacist or the provider if other medications are taken at any point in time while she is on POPs, to determine if an interaction is likely and if a backup method is needed.

Return of fertility

Because of the rapid return of fertility, abstaining from vaginal intercourse or immediately starting another method of birth control is needed once POPs are discontinued. If fertility is desired, POPs can be stopped at any time since it provides a continuous dose of a single hormone.

Available options

In the United States only the norethindrone POP has been approved. In other countries POPs containing levonorgestrel, desogestrel, or other progestogens are available. See Table 4.3 for a (nonexhaustive) list of products available

Table 4.3 Examples of POPs available worldwide

Progestogen	Country	Brand name	Company
Norethindrone (NET) 0.35µg	US	Micronor	Ortho
	US	Nor-QD	Watson
	US	Nora-BE	Watson
	US	Jolivette	Watson
	US	Camila	Barr
	US	Errin	Barr
	UK	Micronor	Janssen-Cilag
	UK	Noriday	Pfizer
Norgestrel (NG) 0.075µg (equivalent to 0.0375µg levonorgestrel)	UK	Neogest	Schering
Levonorgestrel 0.030µg	UK	Norgeston	Bayer
	Australia	Microlut	Bayer
Lynestrenol 0.5000µg	Internationally, non-US	Exluton	Organon
Ethynodiol diacetate 0.500µg	UK	Femulen	Pfizer
Desogestrel 0.075µg	UK	Cerazette	Organon

worldwide. The standard dosing package consists of 28 identical pills.

Of note, the POP Plan B, which is levonorgestrel in a dose of 1.5 mg, has a special indication as emergency contraception and is discussed in Chapter 13.

New products

No new POP that has been approved in the past few years. The most recent new product is a 75 μg desogestrel-only POP. This product is not available in the United States.

Supplying the method: counseling points

The efficacy of the method relies on ingestion every 24 hours, with no variation of more than 3 hours in the dosing interval. Women using the POP must understand that it is essential to be very compliant with this aspect.

The bleeding pattern is often unpredictable and irregular. This is not a medical concern, and does not indicate a lack of efficacy. Women who receive advanced counseling regarding bleeding changes are more likely to accept this and continue the method.

Management of problems

Bleeding pattern changes are the most frequently encountered problem when using POPs. They are not a medical concern but can be a significant nuisance. Approaches include reassurance, since patterns typically improve with time. Nonsteroidal anti-inflammatory agents (NSAIDs) may reduce heavy bleeding.

Adverse effects may be an indication for discontinuation of POPs. See the WHO MEC for details.

Selected references

ACOG Practice Bulletin No. 73. Use of hormonal contraception in women with coexisting medical conditions. Obstet Gynecol 2006; 107(6):1453–72.

ACOG Practice Bulletin No. 109. Noncontraceptive uses of hormonal contraceptives. Obstet Gynecol 2010;115(1):206–18.

Ahrendt HJ, Karckt U, Pichl T, Mueller T, Ernst U. The effects of an oestrogen-free, desogestrel-containing oral contraceptive in women with cyclical symptoms: results from two studies on oestrogen-related symptoms and dysmenorrhoea. Eur J Contracept Reprod Health Care 2007;12(4):354–61.

Ball MJ, Ashwell E, Gillmer MD. Progestagen-only oral contraceptives: comparison of the metabolic effects of levonorgestrel and norethisterone. Contraception 1991;44(3):223–33.

Belsey EM. Vaginal bleeding patterns among women using one natural and eight hormonal methods of contraception. Contraception 1988;38(2):181–206.

Benagiano G, Primiero FM. Seventy-five microgram desogestrel minipill, a new perspective in estrogen-free contraception. Ann N Y Acad Sci 2003;997:163–73.

Bjarnadottir RI, Gottfredsdottir H, Sigurdardottir K, Geirsson RT, Dieben TO. Comparative study of the effects of a progestogen-only pill containing desogestrel and an intrauterine contraceptive device in lactating women. Br J Obstet Gynaecol 2001;108(11):1174–80.

Caird LE, Reid-Thomas V, Hannan WJ, Gow S, Glasier AF. Oral progestogen-only contraception may protect against loss of bone mass in breast-feeding women. Clin Endocrinol (Oxf) 1994;41(6):739–45.

Collaborative Group on Hormonal Factors in Breast Cancer. Breast cancer and hormonal contraceptives: collaborative reanalysis of individual data on 53 297 women with breast cancer and 100 239 women without breast cancer from 54 epidemiological studies. Lancet 1996;347(9017):1713–27.

Culwell KR, Curtis KM, del Carmen Cravioto M. Safety of contraceptive method use among women with systemic lupus erythematosus: a systematic review. Obstet Gynecol 2009;114(2 Pt 1):341–53.

Curtis KM, Martins SL. Progestogen-only contraception and bone mineral density: a systematic review. Contraception 2006;73(5):470–87.

Curtis KM, Ravi A, Gaffield ML. Progestogen-only contraceptive use in obese women. Contraception 2009;80(4):346–54.

Edelman AB, Carlson NE, Cherala G, et al. Impact of obesity on oral contraceptive pharmacokinetics and hypothalamic-pituitary-ovarian activity. Contraception 2009;80(2):119–27.

Haile RW, Thomas DC, Mguire V, et al. BRCA1 and BRCA2 mutation carriers, oral contraceptive use, and breast cancer before age 50. Cancer Epidemiol Biomarkers Prev 2006;15(10): 1863–70.

Hannaford PC, Selvaraj S, Elliott AM, Angus V, Iversen L, Lee AJ. Cancer risk among users of oral contraceptives: cohort data from the Royal College of General Practitioner's oral contraception study. BMJ 2007;335(7621):651.

Heinemann LA, Assmann A, DoMinh T, Garbe E. Oral progestogen-only contraceptives and cardiovascular risk: results from the Transnational Study on Oral Contraceptives and the Health of Young Women. Eur J Contracep Reprod Health Care 1999;4(2):67–73.

Irvine GA, Campbell-Brown MB, Lumsden MA, Heikkila A, Walker JJ, Cameron IT. Randomised comparative trial of the levonorgestrel intrauterine system and norethisterone for treatment of idiopathic menorrhagia. Br J Obstet Gynaecol 1998;105(6):592–8.

Jensen JT, Speroff L. Health benefits of oral contraceptives. Obstet Gynecol Clin North Am 2000;27(4):705–21.

Kivela A, Ruuskanen M, Agren U, Dieben T. The effects of two progestogen-only pills containing either desogestrel (75 microgram/day) or levonorgestrel (30 microgram/day) on carbohydrate metabolism and adrenal and thyroid function. Eur J Contracep Reprod Health Care 2001;6(2):71–7.

Korver T, Klipping C, Heger-Mahn D, Duijkers I, van Osta G, Dieben T. Maintenance of ovulation inhibition with the 75-microg desogestrel-only contraceptive pill (Cerazette) after scheduled 12-h delays in tablet intake. Contraception 2005;71(1):8–13.

Kumle M, Weiderpass E, Braaten T, Persson I, Adami HO, Lund E. Use of oral contraceptives and breast cancer risk: The Norwegian-Swedish Women's Lifestyle and Health Cohort Study. Cancer Epidemiol Biomarkers Prev 2002; 11(11):1375–81.

International Agency for Research on Cancer. Hormonal contraceptives, progestogens only. Vol 72. Lyon: IARC Press; 1999.

Lee E, Ma H, McKean-Cowdin R, et al. Effect of reproductive factors and oral contraceptives on breast cancer risk in BRCA1/2 mutation carriers and noncarriers: results from a population-based study. Cancer Epidemiol Biomarkers Prev 2008;17(11):3170–8.

Lidegaard O, Lokkegaard E, Svendsen AL, Agger C. Hormonal contraception and risk of venous thromboembolism: national follow-up study. BMJ 2009;339:b2890.

Lopez LM, Grimes DA, Schulz KF. Steroidal contraceptives: effect on carbohydrate metabolism in women without diabetes mellitus. Cochrane Database Syst Rev 2009(4):CD006133.

Marchbanks PA, McDonald JA, Wilson HG, et al. Oral contraceptives and the risk of breast cancer. N Engl J Med 2002;346(26):2025–32.

Narod SA, Dube MP, Klijn J, et al. Oral contraceptives and the risk of breast cancer in BRCA1 and BRCA2 mutation carriers. J Natl Cancer Inst 2002;94(23):1773–9.

National Survey of Family Growth. User guide. Available from: http://www.cdc.gov/nchs/nsfg/nsfg_2006_2008_puf.htm. Accessed 10/28/2010.

Nelson AL, Le MH, Musherraf Z, Vanberckelaer A. Intermediate-term glucose tolerance in women with a history of gestational diabetes: natural history and potential associations with breast-feeding and contraception. Am J Obstet Gynecol 2008;198(6):699 e691–7; discussion 699 e697–8.

Pakarinen P, Lahteenmaki P, Rutanen EM. The effect of intrauterine and oral levonorgestrel administration on serum concentrations of sex hormone-binding globulin, insulin and insulin-like growth factor binding protein-1. Acta Obstet Gynecol Scand 1999;78(5):423–8.

Rice CF, Killick SR, Dieben T, Coelingh Bennink H. A comparison of the inhibition of ovulation achieved by desogestrel 75 micrograms and levonorgestrel 30 micrograms daily. Hum Reprod 1999;14(4):982–5.

Tayob Y, Adams J, Jacobs HS, Guillebaud J. Ultrasound demonstration of increased frequency of functional ovarian cysts in women using progestogen-only oral contraception. Br J Obstet Gynaecol 1985;92(10):1003–9.

Trussell J. Contraceptive failure in the United States. Contraception 2004;70(2):89–96.

Truitt ST, Fraser AB, Grimes DA, Gallo MF, Schulz KF. Combined hormonal versus nonhormonal versus progestin-only contraception in lactation. Cochrane Database Syst Rev 2003(2):CD003988.

Vessey M. Oral contraceptive failures and body weight: findings in a large cohort study. J Fam Plann Reprod Health Care 2001;27(2):90–1.

Vessey M, Yeates D. Oral contraceptives and benign breast disease: an update of findings in a large cohort study. Contraception 2007; 76(6):418–24.

Weiderpass E, Adami HO, Baron JA, Magnusson C, Lindgren A, Persson I. Use of oral contraceptives and endometrial cancer risk (Sweden). Cancer Causes Control 1999;10(4):277–84.

WHO. Cardiovascular disease and use of oral and injectable progestogen-only contraceptives and combined injectable contraceptives. Results of an international, multicenter, case-control study. World Health Organization Collaborative Study of Cardiovascular Disease and Steroid Hormone Contraception. Contraception 1998;57(5):315–24.

WHO. Medical eligibility criteria for contraceptive use, 4th ed. Geneva: World Health Organization; 2009. Available from: http://www.who.int/reproductivehealth/publications/family_planning/9789241563888/en/index.html

5

Contraceptive Implants

Nerys Benfield and Philip D. Darney

Department of Obstetrics Gynecology and Reproductive Sciences, University of California, San Francisco and San Francisco General Hospital, San Francisco, CA, USA

Introduction

Implanon, a one-rod etonogestrel (ENG) system, is the only subdermal implant approved in the United States. Clinicians may encounter other systems in use worldwide—the pharmacological profile and physical effects of all the implantable contraceptives are similar. Implants require minor operative procedures for placement and for discontinuation, so clinicians have a special responsibility to become skilled in these operations in order to make sure that these safe and effective methods are readily available to their patients.

Disturbances of menstrual patterns are frequent and since many patients are not familiar with implant contraception, appropriate and informed counseling is crucial.

Method of action

Implants are highly effective progestin-only contraceptives that come in the form of one or more subdermally placed rods. The progestin diffuses from the implant into the surrounding tissues, providing an initial level in the circulation that is lower than with oral or injected methods. Implants have multiple modes of action:

- Supression of ovulation: The ENG implant initially releases 60 μg/day of etonorgestrel and around 30 μg/day after 2 years of use. This progestin centrally suppresses the luteinizing hormone (LH) surge necessary for ovulation. While follicular development does occur, thus avoiding clinically significant hypoestrogenism, Implanon consistently suppresses ovulation for a least 2.5 years. Norplant frequently suppresses ovulation during the first 2 years of use. Only about 10% of women are ovulatory during the first 2 years but this number increases to 50% by 5 years.
- The steady release of progestin has a prolonged effect on the cervical mucus which thickens and decreases in amount, forming a barrier to sperm penetration.
- The progestin causes atrophy of the endometrium which could prevent implantation should fertilization occur.

> **EVIDENCE AT A GLANCE**
>
> With this combination of effects, implant contraceptives are extremely effective. A recent Cochrane meta-analysis of implant clinical trials showed no pregnancies with either Norplant or ENG implants in 45,000 women-months of use.

Good candidates

Contraceptive implants are a good choice for women of reproductive age who desire convenient, long-term, highly effective, continuous contraception. Implants should be considered in the following conditions:

- Women who want to *delay the next pregnancy* for at least 2–3 years or have completed childbearing.

- Women who experience *estrogen-related side effects* on combination methods.
- Women with *contraindications to combination oral contraceptives (COCs) related to the estrogen* component. This includes women with hypertension, migraines, known thrombogenic mutations, smoking, or multiple risk factors for cardiovascular disease.
- Women with *chronic illnesses*, in which health will be threatened by pregnancy and other contraceptives may have deleterious effects. This includes diabetes with or without vascular disease, nephropathy, retinopathy or neuropathy, sickle cell disease, depression, lupus, atrial fibrillation, pulmonary hypertension, and thalassemia, Aside from their need for highly effective contraception, there are no clinically significant metabolic changes associated with the sustained, low doses of progestin delivered by implants. Norplant and ENG implant do not have important clinical effects on the lipoprotein profile, carbohydrate metabolism, thyroid and adrenal function, liver function, or the clotting mechanism. Implants are a particularly good choice for diabetics, or for women at risk for metabolic, cardiovascular, or thromboembolic disorders. Although it is known that progestins can effect carbohydrate metabolism, these effects are not seen with the low doses found in implants. In a cohort study of Norplant users over 5 years, no increase was observed in diabetes, depression, lupus, or cardiovascular diseases. Studies on Norplant users report no clinically important effects on carbohydrate metabolism or insulin sensitivity.
- Implants can also be a good choice for *obese women*. Studies of Norplant show that the greater the weight of the user, the lower the levonorgestrel concentrations during use. But even for heavy women, the release rate is high enough to prevent pregnancy at least as reliably as oral contraceptives. In ENG implant users, etonogestrel concentrations do not decline below contraceptive levels as body weight increases, nor is there an increased risk of difficult insertions or removals with increasing body mass index (BMI).
- *Lactating women*: As progestin-only methods, implant contraceptives are a good choice for breast-feeding women. The World Health Organization Medical Eligibility Criteria (WHO MEC) recommend insertion at 6 weeks postpartum in lactating women. Studies show no effects on breast milk quality or quantity, and infants of mothers with implants grow normally. Implants also seem to be a good choice for immediate postpartum administration. A small study comparing immediate postpartum ENG implant to depot medroxyprogestereone acetate (DMPA) at 6 weeks showed no impact on continuation of exclusive breast-feeding and normal infant weight gain.
- *Immediate postpartum insertion in non-breast-feeding women* may offer a significant advantage to some women rather than waiting the 3 weeks prior to starting combination OCs.
- Women with *major surgery with prolonged immobilization*.

Poor candidates

There are only a few absolute contraindications to implant use; they include:

- *Active* thrombophlebitis or thromboembolic disease
- Undiagnosed genital bleeding prior to evaluation
- Severe decompensated cirrhosis, active hepatitis
- Benign or malignant liver tumors
- Breast cancer
- Women on certain anticonvulsants or rifampicin.

Medical eligibility criteria

In general the WHO MEC demonstrate that implant contraceptives are extremely safe and place very few restrictions to their use, as listed in Table 5.1.

Advantages

Efficacy

Implant contraceptives are as effective as sterilization and IUDs, and more effective than oral, patch, vaginal ring, or barrier contraceptives.

Table 5.1 WHO MEC for implant contraceptives

Category 4[a]	Current breast cancer
Category 3[b]	<6 weeks breast-feeding Current DVT/PE Current worsening of ischaemic heart disease while using ENG implant or stroke Current worsening of migraine with aura while using ENG implant Unexplained vaginal bleeding before evaluation Active hepatic or severe decompensated cirrhosis Benign or malignant liver tumors Rifampin or certain anticonvulsants including phenytoin, barbiturates carbamazepine, primidone, topiramate, oxcarbazepine Breast cancer history with no current disease for 5 years
Good clinical judgment, appropriate medical management and **thoughtful follow-up** should be used in women with the following conditions:	

	Heavy cigarette smoking in women >35 years
	Hypercholesterolemia
	Hypertension
	History of cardiovascular disease, including myocardial infarction, cerebral
	    vascular accident, coronary artery disease, angina, a previous thromboembolic
	    event, artificial heart valves
	Gallbladder disease[c]
	History of ectopic pregnancy
	Severe depression (see Chapter 20)
	Severe migraine headaches
	Certain HIV antiretroviral medications (see Chapter 23)
	Severe acne or hirsutism (see Chapter 22)

[a]Category 4: Condition which represents an unacceptable health risk if the contraceptive method is used.
[b]Category 3: Condition where the theoretical or proven risks usually outweigh the advantages of using the method.
[c]A slight increase in gallbladder disease has been noted in Norplant users. The association is weak and may reflect pre-existing disease as there is no clear biologic mechanism.

Important reasons for the very low failure rate associated with the implant are its high efficacy and the fact that its use requires very little effort on part of the user after placement.

In 11 international clinical trials of 942 women using ENG implant, *no* pregnancies occurred over 2–3 years. In studies of Norplant conducted in 11 countries, totaling 12,133 woman-years of use, the pregnancy rate was 0.2 pregnancies per 100 woman–years, and all but one of the pregnancies that occurred were present at the time of implant insertion.

Rapid reversibility

Unlike injectable contraceptives, the contraceptive effectiveness of implants rapidly reverses after removal. Return of fertility occurs within a few weeks, in contrast to the 6- to 18-month delay in ovulation that can follow DMPA. Most women resume normal ovulatory cycles during the first month after removal, and pregnancy rates during the first year after removal are comparable with those of overall populations of women trying to become pregnant. Implantable contraceptives therefore allow women to more accurately time their return to fertility.

High degree of safety

Overall, the implant has adverse event rates (including death, cardiovascular events, neoplastic disease, anemia, hypertension, bone density changes, gallbladder disease, diabetes, thrombocytopenia, and pelvic inflammatory disease) comparable with women not using implants. There are few WHO MEC restrictions (see Table 5.1)

Noncontraceptive benefits

Exposure of endometriosis to progestin-only contraceptive methods is an effective method to manage the pain associated with this condition. The use of the ENG implant specifically has been reported to reduce endometriosis pain. The ENG implant is also reported to reduce menstrual pain in up to 88% of users previously experiencing dysmenorrhea.

Other possible noncontraceptive benefits are discussed in Chapter 4.

Risks and side effects

The low systemic concentrations of progestins from implant contraceptives cause few side effects and those that do occur generally decrease with duration of use.

Irregular bleeding

The most bothersome side effect of implantable contraceptives is irregular bleeding, which is the most common reason for discontinuation, especially during the first year of use. Because implants allow for follicular development but not ovulation, endogenous estrogen production is nearly normal. Progestin, however, is not regularly withdrawn (as in a normal cycle) to allow endometrial sloughing. Consequently, the endometrium sheds at unpredictable intervals and menstrual bleeding patterns can be highly variable.

With the ENG implant, many women experience prolonged irregular, but rarely heavy, bleeding in the first year that can continue for the duration of use. Studies of Norplant show that alteration of menstrual patterns will occur during the first year of use in approximately 80% of users, later decreasing to about 40%.

Although amenorrhea occurs in approximately 20% of women in the first year, the rate declines with use to 13% by year 3.

> **⚠ CAUTION**
>
> Discontinuation rates secondary to irregular bleeding can be quite high, up to 30%, so **it is critical to discuss these changes** with the potential user.

> **★ TIPS & TRICKS**
>
> - Implant users who can no longer tolerate prolonged bleeding will benefit from short course of oral estrogen; conjugated estrogens 1.25 mg, or estradiol 2 m, daily for 7 days.
> - A second approach is to administer an estrogen–progestin oral contraceptive for 1–3 months.
> - Studies have also shown some benefit with mifepristone, doxycycline, and NSAIDs, but estrogen is probably the most effective treatment.

Headaches

A recent meta-analysis of 11 clinical trials showed the most common nonmenstrual side effect was headache, reported by 25% of patients. Approximately 20% of women who discontinue use do so because of headache. This is similar to the complaints of headaches reported by women using oral contraceptives, and patients can be reassured that the incidence tends to decrease with use.

Weight changes

During ENG implant trials 13% of women complained of weight gain (the second most common complaint). Although an increase in appetite can be attributed to the androgenic activity of progestins, the dose in implantable contraceptives is very low and the evidence for weight gain is variable.

Among women using Norplant in the Dominican Republic, 75% of those who changed weight lost weight, whereas in San Francisco, two-thirds gained weight. A 5-year follow-up of 75 women with Norplant implants could document no increase in BMI. In a meta-analysis of ENG implant trials, 70% of women did gain some weight over the course of 3 years but it is difficult to attribute the gain directly to the contraceptive. In women receiving an implant immediately postpartum there has been shown to be no differences in postpregnancy weight loss.

Breast effects

Breast pain was reported by 12.8% of women using the ENG implant. Studies of Norplant showed that breast pain tends to decrease with increasing duration of use, and patients should be reassured.

Galactorrhea is reported to occur and is more common among women who have had insertion of the implants on discontinuation of lactation. Pregnancy and other possible causes should be ruled out. Decreasing the amount of breast stimulation can help to alleviate the symptom, but if amenorrhea accompanies persistent galactorrhea, a prolactin level should be obtained.

Acne

Acne is the most common skin complaint among implant users and was reported by 13% of ENG implant users, though more women reported improvement of acne than worsening.

Ovarian cysts

Unlike oral contraception, the low serum progestin levels maintained by implants do not suppress follicle stimulating hormone (FSH), which continues to stimulate ovarian follicle growth in most users. Adnexal masses are approximately eight times more frequent in Norplant users compared with normally cycling women.

Potential risks

Impact on bone density

Implant contraceptives have no significant effect of on bone density. Measurements of bone density in young women show that the ENG implant does not affect the teenage gain in bone. In older women, no significant changes in bone density, as measured by DEXA scans of the spine and femur, have been seen.

Ectopic pregnancy

Like all contraceptives, implants decrease the risk of pregnancy, including ectopics. When pregnancy does occur, though, ectopic pregnancy should be suspected because approximately 30% of Norplant pregnancies are ectopic.

Patient counseling

When discussing contraceptive options, the first step is to assess the patient's desire for long-term reversible contraception by assessing her future fertility plans. Personal and family medical history-taking should then concentrate on any factors that might contraindicate use of implants. A detailed medication list is also important to determine if there are any medications that might affect metabolism of the hormonal agent.

The key points for counseling the potential implant user are to discuss the insertion and removal, and make sure the patient is aware of potential side effects, especially *bleeding disruptions*. All users must be aware of the possible *menstrual changes*. It is important to stress that all of these changes are expected, and that most women revert back to a more normal pattern with increasing duration of use. *Other bothersome side effects* include headache, acne, and breast pain.

Discontinuation rates for implant methods can be up to 50% at 3 years with ENG implant and 70% at 5 years with Norplant. While many of these discontinuations are due to desire for childbearing, good counseling about life with an implant can prepare patients for potential issues. Stressing the benefits of the methods, such as efficacy and convenience, will help support the patient in her decision.

Because the insertion and removal of implants require minor surgical procedures, *initiation and discontinuation costs* are higher than with other methods. The cost of implants plus fees for insertion may seem high to patients unless they compare it with the cost of using other methods for a comparable time (see Chapter 2). A recent cost-effectiveness analysis found that ENG implant was the most cost-effective method of contraception compared to DMPA, copper IUD, and Mirena, and was more cost-effective than oral contraceptives at 12 months of use. Making patients aware of long-term cost and time savings with implantable contraceptives can help support their decision to use the method.

Available options

There are three major implant systems around the world today—ENG implant, Norplant, and Jadelle. In the United States only the ENG implant is available.

The *ENG implant* is a single flexible rod 4 cm long and 2 mm in diameter containing 68 mg of etonogestrel, the active metabolite of desogestrel, dispersed in a core of ethylene vinyl acetate wrapped with a membrane of the same material. It was approved in the United States in 2006. The hormone is released at an initial rate of about 67 µg/day, decreasing to 30 µg after 2 years; con-centrations that inhibit ovulation are achieved within 8 hours of insertion. The ENG implant has only one rod, rather than Norplant's six, which simplifies insertion and removal. The preloaded applicator also facilitates precise placement.

EVIDENCE AT A GLANCE

ENG implant suppresses ovulation for at least 2.5 years, and provides highly effective contraception for at least 3 years.

Norplant was developed by the Population Council in 1983 but was unfortunately withdrawn from the U.S. market in 2002 for business reasons. The Norplant system consists of six capsules made of flexible silastic tubing, measuring 34 mm in length and 2.4 mm in diameter and containing 36 mg crystalline levonorgestrel each for a total of 216 mg levonorgestrel, which is very stable and has remained unchanged in capsules examined after more than 9 years of use.

Jadelle was also developed by the Population Council and approved by the U.S. Food and Drug Authority (FDA) in 1996 but has never been marketed in this country. The Jadelle's rods are wrapped in silastic tubing, measure 43 mm long and 2.5 mm in diameter, and contain a total of 150 mg levonorgestrel. Long-term clinical trials indicate that the performance and side effects are similar to Norplant, but removal is faster. A similar system, Sinoplant, is used in China.

Uniplant is a single implant contraceptive, containing 55 mg nomegestrol acetate in a 4 cm silicone capsule with a 100 µg/day release rate. It provides contraception for 1 year.

There are two *nestorone-containing implants*. Nestorone is a single silicone implant and is effective for 2 years. Elcometrine lasts 6 months. This progestin is inactive when ingested orally, possibly making these methods a preferred option for breast-feeding mothers given that there should be no activity of any nestorone transferred through breast milk.

New products

No new implantable contraceptives are currently being developed for use in the United States.

Supplying the method

Counseling and screening

Implants can be inserted at any time during the menstrual cycle as long as pregnancy can be ruled out. They have an almost immediate contraceptive effect when inserted within the first 7 days of a menstrual cycle. When insertion is after day 7, a back-up method is necessary for 3 days, while cervical mucus becomes viscid. Implants can be inserted immediately postpartum.

The nondominant, inner upper arm is the best site for placement because it is easily accessible to the clinician with minimal exposure of the patient, is well protected during most normal activities, and is not highly visible. Migration of implants from this site is rare.

Insertion and removal of implants will be a new experience for most women, who approach it with varying degrees of apprehension and anxiety. Women should be told that the incisions used for the procedures are very small and heal quickly, and that normal activity cannot damage or displace the implants. Potential users should be screened to rule out allergies to the anesthetics, cleaning solutions, or other products used during the insertion.

Insertion is carried out under local anesthesia in the office or clinic, and is rapid: in clinical trials, the average insertion time for ENG implant was 1.1 minutes. Insertion is typically painless, with pain at the insertion site reported by 3% of women, and complications seen in less than 1%. Most women feel only a mild burning with the local anesthetic injection and some pressure.

Because ENG implant is the only implant used in the United States we will discuss its insertion and removal here, but techniques are similar for all the subdermal implants.

Placement

Implantable contraceptives are unique in that women cannot initiate or discontinue these methods without the assistance of a clinician. Before insertion, the patient should read and sign a written consent for the surgical placement of the implants. The consent reviews the potential complications of the procedure that include reaction to the local anesthetic, infection, expulsion of the implants, superficial phlebitis, bruising, and the possibility of a subsequent difficult removal—although the incidence of complicated removals is low, at approximately 5% for Norplant and 1% for ENG implant. It is recommended that the patient touch and feel the implant in an arm model prior to placement.

The scars from insertion and removal are small and not easily seen. Although most women become unaware of the implants, it is important to discuss that a few women report sensing the implants if they have been touched or manipulated for a prolonged period of time, or after vigorous exercise. Other people may notice the implants (as reported by 20% of U.S. patients), and implants tend to be more visible in slender women with good muscle tone. Darker-skinned users may notice further darkening of the skin directly over the implants, which resolves after removal.

Insertion

Positioning and technique

The patient is in supine position, exposing the upper inner arm by rotating the arm out with a bend at the elbow. The insertion site is selected approximately 6–8 cm proximal to the medial epicondyle of the humerus in the groove between the biceps and triceps, and the area is cleaned. Marking the skin at the insertion site can be helpful.

- Local anesthesia is injected to raise a weal at the insertion site and under the skin along the planned track of the insertion needle.
- The presence of ENG implant must be verified by seeing the implant at the tip of the needle, tapping the applicator down if necessary. Once the cap is opened, it is very important to keep the tip of the inserter pointed upwards to prevent the implant from falling out.
- The insertion needle is pushed directly through the skin at no greater than a 20° angle and advanced to its full length as superficially as possible under the skin by tenting the skin with the tip of the needle.
- Once the needle has been fully advanced, break the seal by pressing the obturator support and turn 90°. Fix the obturator with one hand and slowly pull the needle out with the other hand.

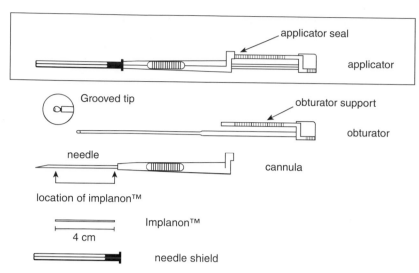

Figure 5.1 Implanon insertion device.

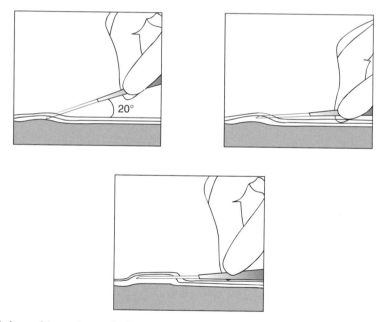

Figure 5.2 Subdermal insertion technique.

Insertion is verified by viewing the grooved tip of the obturator in the needle and palpating the implant in place. Patients should also palpate their own implants and be counseled to keep the area clean and bandage in place for 24–48 hours.

Complications at insertion are very rare but include infection, hematoma, local irritation or rash, expulsion, and allergic reactions. The incidence of complications is minimized by clinician training and experience, and the use of good technique. Any bruising that might occur can be minimized by wrapping the arm to form a pressure bandage. Local irritations typically resolve spontaneously and are often due to allergies to adhesives. Good screening can avoid these issues.

Removal

Implant removal is another small office procedure. Practicing on a model will make the first few removals more comfortable for the patient and provider. In a recent meta-analysis, the mean time for ENG implant removal was 2.6 minutes and for Norplant it was 10.2 minutes. Of course, proper insertion is the key to easy removal. Even with Norplant, most removals are not painful (80% of patients reported pain as "none" or "slight") although patients do tend to feel pressure or tugging with local anesthesia.

Positioning and technique

The patient is positioned as for insertion, the implant is palpated and the area is cleaned. With sterile gloves the incision site is carefully selected just at the distal tip of the rod. This is the most critical step for easy removal.

- Local anesthetic is injected at the incision site and a small 2–3 mm incision is made with an 11-blade scalpel.
- The implant is then pushed towards the incision and the fibrous sheath surrounding the implant is scraped away with the tip of the scalpel, taking care not to cut the implant.
- Once the sheath is broken the implant can be pushed out of the incision and grasped with a clamp or fingers to pull it out.
- The incision is then closed with an adhesive strip and dressed. The technique is the same for multirod systems, making the incision as close to the tips of all rods as possible.
- Sometimes more manipulation with clamps is required to access all the implants.

> ✋ **CAUTION**
>
> As noted earlier, return to fertility is rapid. Patients not wishing to conceive are advised to start an alternate method of contraception on the day of removal.

Management of problems

Bleeding problems

Implant users who can no longer tolerate prolonged bleeding will benefit from a short course of oral estrogen: conjugated estrogens (1.25 mg) or estradiol (2 mg) daily for 7 days. A second approach is to administer an estrogen–progestin oral contraceptive for 1–3 months. Studies have also shown some benefit with mifepristone, doxycycline, and NSAIDs, but estrogen is probably the most effective treatment.

Complicated insertion and removal

Rates of complications during insertion or removal are very low. Infection occurs in less than 1% of cases, and most can be treated with a course of oral antibiotics. Some, though, may require removal of the device if unresponsive to treatment. Infections can also increase the chance of implant expulsion so always continue to palpate for the implant throughout treatment.

For a nonpalpable implant, ultrasound using a linear array transducer (>7 mHz) should be used to localize the implant by applying the transducer to the upper arm perpendicular to the humerus to identify the shadow of the implant. The full implant is then viewed by repositioning the transducer and measuring the depth. The skin should then be marked, after which an incision can be made in the appropriate area and gentle probing for the implant performed. If the implant cannot be localized with ultrasound then MRI should be used.

For implants that are very deeply embedded, one removal technique is to make an incision above the mid-portion of the implant as described by imaging, and use vasectomy forceps to grasp the implant, bring to the skin, and remove from the sheath.

If removal of the implant is very difficult, painful, or prolonged, the procedure should be interrupted and the patient should return in a few weeks to complete the removal once the bleeding and swelling have subsided, at which time the focus should be on careful placement of the incision.

Selected references

Abdel-Aleem H, d'Arcangues C, Vogelsong KK, Gülmezoglu AM. Treatment of vaginal bleeding irregularities induced by progestin only contraceptives. Cochrane Database Syst Rev, 2007(3):CD003449.

Blumenthal P, Gemzell-Danielsson K, Marintcheva-Petrova M. Tolerability and clinical safety of Implanon. Eur J Contracept Reprod Health Care 2008;13(S1):29–36.

Brache V, Faundes A, Alvarez F, Cochon L. Nonmenstrual adverse events during use of implantable contraceptives for women: data from clinical trials. Contraception 2002;65: 63–74.

Croxatto HB, Mäkäräinen L. The pharmacodynamics and efficacy of Implanon. Contraception 1998;58:91–7S.

Darney P, Patel A, Rosen K, Shapiro LS, Kaunitz AM. Safety and efficacy of a single-rod etonogrestrel implant (Implanon): results from 11 international clinical trials. Fertil Steril 2009;91:1646–53.

Dorflinger L. Metabolic effects of implantable steroid contraceptives for women. Contraception 2002;65:47–62.

Huber J, Wenzl R. Pharmacokinetics of Implanon. An integrated analysis. Contraception 1998; 58(Suppl):85–90S.

Levine JP, Sinfonsky F, Christ M. Assessment of Implanon insertion and removal. Contraception 2008;78:409–17.

Meirik O, Fraser IS. d'Arcangues C, for the WHO Consultation on Implantable Contraceptives for Women. Implantable contraceptives for women. Hum Reprod Update 2003;9:49–59.

Power J, French R, Cowan F. Subdermal implantable contraceptives versus other forms of reversible contraceptives or other implants as effective methods for preventing pregnancy. Cochrane Library 2007;18(3):CD001326.

Reinprayoon D, Taneepanichskul S, Bunyavejchevin S, et al. Effects of the etonogestrel-releasing contraceptive implant (Implanon) on parameters of breastfeeding compared to those of an intrauterine device. Contraception 2000;62:239–46.

Sivin I. International experience with Norplant and Norplant-2 contraceptives. Stud Fam Plann 1988;19:81–94.

6

Ins and Outs of the Contraceptive Vaginal Ring

Frans J.M.E. Roumen

Department of Obstetrics and Gynaecology, Atrium Medical Centre Parkstad, Heerlen, The Netherlands

Method of action and effectiveness

The contraceptive vaginal ring (CVR) is a soft, pliable, and transparent plastic ring-shaped device measuring 5.4 cm (2.1 in) in diameter (Figure 6.1). The ring is made of the copolymer ethylene vinylacetate, in which the hormones ethinyl estradiol (EE, 2.7 mg) and etonogestrel (ENG, 11.7 mg) are equally dispersed. ENG is 3-ketodesogestrel, which is the active metabolite of the progestin desogestrel. Due to its composition, the ring steadily releases 15 µg EE and 120 µg ENG daily.

The CVR is easily inserted by the woman into her vagina where the hormones are continuously absorbed through the epithelium, resulting in low and steady serum levels for a 3-week period. Then the ring is removed by the woman for a 1-week ring-free period.

Suppression of ovulation is the basic working mechanism of the CVR, comparable to that with combined oral contraceptives (COCs). Ovulation, as determined by follicle changes (assessed by ultrasound) and progesterone levels, was suppressed throughout a 5-week duration of CVR use, suggesting that one ring remains effective for an additional 2 weeks after the recommended 3-week interval.

The effectiveness of the CVR in large-scale clinical and randomized controlled studies has been shown to be similar to that of other combined hormonal contraceptive methods, with a pregnancy rate of about 1% (Table 6.1). These results were confirmed in observational phase IV studies reflecting the effectiveness of the CVR in typical common real-world practice.

> **EVIDENCE AT A GLANCE**
>
> Serum levels of ethinyl estradiol (EE) and etonogestrel (ENG) in ring users are not altered by concurrent use of a spermicide, nor by the use of tampons. Concurrent use of antibiotics (amoxicillin and doxycycline) with the ring also do not alter serum hormone levels. Concomitant use of miconazole, an antifungal, has been shown to increase release of both hormones. It is unlikely, however, that this increased release will interfere with effective ovulation suppression.

Good candidates

Basically, the CVR represents a useful option for all women looking for an effective, reliable, convenient, and discreet contraceptive. It is an excellent option for women who frequently forget their pill, and for women who are tired of taking an oral contraceptive pill daily, as the ring has to be inserted and removed only once a month. This is especially an advantage for women with irregular lives or working hours, like students, shift workers, and frequent travelers.

Women who want to be self-supporting without having to depend on a healthcare provider for administration of their contraceptive

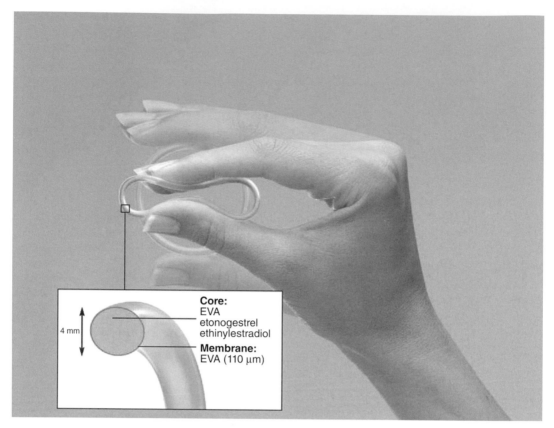

Figure 6.1 The contraceptive vaginal ring is a soft, pliable, and transparent plastic ring-shaped device measuring 5.4 cm (2.1 in) in diameter. The ring is made of the copolymer ethylene vinylacetate (EVA), in which the hormones ethinylestradiol (EE, 2.7 mg) and etonogestrel (ENG, 11.7 mg) are equally dispersed. The ring is easily inserted by the woman into her vagina and used for 3 weeks in a row. Due to the composition of the ring, it steadily releases 15 µg EE and 120 µg ENG daily.

Table 6.1 Contraceptive efficacy with the contraceptive vaginal ring in two noncomparative studies, and in two randomized controlled trials comparing the ring with two different pills: 150LNG/30EE and DRSP/30EE (intent-to-treat population)

Study	Method (number of participants)	Pearl index	95% CI
Roumen et al. 2001	Vaginal ring (n = 1145)	0.65	0.24–1.41
Dieben et al. 2002	Vaginal ring (n = 2322)	1.18	0.73–1.80
Oddsson et al. 2005	Vaginal ring (n = 512)	1.23	0.40–2.86
	150LNG/30EE pill (n = 518)	1.19	0.39–2.79
Ahrendt et al. 2006	Vaginal ring (n = 499)	0.25	0.01–1.36
	DRSP/30EE pill (n = 484)	0.99	0.27–2.53

CI, confidence interval; DRSP, drospirenone; EE, ethinyl estradiol; LNG, levonogestrel.

method (as is required for intrauterine devices, injections, or implants) will be very satisfied with the CVR, as it offers optimal freedom for the user.

In contrast with the serum hormone peaks and troughs of the pill, the CVR delivers nearly steady-state serum hormone levels. The resulting superior cycle control is an attractive argument for women with bleeding complaints during pill use. Women who feel that the low daily exposure to estrogen is less harmful for their general health and may result in less estrogen-related side effects are also good candidates for the CVR.

Poor candidates

As the CVR is a combined hormonal contraceptive, it has essentially the same general contraindications as the COC (see Chapter 3). Other poor candidates are women with an allergy or hypersensitivity to any of the components of the ring, and women with a phobia about touching their own genitals.

Relative contraindications for CVR use are a prolapsed uterus, cystocele or rectocele, severe constipation, history of toxic shock syndrome, and any condition that causes the vagina to be easily irritated.

> ✋ **CAUTION**
>
> Cigarette smoking increases the risk of serious cardiovascular side effects in combination with combined contraceptives like the CVR. This risk increases even more if the woman is over age 35 and if she smokes 15 or more cigarettes a day. Women who use combination hormonal contraceptives, including the CVR, are strongly advised not to smoke.

Medical eligibility criteria

The CVR delivers a low dose of combined hormones ENG and EE, resulting in the same working mechanism and the same absolute and relative contraindications as the COC. Therefore, medical eligibility criteria for the CVR are exactly the same as for low-dose COCs. For an overview the reader is referred to Chapter 3.

> ✋ **CAUTION**
>
> The CVR does not protect against HIV infection (AIDS) and other sexually transmitted infections (STIs) such as chlamydia, genital herpes, genital warts, gonorrhea, hepatitis B, and syphilis. If there is risk of AIDS or other STIs (including during pregnancy or postpartum), the correct and consistent use of condoms is recommended, either alone or with another contraceptive method. Male latex condoms are proven to protect against STI/HIV.

Advantages

The sustained delivery of ENG and EE through the vaginal epithelium into the circulation is the unique difference between the contraceptive vaginal ring and the oral contraceptive pill, resulting in lower maximal serum concentrations (C_{max}) and more steady serum levels with the CVR. The values of C_{max} of ENG and EE with the CVR were approximately 40% and 30%, respectively, of those for a COC containing 150 μg desogestrel (DSG) and 30 μg EE. In a comparative study, C_{max} of EE for the ring, contraceptive patch, and COCs were 37.1 pg/mL, 105 pg/mL, and 168 pg/mL, respectively.

The systemic exposure to ENG was similar for both routes of administration, but the difference in daily dose of EE (15 μg vs 30 μg) means that the systemic exposure of EE was twice as high for the COC compared with the CVR. In the comparative study, the systemic exposure to EE was 3.4 times lower in ring users than in patch users and 2.1 times lower than in COC users. The lower exposure to EE with the CVR may explain the significantly lower levels of sex hormone binding globulin (SHBG).

The sustained delivery of hormones by the CVR is associated with good cycle control. In an efficacy study of 2,322 women over 13 cycles, scheduled bleeding was reported with the CVR in 98.5% of all 16,912 cycles. Irregular/breakthrough bleeding or spotting (excluding early withdrawal bleeding) occurred in 5.5% of all cycles, and decreased with continued use. The median onset of withdrawal bleeding was 3 days after ring

Table 6.2 The incidence of intended bleeding (defined as cycles with a withdrawal bleeding, no early or continued withdrawal bleeding, and no irregular bleeding) during vaginal ring and pill use in one non-comparative study and two randomized controlled trials

Study	Method (number of participants)	Cycles with intended bleeding (%)	p value
Dieben et al. 2002	Vaginal ring (n = 2322)	63.0	
Oddsson et al. 2005 (13 cycles)	Vaginal ring (n = 512) 150LNG/30EE pill (n = 518)	58.8–72.8 43.4–57.9	<0.005 for all cycles
Milsom et al. 2006 (13 cycles)	Vaginal ring (n = 499) DRSP/30EE pill (n = 484)	55.2–68.5 35.6–56.6	<0.01 for all cycles

DRSP, drospirenone; EE, ethinyl estradiol; LNG, levonogestrel.

removal and the mean duration of withdrawal bleeding was 4.5–5.2 days. Early withdrawal bleeding (bleeding that occurs prior to ring removal after the third week) was reported in 6.1% of cycles, and late withdrawal bleeding (bleeding that continues past the ring-free week) occurred in 23.9% of cycles.

Cycle control has been reported to be superior with the CVR compared with a COC in many studies, and the incidence of intended bleeding with the CVR is significantly higher (Table 6.2).

EVIDENCE AT A GLANCE

Many other studies have confirmed that, with a daily value of 15 µg of EE, the CVR has a lower incidence of unscheduled bleeding compared with that which occurs with use of COCs containing higher amounts of EE.

Noncontraceptive benefits

Many noncontraceptive benefits of the COC (See Chapter 3) are also found during CVR use, like decreased blood loss and anemia; decreased dysmenorrhea and cycle-related complaints such as premenstrual mood swings; less ovarian cysts and endometriosis; less increase of uterine myomas; decreased incidence of endometrial and ovarian carcinoma; decreased incidence of pelvic inflammatory disease (PID); fewer benign breast diseases, less androgen synthesis, acne and hirsutism; less osteoporosis; and decreased incidence of colorectal carcinoma.

Risks and side effects

The risk profile of the CVR is generally the same as that of COCs. For an overview the reader is referred to Chapter 3.

EVIDENCE AT A GLANCE

The side effect profile of the CVR is similar to that of COCs, except for a lower incidence of nausea and a higher rate of vaginal symptoms (Table 6.3). Discontinuation of the CVR is mainly associated with local adverse events.

In a CVR–COC crossover study, 71.9% of women reported that the ring never slipped, and 9.4% of women reported ring slippage at least weekly or more. In a randomized controlled trial comparing the CVR and the patch, the ring was expelled at least once during any 3-week period in 20.4% of women.

No significant difference between CVR users and COC users were detected in yeast colony counts, Nugent score, vaginal white blood cell count, vaginal pH, and discharge weight. However, more CVR users reported vaginal wetness during use and had larger numbers of lactobacillus colonies with hydrogen peroxide production compared with COC users. Use of the CVR was associated with more frequent vaginal discharge compared with the contraceptive patch (17% vs 8%), but was not associated with a higher likelihood of bacterial vaginosis.

Weight gain does not appear to be associated with use of the CVR. In noncomparative studies,

Table 6.3 Percentage of women reporting adverse events with the contraceptive vaginal ring and a pill in two noncomparative studies and two randomized controlled trials

Adverse event	Method	Vaginal ring (n = 2322) (Europe[a], America[b])	Vaginal ring (n = 512) vs 150LNG/30EE pill (n = 518)[c]	Vaginal ring (n = 499) vs DRSP/30EE pill (n = 484)[d]
Breast tenderness	Vaginal ring	2.6 (1.9–3.3)	3.1	3.2
	Pill		*1.3*	*4.7*
Headache	Vaginal ring	5.8 (6.6–5.0)	7.2	6.8
	Pill		*5.8*	*7.6*
Nausea	Vaginal ring	3.2 (2.8–3.6)	2.7	0.8
	Pill		*4.0*	*3.7*
Leukorrhea	Vaginal ring	4.8 (5.3–4.2)	3.5	3.2
	Pill		*0.2*	*1.0*
Vaginal discomfort	Vaginal ring	2.4 (2.2–2.6)	—	1.4
	Pill		—	*0.0*
Vaginitis	Vaginal ring	5.6 (5.0–6.2)	3.9	4.6
	Pill		*1.0*	*2.1*
Ring-related adverse events[e]	Vaginal ring	4.4 (3.8–5.0)	4.7	6.6
	Pill		*0.0*	*0.4[f]*

DRSP, drospirenone; EE, ethinyl estradiol; LNG, levonogestrel.
[a]Roumen et al. 2001.
[b]Dieben et al. 2002.
[c]Oddsson et al. 2005.
[d]Ahrendt et al. 2006.
[e]Ring-related adverse events include foreign body sensation, coital problems, and expulsions.
[f]Dyspareunia.

the ring was associated with a mean body weight increase of 0.43–0.84 kg over 13 cycles of treatment. In a trial of 201 women randomized to either the CVR or a COC for three cycles, there was little weight change and no difference in weight change between the two groups at the end of the study.

EVIDENCE AT A GLANCE

The use of some combined hormonal contraceptives has been shown to alter biomarkers of venous thromboembolism risk. The risk of getting blood clots may be greater with the type of progestin in the contraceptive vaginal ring (CVR) than with some other progestins in certain low-dose birth control pills. At the moment, however, it is unknown if the risk of venous thromboembolism is different with ring use than with the use of certain birth control pills. Literature reports indicate that thrombophilic effects of the CVR are minimal and comparable to those of the COC.

In one small crossover study no difference was found between 15 µg EE delivered by oral tablet or CVR on markers of hemostasis. In another study, users of oral contraception who switched to the ring showed beneficial changes in biomarkers of thrombosis. A third study, however, showed that the CVR led to higher activated protein C resistance (APCr) than the COC.

The Transatlantic Active Surveillance on Cardiovascular Safety of NuvaRing (TASC) study is recruiting participants to characterize and compare the risks of short- and long-term use of the combined CVR with marketed COCs.

Key history and physical elements

Oral administration ("the pill") is the most widely used method of contraceptive delivery worldwide; however, despite reductions in estrogen dosage and development of less androgenic progestogens, the effectiveness of COCs is reduced by lack of compliance and adverse effects. Gastrointestinal and first-pass hepatic metabolism results in substantial fluctuations of daily serum hormone levels. Accordingly, higher steroid doses of oral formulations than parenteral agents are needed to maintain effective serum concentrations, which may result in greater hormone-related adverse events. Additionally, the need for daily user compliance may reduce the effectiveness of COCs with typical use due to failure to take every pill as scheduled.

These limitations can be overcome with nonoral and nondaily contraceptives. It has been known for decades that when hormones and other agents are placed in the vagina, they are absorbed through the vaginal epithelium into the circulation. Unlike most other nonoral contraceptives, such as an injection, an implant, or an intrauterine device, the CVR does not need to be administered by a healthcare provider, thus offering optimal freedom for the user. The only other nonoral alternative to COCs that offers similar ease of use is the contraceptive patch.

Because the delivery of medication via the CVR is not subject to gastrointestinal effects on absorption and because the steroids are absorbed at a continuous rate through the vaginal wall, lower doses of hormones can be used and released in a more sustained and prolonged manner than orally, providing more stable serum concentrations.

Patient counseling

Currently available combined hormonal contraceptives are the daily pill, the weekly patch, and the monthly ring. These methods prevent unwanted pregnancy by inhibiting ovulation and increasing the viscosity of cervical mucus. When used properly, these methods are highly effective.

For the individual woman seeking a combined hormonal contraceptive method, other criteria are important in the decision-making about which contraceptive is the most suitable for her, such as concerns about forgetting the method, tolerability and safety, and intimacy aspects. Generally, concerns about the pill are the need to take it every day and the consequences of a missed pill; concerns about the transdermal system are the possibility of detachment or skin irritation, its visibility or lack of discretion; and concerns about the ring are doubts about its comfort, fear of using a foreign body, and dislike of vaginal manipulation.

A special concern regarding the vaginal ring method is the feeling of the ring during intercourse. In the combined data of the noncomparative European and North American studies, the proportion of women who reported at least occasionally feeling the ring during intercourse was 18% and higher in the discontinuers (23%) than the completers (15%). The percentage of partners feeling the ring during intercourse was 32% (discontinuers 37%, completers 29%). Most partners, however, in both the completers (83%) and the discontinuers (83%) groups did not object to women using the ring.

Discontinuation can be used as measure of tolerability and user satisfaction. In most studies of the ring compared with COCs, discontinuation rates tended to be similar between ring users and COC users. In studies comparing the CVR with the transdermal patch, significantly more women continued ring use than patch use. Preference for the ring was higher than for the patch. Generally, acceptability of the ring in women and their partners is as high as with the COC with the same global improvement of sexual function.

Compared to women not using any contraception, both COC and ring users reported significant improvements in anxiety, sexual pleasure, frequency and intensity of orgasm, satisfaction, sexual interest, and complicity. The ring was associated with an increase in sexual fantasy. Also the partners of both COC and ring users reported significant improvements in anxiety, pleasure and satisfaction, and frequency and intensity of orgasm. Increases in sexual interest, complicity, and sexual fantasy were observed only in partners of women using the ring.

In an open-label randomized trial to assess sexual function of first-time users of the CVR or transdermal patch, a slight decrease was seen in scores on the Female Sexual Function Index with the ring and a slight increase with the patch.

Available options

The ENG–EE formulation, the only currently commercially available CVR, was developed under the brand name NuvaRing® (NV Organon, Oss, The Netherlands). The only other available nonoral method of combined hormonal contraception that can be applied by the woman herself is the transdermal patch (Ortho Evra; see Chapter 7). The patch releases 20 μg of EE and 150 μg of norelgestromin, which is metabolized to norgestimate.

> **EVIDENCE AT A GLANCE**
>
> Pharmacokinetic properties of the patch are different from those of the vaginal ring, as are tolerability and acceptability.

New products

Phase 3 studies are in progress with a 1-year ring delivering 15 μg of EE and 150 μg of nestorone, to be used for 13 cycles. Progestin-only vaginal rings are also in the developmental phase, especially a 3-month ring to be used during lactation.

Supplying the method: counseling points

How to use the vaginal ring?

After insertion, the ring must be kept in place for 3 consecutive weeks. After removal, usually a withdrawal bleeding will occur. A new ring is inserted after a 1-week break.

When to start the vaginal ring?

- If no hormonal contraceptive is used in the preceding cycle, the CVR is inserted on cycle day 1. No additional contraceptive method is necessary. Starting on cycle days 2–5 is also possible, but in this case an extra method of birth control during the first 7 days of ring use is necessary.
- If the woman switches from a COC or patch (containing both progestin and estrogen), she can insert the ring on any day, but at the latest on the day following the usual hormone-free

interval. No extra birth control method is needed.
- If the woman changes from a progestagen-only method (minipill, implant, or injection) or from a progestagen-releasing intrauterine system (IUS), she may switch on any day from a minipill, on the day of removal of an implant or the IUS, and on the day when the next injection would be due. In all of these cases, an extra method of birth control for the first seven days of ring use is advised.
- If the CVR use is started within 5 days after a complete first trimester abortion or miscarriage, no extra method of contraception is needed.

How to insert the vaginal ring?

Press the opposite sides of the ring together between thumb and index finger, and gently push the folded ring into the vagina. The exact position of the ring in the vagina is not important for it to work. Although some women may be aware of the ring in the vagina, most women do not feel it once it is in place. If she feels discomfort, the ring is probably not inserted back far enough in the vagina. The ring can be gently pushed further into the vagina with a finger (Figure 6.2).

How to remove the vaginal ring?

The ring can be removed by hooking the index finger under the forward rim or by holding the rim between the index and middle finger and pulling it out. The ring must be removed 3 weeks after insertion on the same day of the week as it was inserted, at about the same time of day. The withdrawal bleeding will usually start 2–3 days after the ring is removed and may not have finished before the next ring is inserted.

When to insert a new ring?

After no more than a 1-week ring-free break, a new ring must be inserted on the same day of the week as it was removed in the last cycle.

> **⚠ CAUTION**
>
> - The CVR must be stored at room temperature, 25 °C (77 °F); the acceptable

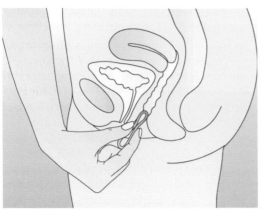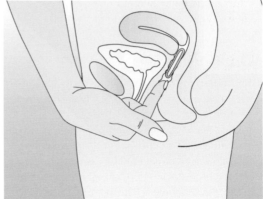

Figure 6.2 The contraceptive vaginal ring is inserted by the woman by pressing the opposite sides of the ring together between thumb and index finger, and gently pushing the folded ring into the vagina. The exact position of the ring in the vagina is not important for it to work. If the woman feels discomfort, the ring is probably not inserted back far enough in the vagina. With a finger the ring can be gently pushed further into the vagina, where it mostly fits in the posterior fornix.

range is 15–30 °C (59–86°F). Storage above 30 °C (86 °F) or in direct sunlight should be avoided. The used ring must be placed in the resealable foil pouch and properly disposed of in a waste receptacle out of the reach of children and pets.

Management of problems

Expulsion (slipping out) of the vaginal ring

The vaginal ring can accidentally slip out of the vagina while removing a tampon, during intercourse, or with a large Valsalva maneuver, particularly with defecation.

- If the ring slips out of the vagina and it has been out for less than 3 hours, the woman is still protected from pregnancy. The ring can be rinsed with cool to lukewarm (not hot) water and reinserted as soon as possible, and at the latest within 3 hours of removal or expulsion (slipping out).
- If the ring is out of the vagina for more than 3 continuous hours during the first or second week of use, its contraceptive effectiveness may be reduced. The ring should be reinserted as soon as possible, and an extra method of birth control, such as male condoms or sper-

micide, should be used until the ring has been used continuously for 7 days.
- If the ring slips out of the vagina for more than 3 continuous hours during the third week of the 3-week use period, the ring must be thrown away. The woman can choose to insert a new ring immediately without experiencing a withdrawal bleeding, or have a withdrawal bleeding and insert a new ring after no more than 7 days. In addition, a barrier method such as condoms or spermicides must be used until the ring has been used continuously for 7 days.
- Women with conditions affecting the vagina, such as a prolapsed uterus, may be more likely to have the ring slip out of the vagina. If the ring slips out repeatedly, it is better to offer her another effective contraceptive method.

Ring removal too late
- If the ring has been left in the vagina for an extra week or less, the woman will remain protected. After removal, a new ring can be inserted after a 1-week ring-free break.
- If the ring has been left in place for more than 4 weeks, pregnancy must be excluded, and an extra method of birth control, such as male condoms or spermicide, must be used until

the new ring has been in place for 7 consecutive days.

Selected references

Ahrendt HJ, Nisand I, Bastianelli C, et al. Efficacy, acceptability and tolerability of the combined contraceptive ring, NuvaRing, compared with an oral contraceptive containing 30 microg of ethinyl estradiol and 3 mg of drospirenone. Contraception 2006;74:451–7.

Creinin MD, Meyn LA, Borgatta L, et al. Multicenter comparison of the contraceptive ring and patch: a randomized controlled trial. Obstet Gynecol 2008;111:267–77.

Dieben TO, Roumen FJ, Apter D. Efficacy, cycle control, and user acceptability of a novel combined contraceptive vaginal ring. Obstet Gynecol 2002;100:585–93.

Gracia CR, Sammel MD, Charlesworth S, Lin H, Barnhart KT, Creinin MD. Sexual function in first-time contraceptive ring and contraceptive patch users. Fertil Steril 2010;93:21–8.

Guida M, Di Spiezio Sardo A, Bramante S, et al. Effects of two types of hormonal contraception—oral versus intravaginal—on the sexual life of women and their partners. Hum Reprod 2005;20:1100–6.

Milsom I, Lete I, Bjertnaes A, et al. Effects on cycle control and bodyweight of the combined contraceptive ring, NuvaRing, versus an oral contraceptive containing 30 microg ethinyl estradiol and 3 mg drospirenone. Hum Reprod 2006;21:2304–11.

Mulders TM, Dieben TO. Use of the novel combined contraceptive vaginal ring NuvaRing for ovulation inhibition. Fertil Steril 2001;75: 865–70.

O'Connell KJ, Osborne LM, Westhoff C. Measured and reported weight change for women using a vaginal contraceptive ring vs. a low-dose oral contraceptive. Contraception 2005;72:323–7.

Oddsson K, Leifels-Fischer B, de Melo NR, et al. Efficacy and safety of a contraceptive vaginal ring (NuvaRing) compared with a combined oral contraceptive: a 1-year randomized trial. Contraception 2005;71:176–82.

Oddsson K, Leifels-Fischer B, Wiel-Masson D, et al. Superior cycle control with a contraceptive vaginal ring compared with an oral contraceptive containing 30 microg ethinylestradiol and 150 microg levonorgestrel: a randomized trial. Hum Reprod 2005;20:557–62.

Roumen FJ, Apter D, Mulders TM, Dieben TO. Efficacy, tolerability and acceptability of a novel contraceptive vaginal ring releasing etonogestrel and ethinyl oestradiol. Hum Reprod 2001;16:469–75.

Timmer CJ, Mulders TM. Pharmacokinetics of etonogestrel and ethinylestradiol released from a combined contraceptive vaginal ring. Clin Pharmacokinet 2000;39:233–42.

van den Heuvel MW, van Bragt AJ, Alnabawy AK, Kaptein MC. Comparison of ethinylestradiol pharmacokinetics in three hormonal contraceptive formulations: the vaginal ring, the transdermal patch and an oral contraceptive. Contraception 2005;72:168–74.

Vercellini P, Barbara G, Somigliana E, Bianchi S, Abbiati A, Fedele L. Comparison of contraceptive ring and patch for the treatment of symptomatic endometriosis. Fertil Steril 2010;93: 2150–61.

Veres S, Miller L, Burington B. A comparison between the vaginal ring and oral contraceptives. Obstet Gynecol 2004;104:555–63.

7

Contraceptive Patch

Anita L. Nelson

Department of Obstetrics and Gynecology, David Geffen School of Medicine at ULCA and Harbor-UCLA Medical Center, Torrance, CA, USA

Introduction

The transdermal patch offers contraceptive efficacy similar to that of birth control pills but has a higher level of correct and consistent use due to its once-a-week administration.

Similar to oral contraceptives (OCs), the contraceptive patch is effective, rapidly reversible, and is probably associated with the same contraceptive and noncontraceptive benefits. Also similar to OCs, if women chose to start the patch on the first day of menses, no contraceptive back-up method is needed. The "quick start" protocol (starting the patch the same day as visit) requires that pregnancy is ruled out and that back-up contraception is used for 7 days. There are only limited studies on extended cycle use where patches are used for more than 3 weeks prior to a patch-free period.

Methods of action and efficacy

Just as with any combined hormonal contraceptive method, the contraceptive patch has two fundamental mechanisms of action. First, the surge of luteinizing hormone (LH) is prevented and ovulation is thereby inhibited. The second mechanism is due to the action of the progestin component which thickens cervical mucus throughout the menstrual cycle to block sperm entrance into the upper genital tract. The progestin component of the patch also thins the endometrial lining and, over time, reduces the amount of blood loss during menses, but may cause temporary increases in unscheduled spotting and bleeding that is associated with early patch use.

Failure rates in typical first-year use for the contraceptive patch are not yet available from the national surveys, so most texts list the first-year typical-use failure rates for the patch as equivalent to those of the pill. In a large study including 22,155 treatment cycles, the overall Pearl Index from the pooled data was 0.88% per woman-year. With correct and consistent patch use, the Pearl Index is reported as low as 0.70%.

One North American trial compared the efficacy of the patch to a triphasic levonorgestrel pill and reported that pregnancy rates were not statistically different between the two methods. (Pearl Index was 1.24 for the patch and 2.18 for the pill). In another study, the failure rate with incorrect patch use was 4.6%; for incorrect pill use, the failure rate was 7.5%.

> ### EVIDENCE AT A GLANCE
>
> In the clinical trials, there was evidence that body mass had a clear adverse effect on the efficacy of the patch. Analyzing pregnancy rates by decile of subject weight, one third of all the pregnancies occurred in the 3% of the study population who weighed at least 90 kg (198 lbs).

Good candidates

The contraceptive patch meets the needs of women who choose to use combined hormonal

Contraception, First Edition. Edited by Donna Shoupe.

Table 7.1 Correct and consistent use reported by users of contraceptive patches vs. oral contraceptive pills: % of cycles with correct and consistent use for 13 cycles

Age group	Transdermal patch	Oral contraceptive
18–19	87.8	67.7
20–24	88.3	74.4
25–24	88.3	79.8
30–34	89.4	85.2
35–39	88.3	82.6
≥40	91.6	84.6
Overall	88.7	79.2

Modified from Archer DF, Cullins V, Creasy GW, Fisher AC. The impact of improved compliance with a weekly contraceptive transdermal system (Ortho Evra) on contraceptive efficacy. *Contraception* 2004;69(3):189–95.

contraceptives. The once-a-week pill/patch application replaces the need for daily administration and makes successful use much easier to achieve. The visibility of the patch also reassures women that they have ongoing protection, thus avoiding the nagging concern: did I take my pill today?

As shown in Table 7.1, study subjects of every age in the patch group reported higher rates of consistent and correct patch use compared to subjects using oral contraceptives. This difference was greatest among women aged 18–19, where 87% of patch users reported correct weekly application for 1 year compared to 67% of daily pill users. A Cochrane systematic review concluded that self-reported compliance was better with the patch than with the pill, but that overall efficacy was similar.

Women with GI absorption challenges may be candidates for transdermal hormonal contraceptives.

Poor candidates

Women who are poor candidates for oral contraceptive use are generally poor candidates for contraceptive patch use (see Chapter 3).

Because the patch relies on intact skin epithelium for predictable hormone absorption, women with skin disorders, either chronic disorders (e.g., psoriasis) or temporary ones (e.g., sunburn), should avoid using contraceptive patches.

Women over 90 kg (198 lbs) had markedly higher pregnancy rates in the clinical trials. The American College of Obstetricians and Gynecologists (ACOG) has recommended that obese (BMI >30) women over age 35 should be offered estrogen-containing methods of birth control only "with caution" because of their increased risk of thromboembolism.

Finally, women needing discreet and private contraception are poor candidates for patch use. There is really no good place for a woman to hide her patch from her partner, and with modern clothing styles, the patch could be visible anyway. It is particularly hard for teens to hide the patch from parental eyes.

Medical eligibility criteria

The medical eligibility criteria for the patch mirrors those of combined hormonal contraceptives (see Chapter 3). One additional consideration is skin problems, as discussed under "Risks and side effects" below.

Table 7.2 contrasts the conditions which the CDC's 2010 Medical Eligibility Criteria (MEC) lists as category 4 and the contraindications listed in the product labeling. Good clinical judgment is recommended in deciding appropriate use of any contraceptive method.

Advantages

The greatest advantage of the patch is its once-a-week application, which makes it much easier for women to use compared to the pill's requirement for daily ingestion.

In one clinical trial, 26.2% patch users discontinued before the end of the 13-cycle study with slightly under half of (11.9%) of those women withdrawing due to adverse events. In the one trial in which patches were provided free of charge, 62% of teens completed all 3 months of study use and 77% planned to continue to use patches. In a 3-month trial of women of all ages comparing patches versus vaginal rings, the continuation rate with the ring was slightly greater (94.6%) than that of the patch (88.2%).

Table 7.2 2010 US Medical Eligibility Criteria category 4 conditions compared to contraindications listed in Ortho Evra package insert

US MEC category 4[a]	Contraindication on product label[b]
History or acute DVT/PE or high risk for recurrence	History of DVT, thrombophlebitis, thromboembolic disease
Major surgery with prolonged immobilization or thrombolic mutations	Major surgery with prolonged immobilization
SLE with positive (or unknown) antiphospholipid antibodies	History of thromboembolic disease
Severe acute viral hepatitis	Acute or chronic hepatocellular disease with abnormal liver function
Hepatocellular adenoma	Hepatic adenoma
Malignant hepatoma	Hepatic carcinoma
Breastfeeding <6 weeks postpartum	
Smoking ≥35 years and ≥15 cigarettes/day	(Black box warning)
Systolic BP ≥ 160; diastolic BP ≥ 100	Severe hypertension
Migraines with aura	Headache with focal neurologic symptoms
Complicated valvular heart disease: HTN with vascular disease	Valvular heart disease with complications
Ischemic heart disease	Coronary artery disease (current or past history)
Stroke	Cerebrovascular disease
DM >20 years or with vascular disease	Diabetes with vascular disease
Current breast cancer	Known or suspected breast cancer or personal history of breast cancer
Severe cirrhosis	Cholestatic jaundice of pregnancy, jaundice with prior hormonal contraceptive use
Cardiomyopathy	Carcinoma of the endometrium or other known or suspected estrogen-dependent neoplasia
Complicated solid organ transplant	Undiagnosed abnormal genital bleeding
	Known or suspected pregnancy
	Hypersensitivity to any component of this product

[a] Center for Disease Control and Prevention US Medical Eligibility Criteria for Contraceptive Use 2010. http://www.cdc.gov/MMWR/PREVIEW/MMWR HTML/RR59F0528A1.HTM/
[b] Physician's Desk Reference (PDR63) 2009 Edition, Montvale, NJ, p. 2438.

The visibility of the patch can be an advantage in some cases, because it makes continued use easier to maintain. Women need to worry less about whether or not they have taken their contraception for the day. Some have also suggested that the visibility of the patch can provide partners reassurance that the woman is not at risk for pregnancy.

Norelgestromin, used in the patch, is a derivative of norgestimate, a progestin with few androgen-related side effects. The patch also offers some noncontraceptive menstrually related and general health benefits, as listed below.

Noncontraceptive benefits

Clinical experience with the patch has been too brief to document many of the long- and intermediate-term health benefits, but it is likely that the patch will have the same long-term health benefits seen with oral contraceptives (see Chapter 3), because the patch's actions are virtually identical to those of oral contraception. These benefits would include less anemia, less risk of endometrial hyperplasia and carcinoma, lower risk of ovarian carcinoma (due to decreased ovulation) and less risk of hospitalization from gonococcus (GC)-related pelvic inflammatory disease (PID). The reduction in the risk of endometrial hyperplasia may be particularly important for women with anovulatory cycling.

The contraceptive patch provides women with predictable withdrawal bleeding. This allows them to anticipate the timing of their bleeding and plan their lives around their bleeding episodes. Bleeding with hormonal contraceptives generally is lighter and of shorter duration than with spontaneous menses.

In a recent study, the Female Sexual Function Index (FSFI) rose among patch users rose in the 3 months while those of the ring decreased slightly. The differences were statistically significant but may not be clinically significant. Another study found that the patch exerted a positive influence on bone turnover in young postadolescent adults.

Risks and side effects

The side effects from patch use are very similar to those associated with combination pill use (see Chapter 3). For women with estrogen-related side effects, patch placement on the lower abdomen may diminish those side complaints. Table 7.3 shows the most common side effects reported during the North American trial in which the patch was compared to a pill.

- Skin site reactions were reported by 20.2% of patch users; 2.6 % stopped patch use as a result of these reactions. Pill users had no such problems.
- Patch users complained more about breast tenderness, discomfort or engorement compared to pill users, but that difference was confined to the first two cycles of use (15.4% vs 3.5% in cycle 1 and 6.6% vs 1.5% in cycle 2).
- Dysmenorrhea was also more frequently reported in the early cycles by patch users than by pill users.

Table 7.3 Most common adverse events: transdermal contraceptive patch versus oral contraceptives

	Patch	Oral contraceptive
Headache	21.9%	22.1%
Site reaction	20.2%	0%
Nausea	20.4%	18.3%
Breast symptoms	18.7%*	5.8%
Dysmenorrhea	13.3%	9.6%
Abdominal pain	8.1%	8.4%

*Only higher in first two cycles.
Modified from Audet MC, Moreau M, Koltun WD, Waldbaum AS, Shangold G, Fisher AC, Creasy GW; ORTHO EVRA/EVRA 004 Study Group. Evaluation of contraceptive efficacy and cycle control of a transdermal contraceptive patch vs an oral contraceptive: a randomized controlled trial. *JAMA* 2001;285(18):2347–54.

The serious health risks associated with the patch are rare and similar to the risks associated with pill use. It is generally accepted that there is an increase risk of thrombosis with the use of contraceptive methods containing ethinyl estradiol (EE) compared to women using no method. It has been suggested that patch users have a higher risk of venous thromboembolism (VTE) than pill users. The concern for additional VTE risk arose in part from a fundamental misunderstanding about the differences in hepatic protein induction by hormones that are orally ingested compared to the impact of hormones that are absorbed transdermally. Peak serum estrogens with the patch are 50% lower than those of the pill, but area-under-the-curve (AUC) analysis showed that total 24-hour serum levels estrogen exposure with the patch was 60% greater than with a 35-µg EE pill, approximately the level that would be expected with use of a 50-µg EE pill. It has clearly been demonstrated that 50-µg EE pills are associated with higher risks of VTE than 35-µg EE pills, so some observers claimed that this 24-hour serum AUC information was prima facia evidence that patches posed higher VTE risks than low-dose pills. However, this conclusion neglects the difference in hepatic estrogen exposure between the oral and transdermal administration. The most important way that any estrogen increases VTE risk is by increasing hepatic production of extrinsic clotting factors (e.g., factors VII, IX) and/or the reducing hepatic production of antithrombin III, etc. Therefore, in judging any method's risk for VTE, the most important element is *hepatic* exposure to EE, not serum levels. The conclusion that serum estrogen levels can be used to predict VTE risk is only valid when comparing similar routes of administration (e.g. oral to oral and transdermal to transdermal). It is *not* valid when comparing an oral to a transdermal method. When estrogen from the pill is absorbed through the intestinal epithelium and into the liver, much of it is conjugated and promptly excreted through the gallbladder and back into the intestine. Only a fraction of the estrogen to which the liver is exposed from the pill is absorbed into the bloodstream for measurement. On the other hand, all of the estrogen to which the patch exposes the liver is reflected in blood tests.

Therefore, in order to determine if the transdermal contraceptive patch has an impact on VTE risk that is different from the modern oral contraceptive, epidemiologic studies are needed (Table 7.4).

- In two epidemiologic studies, there was no statistically significant difference between the patch and pill users (95% confidence intervals included 1). Comparing the risk of nonfatal VTE in new start users of the patch compared to users of a 30-µg EE plus levonorgestrel pill, it was found in two different data sets that for women under age 40, the risk of idiopathic VTE with patch use is not materially different than that of pill users.

- In a postmarketing study comparing the patch to a 30-µg EE plus levonorgestrel pill, the absolute number of nonfatal VTEs was 19.9/100,000 woman–years for the OC and 25.2 cases/100,000 woman–years for the patch, again demonstrating the relative rarity of this adverse event. In a final study, the patch users had an apparently higher VTE risk. However, when only new initiators of patch were compared to new initiators of the pill, the increased risk was no longer statistically significant.

When taken together, these studies provide evidence that transdermal patch users have a similar VTE risk to users of a 30–35-µg EE plus levonorgestrel pill. Most assuredly, patch use confers a significantly lower VTE risk than does pregnancy. However, the manufacturer has altered its product labeling to include a warning about a possible increased risk of thromboembolic events. Clinician enthusiasm for prescribing this patch may have been irreversibly dampened by the medical/legal actions that were taken before the results of large-scale studies were made available.

Table 7.4 Risks of venous thromboembolism transdermal patch versus OCs: epidemiologic studies

Patch vs NGM/35 EE pill	0.9 (95% CI 0.5–1.6)[a]
Patch vs NGM/35 EE pill	1.1 (95% CI 0.6–2.1)[b]
Patch vs norgestimate pill	2.2 (95% CI 1.3–3.8)[c]
New start users	2.2 (9.5% CI 0.8–6.1)[c]
Patch vs LNG/EE pill	2.0 (95% CI 0.9–4.1)[d]

[a] Jick SS et al. Contraception 2006; 73(3): 223–8
[b] Jick S et al. Contraception 2007; 76(1): 4–7
[c] Cole JA et al. Obstet Gynecol 2007; 109(2): 339–46
[d] Jick SS et al. Contraception. 2010; 81(1): 16–21.

Key history and physical examination

It is important to obtain a thorough history before prescribing any combined hormonal contraceptive. There are relatively few absolute contraindications to estrogen use (see Table 7.2) and identification of women for whom the patch should not be offered is generally straightforward.

Only a few elements of physical examination are needed before prescribing the contraceptive patch. It is necessary to measure the patient's weight and blood pressure. Beyond that, there is no need to perform physical examination before prescribing contraceptive patches.

Routine well-woman care, including routine screening for sexually transmitted infections

(STIs) in younger women (<26 years) and screening for breast and cervical neoplasia in older women (>21 years), is important for the woman's general health, but should not be required as a precondition for access to hormonal contraception.

Patient counseling

Although the patch is relatively easy to use, you should carefully counsel women concretely about all aspects of patch use to enable them to be correct and consistent users.

The package insert recommends that a woman place her first patch on the first day of her menses. The day of the week on which the first patch is placed becomes the woman's "patch day." She should remove her existing patch on her next "patch day" and place the new patch on a different site.

The patch may be placed in any of four sites: upper arm, lower abdomen, buttock, or upper torso (except breasts). Hormonal absorption from the lower abdomen is approximately 20% lower than it is from any of the other three sites, although circulating levels from abdominally placed patches are still within therapeutic ranges. The intended skin application site should be clean and dry. No creams or lotions (including sun screen products) can be placed within several centimeters of the target patch area. Any patch site can be reused after a 7-day rest, if it is not irritated.

To apply the patch, remove one side of the peel-off layer and press that half of the patch against the skin. Fold over the free (unattached) half of the patch to expose the other peel-off layer. Remove that plastic and smoothly press the patch from the middle out to the edge of the second half. Press firmly around the perimeter of the patch to insure that the edges of the patch are snugly stuck to the skin. The patch user should be advised to confirm that her patch is completely adherent each day, particularly after bathing or exercising.

No back-up contraception is needed if a woman places her first patch on the first day of her menses ("first day start") or if she is still covered by another method, e.g. when she is switching from depot medroxyprogesterone acetate (DMPA) or from OCs. Women who start on other days (Quick Start) should use back-up methods for the first 7 days.

Sometimes a sticky gray film may remain at the site from which the old patch was removed. Lotions, creams, baby oil, and even vegetable oil easily remove this adhesive residue. Patients should be advised to avoid using stronger agents (such as nail polish remover, cleanser) or forceful abrasion to remove the residue. Because the used patch still contains considerable amounts of hormones, it should be folded in half (adhesive side in) and disposed of in the solid waste, not flushed down the toilet.

After 3 weeks of consecutive patch use, the woman should delay placing another patch for 7 days (for a "patch-free week") during which time she should expect her withdrawal bleeding.

☆ TIPS & TRICKS

Routine instructions for 4-week cycle
Starting:
- Apply first patch within first 5 days of first day of bleeding (no back-up needed)

or

- Quick Start—place the patch now, use condoms for 7–9 days. Take emergency contraception (EC) now if you have had any unprotected sex within the last 5 days.

Changing:
- Remove the patch 7 days later. Put #2 patch on a different spot. Remove residual adhesive with baby oil or cooking oil.
- Remove #2 patch 7 days later. Put #3 patch on a spot different than #2 was placed. Remove old adhesive.
- Remove #3 patch 7 days later. Remove old adhesive.
- Restart next cycle of patches 7 days after you removed #3 patch. Then follow changing instructions.

Other consultation tips

Quick Start

Quick Start (a.k.a. same day start) patch use, in which the patient starts her first patch on days other than as recommended by package label, has been reported to be acceptable if all of the following steps are followed:

- Provide emergency contraception if the woman has had unprotected intercourse in the previous 5 days.
- Advise the patient to place her first patch the day of the visit.
- Have the patient use condoms or some other back-up method for the first 7–9 days of patch use.

Remind the patient that her next bleeding episode will not occur until she is on her patch-free week.

Pregnancy testing is not needed unless the patient's last menses was not normal, she has symptoms or concerns about pregnancy, or she is in the luteal phase in her cycle with a history of earlier unprotected intercourse. Women who do not have scheduled bleeding during the patch-free week should also have pregnancy ruled out.

Extended cycle use

Extended cycle use of Ortho Evra has been reported in one 91-day study. Consecutive weekly applications of patches were done for 12 weeks (84 days), followed by a patch-free week. This extended cycle use reduced the median number of bleeding days compared to conventional use (6 days vs 14 days) and was associated with fewer bleeding episodes (2 vs 3). However, it should be noted that serum estradiol levels increased over time in the 91-day trial.

Another report found that extended cycle patch use was an effective approach to suppressing estrogen withdrawal headaches. There are no published studies of longer term use or of repeated 84/7 cycles with the contraceptive patch.

Counseling women that they have the freedom to add extra weeks of patches occasionally to delay the onset of their withdrawal bleeding to meet personal scheduling needs is clearly a safe practice, which women should appreciate.

Available options

Ortho Evra is the only version of the contraceptive patch currently available in the United States. A lower dose patch is used in Europe.

Ortho Evra (Ortho-McNeil Janssen Pharmaceuticals, Rariton, NJ) measures 20 cm² (4 × 5 cm) and delivers 150 µg of the progestin norel-gestromin (NGMN) and 20 µg of the estrogen EE each day. NGMN is an active metabolite of the well-known progestin norgestimate, which was used in the first OC approved by the U.S. Food and Drug Authority (FDA) for the treatment of mild to moderate acne. EE is the estrogen that has been used in virtually every low-dose birth control pill in the U.S. since the 1980s. The U.S. patch called Ortho Evra contains 0.75 mg EE and 6 mg NGMN to produce these release rates. The Canadian and European version of the contraceptive patch, called Evra, releases the same amount of hormones daily, but contains only 0.6 mg EE.

The design requirements for a contraceptive patch were quite demanding compared to those for earlier patches used for postmenopausal hormone therapies. The contraceptive patch had to be relatively small and very thin, to meet the demands of young women who would not tolerate bulges beneath their tight-fitting clothes. The adhesive also had to be quite strong, because these patches were to be used by very active women. The solution was quite clever—the medication was mixed with the adhesive. A backing layer, made of a beige flexible polyethylene, provides structural support and provides protection to the inner layer. The third layer is a removable peel-back layer that covers the adhesive layer and is removed before placement of the patch.

New products

Because of the sustained interest in transdermal contraceptives, newer patches may be developed in the future but perhaps with different progestins and lower doses of estrogen. One such patch measuring 10 cm² that releases 50 µg gestodene and 18 µg EE daily was shown to suppress ovulation in a phase II trials. A variant of that patch with 0.55 mg EE and 2.1 mg gestodene is currently in clinical trial.

Another possibility may be a progestin-only patch which could be safely used by virtually every woman except those with skin conditions or recent breast cancer.

Managing problems: what ifs …?

During the clinical trials, complete detachment of the patch from the skin occurred in 1.8% of patches; partial detachment was reported in 2.9% of cycles. To insure that the patch would work even on damp skin, it was tested and found to be adherent in humid climates and in saunas, swimming pools, and whirlpools. However, in real life rates of patch detachment may be higher, underscoring the need to counsel women carefully about correct patch placement techniques. In one postmarketing study of patch use by teen women, 35.7% of them reported complete or partial detachment of at least one patch in the 3-month study period.

The package insert clearly explains to patients what patients should do if they have any detachment problems. If the patch partially detaches for less than 24 hours, attempts should be made to reattach it with digital pressure. The patch should never be taped in place, since taping adversely affects the hormone release rate. If the patch will not reattach, it should be completely removed and a new patch should be applied at a different site.

Completely detached patches also require use of a new patch in a new site. The patient may decide to replace that new patch on her usual "patch day" or she can adopt a new "patch day" and use the new patch for the full 7 days. If the patch has been detached for an unknown period of time or for more than 24 hours, the patient should be advised to use a back-up method for 7 days.

If the patient loses the patch early in the first weeks and has unprotected intercourse, she should consider adding emergency contraception (EC), particularly if she had any delay in starting her patch.

Patients may be reimbursed by the manufacturer for a finite number of patches they purchase from the pharmacy to cover their immediate needs following detachment.

★ **TIPS & TRICKS**

In the real world, women may forget to remove their patches on time. Each patch contains an extra 2-day reservoir of drug to help reduce the impact of late removals. Other random "to do's" and "what ifs" are summarized in the box below.

If a woman is late removing her third patch, she should remove it immediately and wait till her next "patch day" to place a new one. Her withdrawal bleeding should start within 1–2 days after patch removal (she should not be concerned by the apparent delay). If she is late removing her first or second patch, she can remove that patch and place the new one immediately. A back-up method or EC is not needed if she is only 1–2 days late changing the patch, but it may be appropriate is there has been a greater delay in changing her patch. If a woman is late starting her first patch, she should protect herself as she would if she were late starting her pills. In fact, she should follow all of the steps listed above in the section on "Quick Start" above.

★ **TIPS & TRICKS**

What ifs
The package insert provides detailed instructions. The ones listed here are simplified and are conservative management recommendations.

What if the patch detaches for less than 24 hours?
- Try to put it back on. Do not use any tape to hold the patch in place.
- If it does not stick, put on a new patch.
- If it does stick, use it until it is time to change the patch.

What if the patch detaches for more than 24 hours?
- Put on a new patch.
- Use EC if you had any unprotected intercourse.
- Use condoms for 7 days.

What if the patch causes irritation?
- Stop using the patch.
- Choose another method.
- Use EC if needed.

What if I forget to start the patch on time?
- Put on the patch ASAP.
- Use EC if you have had any unprotected sex in the last 5 days.

- Use condoms for the next 7–9 days.
- Get a pregnancy test if you do not bleed during the next patch-free week.

What if I forget to change the 1st or 2nd patch on time?

- If you are less than 48 hours late, take off this patch and put a new one on ASAP.
- If you are 3 or more days late, take off this patch and put a new one.
- Use condoms for 7 days. Think about using EC if you had sex during the time the patch was used up.

What if I forget to take off the 3rd patch on time?

- Take if off now.
- Put on the first patch in the next packet on your next "patch change" day.

Summary

Transdermal contraception provides a convenient option for women who desire to use combined hormonal contraception but worry about daily administration. Providing women concrete directions about when to start the patch, when to change it, and what to do if it detaches, will address most of the issues associated with correct use. However, since error is possible, it is also helpful to advise women about what to do if they are late starting their patch, late changing it, or fail to notice that they have lost it. EC is always a very comforting option, see Tips & Tricks: What ifs … above.

Selected references

Abrams LS, Skee DM, Natarajan J, et al. Pharmacokinetics of norelgestromin and ethinyl estradiol delivered by a contraceptive patch (Ortho Evra/Evra) under conditions of heat, humidity, and exercise. J Clin Pharmacol 2001;41(12): 1301–9.

ACOG Practice Bulletin No. 73. Use of hormonal contraception in women with coexisting medical conditions. Obstet Gynecol 2006; 107(6):1453–72.

Archer DF, Cullins V, Creasy GW, Fisher AC. The impact of improved compliance with a weekly contraceptive transdermal system (Ortho Evra) on contraceptive efficacy. Contraception 2004;69(3):189–95.

Center for Disease Control and Prevention US Medical Eligibility Criteria for Contraceptive Use 2010. http://www.cdc.gov/MMWR/PREVIEW/MMWR HTML/RR59F0528A1.HTM/.

Cole JA, Norman H, Doherty M, Walker AM. Venous thromboembolism, myocardial infarction, and stroke among transdermal contraceptive system users. Obstet Gynecol 2007; 109(2 Pt 1):339–46. Erratum in: Obstet Gynecol 2008;111(6):1449.

Creinin MD, Meyn LA, Borgatta L, et al. Multicenter comparison of the contraceptive ring and patch: a randomized controlled trial. Obstet Gynecol 2008;111(2 Pt 1):267–77.

Food and Drug Administration. FDA update labeling for OrthoEvra contraceptive patch. Available at: http://www.fda.gov/NewsEvents/Newsroom/PressAnnouncements/2008/ucm 116842.htm Last accessed 01/04/10.

Gallo MF, Grimes DA, Schulz KF. Skin patch and vaginal ring versus combined oral contraceptives for contraception. Cochrane Database Syst Rev 2003;(1):CD003552. Update in Cochrane Database Syst Rev 2008;(1):CD003552.

Goa KL, Warner GT, Easthope SE. Transdermal ethinylestradiol/norelgestromin: a review of its use in hormonal contraception. Treat Endocrinol 2003;2(3):191–206.

Gracia CR, Sammel MD, Charlesworth S, Lin H, Barnhart KT, Creinin MD. Sexual function in first-time contraceptive ring and contraceptive patch users. Fertil Steril 2010;93(1):21–8.

Heger-Mahn D, Warlimont C, Faustmann T, Gerlinger C, Klipping C. Combined ethinylestradiol/gestodene contraceptive patch: two-center, open-label study of ovulation inhibition, acceptability and safety over two cycles in female volunteers. Eur J Contracept Reprod Health Care 2004;9(3):173–81.

Jick SS, Hagberg KW, Hernandez RK, Kaye JA. Postmarketing study of ORTHO EVRA and levonorgestrel oral contraceptives containing hormonal contraceptives with 30 mcg of ethinyl estradiol in relation to nonfatal venous thromboembolism. Contraception 2010;81(1): 16–21.

Jick SS, Kaye JA, Russmann S, Jick H. Risk of nonfatal venous thromboembolism in women using a contraceptive transdermal patch and oral contraceptives containing norgestimate and 35 microg of ethinyl estradiol. Contraception 2006;73(3):223–8.

Jick S, Kaye JA, Li L, Jick H. Further results on the risk of nonfatal venous thromboembolism in users of the contraceptive transdermal patch compared to users of oral contraceptives containing norgestimate and 35 microg of ethinyl estradiol. Contraception 2007;76(1):4–7.

LaGuardia KD, Fisher AC, Bainbridge JD, LoCoco JM, Friedman AJ. Suppression of estrogen-withdrawal headache with extended transdermal contraception. Fertil Steril 2005;83(6):1875–7.

Massaro M, Di Carlo C, Gargano V, Formisano C, Bifulco G, Nappi C. Effects of the contraceptive patch and the vaginal ring on bone metabolism and bone mineral density: a prospective, controlled, randomized study. Contraception 2010;81(3):209–14.

Multicenter, open-label, uncontrolled study to investigate the efficacy and safety of the transdermal contraceptive patch containing 0.55 mg ethinyl estradiol and 2.1 mg gestodene in a 21-day regimen for 13 cycles in 1650 healthy female subjects. ClinicalTrials.gov identifier NCT00910637. Available at: http://www.clinicaltrials.gov/ct2/show/NCT00910637. Accessed 7/1/09.

Murthy AS, Creinin MD, Harwood B, Schreiber CA. Same-day initiation of the transdermal hormonal delivery system (contraceptive patch) versus traditional initiation methods. Contraception 2005;72(5):333–6.

Rubinstein ML, Halpern-Felsher BL, Irwin CE Jr. An evaluation of the use of the transdermal contraceptive patch in adolescents. J Adolesc Health 2004;34(5):395–401.

Sibai BM, Odlind V, Meador ML, Shangold GA, Fisher AC, Creasy GW. A comparative and pooled analysis of the safety and tolerability of the contraceptive patch (Ortho Evra/Evra). Fertil Steril 2002;77(2 Suppl 2):S19–26.

Stewart FH, Harper CC, Ellertson CE, Grimes DA, Sawaya GF, Trussell J. Clinical breast and pelvic examination requirements for hormonal contraception: Current practice vs evidence. JAMA 2001;285(17):2232–9.

Stewart FH, Kaunitz AM, Laguardia KD, Karvois DL, Fisher AC, Friedman AJ. Extended use of transdermal norelgestromin/ethinyl estradiol: a randomized trial. Obstet Gynecol 2005;105(6):1389–96.

van den Heuvel MW, van Bragt AJM, Alnabawy A, Kaptein MC. Comparison of ethinyl estradiol pharmacokinetics in three hormonal contraceptive formulations: the vaginal ring, the transdermal patch, and an oral contraceptive. Contraception 2005;72:168–74.

Zacur HA, Hedon B, Mansour D, Shangold GA, Fisher AC, Creasy GW. Integrated summary of Ortho Evra/Evra contraceptive patch adhesion in varied climates and conditions. Fertil Steril 2002;77(2 Suppl 2):S32–5.

8

Progestin Injectables

Susanna Meredith and Andrew M. Kaunitz

Department of Obstetrics and Gynecology, University of Florida College of Medicine, Jacksonville, FL, USA

History of DMPA in the United States

Since its introduction in 1960, depot medroxy-progesterone acetate (DMPA, Depo-Provera) has been used for a variety of gynecological conditions including endometriosis and abnormal menstrual bleeding. After 20 years of regulatory review, the U.S. Food and Drug Administration (FDA) approved DMPA in 1992 for use as a contraceptive. Approval had been delayed because a concern over an increased risk of breast cancer as reported in studies on beagle dogs. However, a multinational World Health Organization (WHO) study in 1991 did not find an increase in the risk of breast cancer in users and DMPA was finally approved as a contraceptive agent in the United States. In 2004, Depo-SubQ provera 104 was approved by the FDA as a contraceptive option and later approved as a treatment for pain related to endometriosis.

Mechanism of action

With use of DMPA, gonadotropin secretion and ovulation are inhibited. The serum levels of the progestin also thicken cervical mucus and reduce tubal motility, thus inhibiting sperm transport through the cervix and fallopian tubes and preventing fertilization.

Efficacy of DMPA

In clinical trials of intramuscular DMPA, failure rates have been very low, ranging from 0.0 to 0.7/100 women–years. Since some women may not return on time, or at all, for repeat injections; typical failure rates with DMPA in the general population are higher and range between 3–5%. Specific typical use failure rates are not available for the newer subcutaneous (SC) formulation, although it is assumed that they are similar to the rates after intramuscular (IM) administration. No contraceptive failures were reported in clinical trials.

Obesity or the use of concomitant medications has not been shown to reduce to efficacy of DMPA.

Good candidates

- Women who want safe, effective contraception and are unable to use estrogen-containing combination methods
- Older women with comorbid conditions or risk factors for cardiovascular disease, migraine headaches, or hypertension. This includes patients over age 35 who smoke, have hypertension, diabetes, or obesity; as well as women of any age with a history of migraines with aura, heart disease, stroke, or previous thromboembolic events. In these patients, many of whom have health considerations that increase risks associated with pregnancy and childbirth, DMPA serves as a safe and effective alternative contraceptive (Table 8.1).
- Women with epilepsy or sickle cell disease.
- Women who dislike or are unable to consistently use daily, weekly, monthly, or coital-related methods.

Table 8.1 Clinical situations where DMPA is an appropriate contraceptive choice

Breast-feeding
Cerebrovascular disease
Congestive heart failure
Coronary artery disease
Diabetes
Hemoglobinopathy
Hypertension
Lipid disorders
Liver disease
Migraine with aura or that intensify with OC use
Obese women over the age of 35
Peripheral vascular disease
Seizure disorder on medications that may reduce efficacy of OC
Smokers over the age of 35
Systemic lupus erythematosus
Thromboembolism

OC, oral contraceptive.

- Women with heavy menses or bleeding problems.
- Women with iron deficiency anemia from heavy menstrual bleeding.
- Women with endometriosis-related pain: dysmenorrhea, chronic pelvic pain, dyspareunia.
- Women who need short-term contraception, awaiting tubal sterilization or immediately following transcervical sterilization (see Chapter 24) or a male partner's vasectomy.
- Breast-feeding women after 6 weeks postpartum. DMPA does enter breast milk in infants of nursing mothers using injectable contraception; however, the quality and quantity of breast milk are not affected. As well, no adverse neonatal effects have been reported among women who used DMPA while breast-feeding.
- Obesity (BMI >30 kg/m^2): DMPA is generally safe and effective for obese women; weight control remains an important concern and should be monitored.
- DMPA is a popular method of contraception among adolescents, with high patient satis-

faction rates. Other methods, including oral contraceptives, have high failure rates in the adolescent population. With typical use, pregnancy rates with DMPA are lower than with oral contraception.

Medical eligibility requirements

See Table 8.2.

Advantages

- Highly effective contraceptive method.
- No need for daily, monthly, or coitally related action.
- No estrogen and therefore no increased risk of deep vein thrombosis, myocardial infarction, pulmonary embolism (PE), or stroke.
- Decreased risk of iron deficiency anemia.
- Probable reduced pelvic inflammatory disease (PID), ectopic pregnancy, and problems associated with uterine fibroids.
- Decreased incidence of dysmenorrhea, ovulation pain, and functional ovarian cysts.
- Decreased pain symptoms associated with endometriosis.
- Decreased risk of endometrial cancer: DMPA lowers the risk of endometrial cancer by 80%.
- Decreased incidence of seizures in women with epilepsy. Contraceptive effectiveness is not affected by enzyme-inducing antiepileptic drugs.
- Decreased incidence and severity of sickle cell crises in women with sickle cell disease.

Noncontraceptive benefits

- DMPA can be used in the treatment of a variety of gynecologic conditions including heavy menstrual bleeding, dysmenorrhea, vasomotor symptoms, and endometriosis-related pain.
- DMPA injections have been shown to be useful in women with iron deficiency anemia, reducing the number of painful crises these women experience as well as their total menstrual blood loss.
- Long-term, use of DMPA has also been associated with a decreased incidence of PID and candidal vulvovaginitis.
- DMPA reduces endometrial hyperplasia and the risk of endometrial carcinoma.

Table 8.2 DMPA: medical eligibility requirements

Category	
1	Epilepsy, >6 weeks postpartum breast-feeding, >21 days postpartum non-breast-feeding, immediately postabortion first or second trimester, obesity, cigarette smoking under or over 35 years of age, family history DVT/PE, major surgery without prolonged immobilization, minor surgery, superficial venous thrombosis, uncomplicated or complicated valvular heart disease (atrial fibrillation, endocarditis), epilepsy, depressive disorders, severe dysmenorrhea, endometriosis, benign ovarian tumors, fibroids, PID, (current or past), increased risk of PID, AIDS, pelvic TB, gestational diabetes. Goiter, hypothyroid, hyperthyroid, carrier viral hepatitis, iron deficiency anemia, griseofulvin and other antibiotics
2	<18, >45, multiple risk factors such as older age, smoking, diabetes, hypertension (adequately evaluated or not), systolic 140–159 or diastolic 90–99, history of DVT/PE, major surgery with prolonged immobilization, known thrombogenic mutations, known hyperlipidemias, migraine without aura any age, irregular or heavy, prolonged bleeding, trophoblast disease, CIN, undiagosed breast mass, AIDS on AVR therapy, non-insulin or insulin-dependent diabetes, symptomatic or asymptomatic gallbladder disease, compensated cirrhosis (mild), rifampin and other anticonvulsants
3	Breastfeeding <6 weeks postpartum, vascular disease systolic ≥160 or diastolic ≥100, vascular disease, current DVT/PE, current and history of ischaemic heart disease, stroke, unexplained vaginal bleeding before evaluation, breast cancer disease free 5 years, nephropathy, neuropathy, retinopathy, diabetes >20 years, active hepatitis, severe decompensated cirrhosis, benign or malignant liver tumors, migraine with aura worsening while on DMPA
4	Current breast cancer

AVR, antiretroviral; CIN, cervical intraepithelial neoplasia; DVT, deep venous thrombosis; PE, pulmonary embolism; PID, pelvic inflammatory disease.
Key:
Category 1: A condition for which there is no restriction of the contraceptive method.
Category 2: A condition where the advantages of the method generally outweigh the theoretical or proven risks.
Category 3: A condition where the theoretical or proven risks usually outweigh the advantages of using the method.
Category 4: A condition which represents an unacceptable health risk if the contraceptive method is used.
Adapted from WHO 2009 (www.who.int/reproductive health/publications/en/).

Risks and side effects

The most common side effects reported by DMPA users include menstrual changes (irregular menstrual bleeding or amenorrhea), and weight gain.

Irregular menstrual bleeding

Menstrual changes occur in almost all DMPA users. These menstrual irregularities can lead to poor continuation rates if women are not adequately counseled by their healthcare provider before the initiation of the medication.

Most users experience periods of unpredictable bleeding or spotting during the first year of use. If a patient finds that unscheduled bleeding or spotting is unacceptable, oral or transdermal estrogen can be prescribed. A Cochrane database trial reported that the addition of estrogen treatment reduces the total number of days of bleeding.

Amenorrhea

More than 50% of users report amenorrhea after 12 months of use and 75% reporting amenorrhea with longer use. For many women, amenorrhea is viewed as a positive effect of the medication, reducing their heavy menstrual bleeding and associated cramping.

Weight gain

Potential weight gain is another concern of patients considering use of DMPA. Studies regarding the association of DMPA and weight gain have had varied results. Several studies, including a randomized control trial, showed no significant weight gain in DMPA users during their first year of use, as compared with other forms of contraception. Other studies have found a 3–6 kg weight gain/year in patients using DMPA. DMPA users who are obese appear to gain more weight than normal weight users.

In the adolescent population, DMPA users were more likely to gain more than 10% of their baseline weight in 1 year of use as compared with users of oral contraceptives. In another study, adolescents reported an average of 6 kg of weight gain with DMPA use. Compared with teens with normal BMI, adolescents who are overweight prior to the initiation of DMPA are more likely to have significant weight gain during use of injectable contraception.

Skeletal health concerns

A major concern regarding the use of DMPA is the relationship between current DMPA use and bone loss. Prolonged DMPA use leads to lowered ovarian estrogen production, in which bone resorption exceeds bone formation, leading to a decrease in total bone mineral density (BMD). The BMD of DMPA users decreases by 0.5–3.5% with 1 year of use and 5.7–7.5% with 2 years of use. Losses in BMD occur only with current use and are reversed after discontinuation of DMPA. The best available evidence does not suggest an increased risk in fractures in patients using DMPA, and the use of DMPA is not in itself an indication for BMD testing.

> ### ✱ TIPS & TRICKS
> * Despite the current black box warning by the FDA regarding DMPA and bone loss recommending restriction of use by adolescents to less than 2 years, the available data does not justify restricting use in women of any age or the duration of DMPA therapy which can be used for decades.

Although some clinicians use supplemental estrogen therapy with DMPA to prevent loss of BMD, the long-term benefits and risks of such supplementation are unknown. Assurance of adequate calcium intake and weight-bearing exercises are important adjuncts to minimize bone loss.

Other side effects

Progestins as a class prevent migraines in some patients. However, DMPA injections have been reported to trigger headaches in susceptible patients.

While a history of depression is not a contraindication to the use of DMPA, progestins can cause or worsen depressive symptoms in patients with history of mood disorders or severe premenstrual syndrome (PMS). Thus, physicians should monitor patients with a history of depression or PMS closely after initiation of DMPA (see Chapter 20).

Despite the fact that administration of DMPA lowers a woman's levels of circulating estradiol, hot flashes and vaginal dryness are not commonly encountered.

DMPA and sexually transmitted infections

DMPA does not protect against the transmission of sexually transmitted infections (STIs). However, the thickened cervical mucus associated with use of progestin contraceptives may reduce the risk of developing PID in patients exposed to a STI.

Patients using DMPA are more likely at baseline to have an STI (including HIV) than women choosing other methods of contraception; however, whether or not DMPA increases the risk of HIV infection remains controversial. Some studies have shown that the use of DMPA increased cervical HIV shedding, possibly facilitating the transmission of the disease, while other studies have shown no association between DMPA and HIV acquisition.

Interactions between DMPA and other drugs

Oral contraceptive pills have been shown to decrease the efficacy of several *protease inhibitors* used to treat HIV. However, in a study of 20 HIV infected women, DMPA did not affect the pharmacokinetics of zidovudine (see Chapter 23).

Many *anticonvulsant medications* induce liver enzymes and thus lower levels of contraceptive steroids in women using oral contraceptives. Some anticonvulsants are also teratogens. Use of DMPA has intrinsic anticonvulsant properties, and reduced efficacy has not been reported when DMPA is used concomitantly with medications which induce liver enzymes. Accordingly, DMPA represent a particularly useful contraceptive choice for women with seizure disorders.

Patient counseling

- Patients should be advised not to rub the site of injection.
- Irregular bleeding or amenorrhea is expected and is not harmful. If bothersome bleeding continues, treatment options include more frequent DMPA injections, short-term OCP use, oral progestins or estrogens.
- The longer DMPA is used, the higher the chance for amenorrhea.
- Limiting caloric intake and increasing exercise is particularly important if weight gain is noted.
- Minor side effects are uncommon and generally mild but may include moodiness, mild depression, headaches, or breast tenderness.
- Adequate calcium intake and weight-bearing exercise may be particularly beneficial in long-term users.
- When DMPA is discontinued, it may take several (or even many) months for regular menses to return.

Available options

DMPA is an aqueous suspension of 17-acetoxy 6-methyl progestin available as an IM or SC formulation. The IM formulation of DMPA is available as a branded or generic formulation in the United States and is administered into the gluteal or deltoid muscle at a dose of 150 mg/1 mL intramuscularly every 3 months or 13 weeks. Depo-subQ provera 104 (available only as a branded formulation) is administered subcutaneously at a dosage of 104 mg/0.65 mL every 12–14 weeks.

The progestin in both formulations maintains serum levels sufficient to prevent ovulation for extended periods of time because the microcrystals in the medication have a low solubility and are absorbed in either the muscle or subcutaneous tissue over several months.

Serum concentrations of DMPA vary among individuals but average 1.0 ng/mL for 3 months with a gradual decline thereafter. The newer 104 SC dosage has a slower, longer sustained absorption requiring only 70% of the dosage of the IM formulation.

In the United States, DMPA IM is available as a generic which costs less than the branded IM formulation or the newer SC formulation that is currently available only in a branded form. As compared with other forms of contraception over 5 years of use, DMPA injections and intrauterine devices are highly cost-effective (see Chapter 2).

Other barriers to use of DMPA include time, travel, expense, and inconvenience of clinic visits. Possible self-administration of the SC medication may improve compliance.

Supplying the method

The IM formulation of DMPA should be administered in the deltoid or gluteal muscle only. Care should be made to avoid the subcutaneous tissue. The SC formulation should be administered in the upper thigh or abdomen, with the exclusion of the periumbilical and umbilical areas, over 5–7 seconds.

Initiation of medication

For new patients, if DMPA is administered between days 1–5 of the menstrual cycle or within the first 5 days postpartum, no back-up method is needed.

If a patient is breast-feeding, many (including WHO MEC) recommend that DMPA should be initiated at 6 weeks postpartum. However, available evidence suggests that immediate postpartum initiation of DMPA in nursing mothers is safe from a maternal as well as a neonatal perspective.

In patients switching from combined (estrogen–progestin) hormonal contraception such as oral contraceptive pills, the contraceptive vaginal ring, or the transdermal patch, the first DMPA injection should be within 7 days after taking the last active pill or after removing the ring or patch.

DMPA can also be initiated after day 5 of the cycle in patients with a negative pregnancy test ("quick start" approach). Quick start or same-day administration requires 7 days of back-up (e.g., condom or spermicide) contraception. Both physicians and patients should realize that a small proportion of women initiating DMPA via the quick start approach may have already ovulated, and may be pregnant even with a negative pregnancy test. In patients who received DMPA inadvertently while pregnant, no increased rate of ectopic pregnancies or congenital anomalies has been reported.

Repeat injections

According to package labeling, DMPA IM or Depo-SubQ provera should be administered within 13 weeks of the last injection. If more than 13 weeks have passed since the last injection, a pregnancy test should be performed prior to administering the injection to exclude pregnancy.

Literature supports a 2-week grace period because ovulation dose not occur for a least 14 weeks following the last injection. WHO supports a 4-week grace period in its most recent family planning guideline, and such standards may be more reasonable in developing countries where pregnancy testing is expensive and not readily available.

In patients who wish to discontinue their DMPA injections and who desire another form of contraception, initiating a new method no later than 12–14 weeks after the last DMPA injection minimizes the risk of pregnancy.

Reversibility

DMPA does not permanently affect fertility; however, women considering use of DMPA should be counseled that injectable contraception is unique among U.S. hormonal contraceptives in that return to ovulation and fertility after discontinuation may be delayed.

Fifty percent of women who discontinued DMPA were able to conceive within 10 months of the last injection; however, fertility may be delayed for several more months in a small minority of patients; such delay most commonly occurs in patients with higher body mass index.

Management of problems

- Irregular bleeding or amenorrhea is expected and is not harmful. If bothersome bleeding continues, treatment options include more frequent DMPA injections, short-term OCP use, oral progestins, or estrogens.
- Limiting caloric intake and increasing exercise particularly important if weight gain is noted.
- Side effects are uncommon, but may include moodiness, mild depression, headaches, or breast tenderness.
- Adequate calcium intake and weight-bearing exercise may be particularly beneficial in long-term users.

Conclusions

DMPA represents a long-acting and safe contraceptive choice for a variety of candidates. Potential users may choose injectable contraception because of the convenience associated with four injections each year, because it contains no estrogen, or because of its noncontraceptive benefits, including reduction/elimination of menstrual blood loss. Clinicians should review the risks, benefits, and alternatives to DMPA with candidates for injectable birth control, focusing on the high likelihood of irregular bleeding during the first year of use, and the delayed return to fertility.

Selected references

Abdel-Aleem H, d'Arcangues C, Vogelsong K, Gulmezoglu AM. Treatment of vaginal bleeding irregularities induced by progestin only contraceptives. Cochrane Database Syst Rev 2007;2:CD003449.

ACOG Committee Opinion No. 415: Depot medroxyprogesterone acetate and bone effects. Obstet Gynecol 2008;112:727.

ACOG Practice Bulletin No. 73: Use of hormonal contraception in women with coexisting medical conditions. Obstet Gynecol 2006;107:1453.

Aweeka FT, Rosenkranz SL, Segal Y, et al. The impact of sex and contraceptive therapy on the plasma and intracellular pharmacokinetics of zidovudine. AIDS 2006;20:1833–41.

Belsey EM. Vaginal bleeding patterns among women using one natural and eight hormonal methods of contraception. Contraception 1988;38:181.

Berenson AB, Rhaman M. Changes in weight, total fat, percent body fat, and central to peripheral fat raio associated with injectable and oral contraceptive use. Am J Obstet Gynecol 2009;200:329.

Bjorn I, Bixo M, Nojd KS, et al. Negative mood changes during hormone replacement therapy: a comparison between two progestogens. Am J Obstet Gynecol 2000;183:1419.

Borgatta L, Murthy A, Chuang C, Beardsley L, Burnhill MS. Pregnancies diagnosed during Depo-Provera use. Contraception 2002;66: 169–72.

Chiou CF, Trussell J, Reeves E. Economic analysis of contraceptive for women. Contraception 2003;68:3.

Crosignani PG, Luciano A, Ray A, Bergqvist A. Subcutaneous depot medroxyprogesterone acetate versus leuprolide acetate in the treatment of endometriosis-associated pain. Hum Reprod 2006;21:248–56.

Cullins VE. Noncontraceptive benefits and therapeutic uses of depot medroxyprogesterone acetate. J Reprod Med 1996;41:428–433.

Curtis KM, Martins SL. Progestogen-only contraception and bone mineral density: a systematic review. Contraception 2006;73:47–87.

Curtis KM, Ravi A, Gaffield ML. Progestogen-only contraceptive use in obese women. Contraception 2009;80:346–54.

Davis AJ. Use of depot medroxyprogesterone acetate contraception in adolescents. J Reprod Med. 1996;41:407–13.

Depo-Provera contraceptive injection package insert. New York, NY: Pfizer Pharmaceuticals, Inc.; 2004.

Espey E, Steinhart J, Ogburn T, Qualls C. Depoprovera associated with weight gain in Navajo women. Contraception 2000;62:55–8.

Fotherby K, Koetsawang S, Mathrubutham M. Pharmacokinetic study of different doses of Depo-Provera. Contraception 1980;22:527.

Gbolade, BA. Depo-Provera and bone density. J Fam Plann Reprod Health Care 2002;28:7.

Jain J, Jakimiuk AJ, Bode FR, Ross D, Kaunitz AM. Contraceptive efficacy and safety of DMPA-SC. Contraception 2004;70:269.

Kaunitz AM. Long-acting injectable contraception with depot medroxyprogesterone acetate. Am J Obstet Gynecol 1994;170:1543.

Kaunitz AM. Menstruation: choosing whether … and when. Contraception 2000;62:277–84.

Kaunitz AM, Arias R, McClung M. Bone density recovery after depot medroxyprogesterone acetate injectable contraception use. Contraception 2008;77:67.

Kost K, Singh S, Vaughan B, et al. Estimates of contraceptive failure from the 2002 National Survey of Family Growth. Contraception 2008;77:10.

Leiman G. Depo-medroxyprogesterone acetate as a contraceptive agent: its effect on weight and blood pressure. Am J Obstet Gynecol 1972;114:97.

Mainwaring R, Hales HA, Stevenson K, et al. Metabolic parameter, bleeding, and weight changes in US women using progestin only contraceptives. Contraception 1995;51:149–53.

Mangan SA, Larsen PG, Hudson S. Overweight teens at increased risk for weight gain while using depot medroxyprogesterone acetate. J Pediatr Adolesc Gynecol 2002;15: 79–82.

Martin VT, Behbehani M. Ovarian hormones and migraine headache: understanding mechanisms and pathogenesis—part 2. Headache 2006;46:365.

Matson SC, Henderson KA, McGrath GJ. Physical findings and symptoms of depot medroxyprogesterone acetate use in adolescent females. J Pediatr Adolesc Gynecol 1997;10:18–23.

Mishell DR, Jr. Pharmacokinetics of depot medroxyprogesterone acetate contraception. J Reprod Med 1996;41:381.

Moore LL, Valuck R, McDougall C, Fink W. A comparative study of one-year weight gain among users of medroxyprogesterone acetate, levonorgestrel implants, and oral contraceptives. Contraception 1995;52:215–19.

Morrison CS, Richardson BA, Mmiro F, et al. Hormonal contraception and the risk of HIV acquisition. AIDS 2007;21:85–95.

Nelson AL, Katz T. Initiation and continuation rates seen in 2-year experience with SameDay injections of DMPA. Contraception 2007;75:84–7.

Paulen ME, Curtis KM. When can a woman have repeat progestogens-only injectable-depot medroxyprogesterone acetate or norethisterone enanthate? Contraception 2009;80:391–408.

Prabhakaran S. Self-administration of injectable contraceptives. Contraception 2008; 77:315–17.

Risser WL, Gefter LR, Barratt MS, Risser JM. Weight changes in adolescents who used hormonal contraception. J Adolesc Health 1999; 24:433–6.

Rodriguez MI, Kaunitz AM. An evidence-based approach to postpartum use of depot medroxyprogesterone acetate in breastfeeding women. Contraception 2009;80:4–6.

Sapire, KE. Letter to the editor: Depo-Provera and carbamazepine. Br J Fam Plann 1990;15;130.

Schwallie PC, Assenzo JR. The effect of depo-medroxyprogesterone acetate on pituitary and ovarian function, and the return of fertility following its discontinuation: a review. Contraception 1974;10:181.

Tolaymat L, Kaunitz AM. Long-acting contraceptives in adolescents. Curr Opinion Obstet Gynecol 2007;19:453.

Trussell J. Contraceptive failure in the United States. Contraception 2004;70:89.

Wang CC, McClelland RS, Overbaugh J, et al. The effect of hormonal contraception on genital tract shedding of HIV-1. AIDS 2004; 18:205–9.

WHO Collaborative Study of Neoplasia and Steroid Contraceptives. Breast cancer and depot-medroxyprogesterone acetate: a multinational study. Lancet 1991;338:833–8.

WHO Collaborative Study of Neoplasia and Steroid Contraceptives. Depot-medroxyprogesterone acetate (DMPA) and risk of endometrial cancer. Int J Cancer 1991;49:186–90.

9

Intrauterine Devices

Daniel R. Mishell Jr

Division of Reproductive Endocrinology and Infertility, Keck School of Medicine, University of Southern California, USA

Introduction

The benefits of intrauterine devices (IUDs) include:

- A high level of effectiveness
- The need for only a single act to begin long-term contraception protection
- Minimal to no systemic side effects.

Despite these advantages, less than 5% of U.S. women of reproductive age use the IUD for contraception, compared to 15–30% in many European countries and 45% in China. Unlike many other types of contraception, this method does not require daily user motivation to ingest a pill, or to consistently and properly use a coitus-related method. As a result of the ease of use, as well as the necessity of a visit to a healthcare provider to discontinue the method, IUDs are often linked to the highest continuation rate among all reversible methods of contraception.

Mechanism of action

⚛ SCIENCE REVISITED

The main contraceptive action of copper-bearing IUDs (Cu-IUDs) is interfering with the sperm's ability to survive and to move through the uterus into the fallopian tubes where fertilization occurs. The levonorgestrel-releasing intrauterine system (LNG-IUS) acts as a foreign body in the uterus prompting release of leukocytes and prostaglandins by the endometrium. Additionally, the LNG released from the IUD thickens the cervical mucus and prevents sperm transport through the cervical canal.

The presence of the IUD in the uterine cavity causes a localized sterile inflammatory reaction. The endometrium reacts with increases in white blood cells and prostaglandins. The leukocytes phagocytize the sperm and the tissue breakdown products are toxic to the spermatozoa and blastocyst. The inflammatory reaction is directly related to both the size of the IUD and the amount of copper. The presence of copper markedly increases the inflammatory reaction and inhibits sperm transport viability in the cervical mucus. Additionally, copper ions are released into the fluids of the uterus and fallopian tubes, further debilitating sperm. Because of these intense spermicidal actions, few if any sperm reach the oviducts.

The LNG-IUS and the Cu-IUD have very low rates of ectopic pregnancies, providing additional evidence that fertilization generally does not occur.

Shortly after removal of either type of IUD, the inflammatory reaction disappears rapidly and fertility is quickly restored. Fertility rates, term delivery rates, and spontaneous abortion as well as ectopic rates are similar to those in women discontinuing barrier methods or using no method.

Efficacy

Unlike other contraceptives that rely on frequent and proper use by the user, the typical-use failure rate for the IUD is similar to the perfect-use failure rates. Failure rates do, however, include, pregnancies in women with unnoticed expulsion. First-year failure rates are less than 1% with the LNG-IUS and the T 380 A Cu-IUD. With correct high-fundal placement, the incidence of partial or complete expulsion is very low and lower pregnancy rates are reported.

With continual use of the IUD, the annual incidence of method failure steadily decreases. After 5 years' use of the LNG-IUS, the cumulative failure rate is about 1.1% and after 12 years of Cu-IUD use, the cumulative failure rate is reported to be as low as 1.7%. With increasing age, the rates of all major adverse events—including expulsion and removal for bleeding or pain—also steadily decreases. Thus, while the IUD can be used in young nulliparous women, it is especially suited for older parous women.

Good candidates

- Multiparous women who want long-term contraception. Nulliparous women are also candidates, although insertion may be more difficult and painful, and expulsion rates are higher.
- Women with medical conditions that make them poor candidates for other methods: those over 35 with risk factors for cardiovascular disease, smoking, long-standing obesity, diabetes, or thromboembolism.
- Women who have bothersome side effects with other methods.
- Women who are not amenable to daily or coital-related methods.
- Women immediately after a first-trimester pregnancy loss.
- Postpartum women, 4 weeks or more postpartum or <48 hours, breast-feeding or not.
- Women on medications that affect liver enzymes and decrease the effectiveness of oral contraceptives.
- Obese women (BMI >30 kg/m^2).
- Women who have completed their families.

Cu-IUD

- Women with liver disease, hepatitis.
- Women with uncomplicated valvular heart disease, hypertension, hyperlipidemia, ischemic heart disease, stroke.

- Women over 35 years of age with migraines, or at any age with focal neurological symptoms or aura.
- Women with gallbladder disease.

LNG-IUS

- Women with dysmenorrhea, menorrhagia, or endometriosis.
- Women with anemia or sickle cell disease.

Poor candidates

- Women who are immunocompromised or have increased susceptibility to pelvic infection.
- Women at increased risk for pelvic inflammatory disease (PID) may be candidates, but clinical judgment should be used to evaluate the risks and benefits. Acute PID with in the last 3 months is a contraindication.
- Women with AIDs unless they are stable on antiretroviral therapy.
- Pregnancy or suspicion of pregnancy (unless used as emergency contraception; see Chapter 13).
- Abnormalities of the uterus resulting in distortion of the uterine cavity.
- Postpartum endometritis or postabortal endometritis in the last 3 months.
- Genital bleeding before evaluation.
- Mucopurulent cervicitis, untreated acute cervicitis or vaginitis or other lower genital tract infection, pelvic TB.
- Previously placed IUD that has not been removed.
- Known or suspected uterine or cervical neoplasm.

Cu-IUD contraindications

- Wilson disease (theoretically, a copper IUD may exacerbate Wilson disease).
- Allergy to any component of the Cu-IUD.
- Current behavior suggesting a high risk for PID.

LNG-IUS contraindications

- Known or suspected carcinoma of the breast.
- Hypersensitivity to any component of the LNG-IUS.
- Acute liver disease or liver tumor (benign or malignant).

Medical eligibility criteria

See Table 9.1.

Advantages

Cu-IUD

The Cu-IUD is approved for contraceptive protection for 10 years, although some studies indicate that it is effective for 12 years. This is one of the most cost-effective methods of contraception (see Chapter 2) and has relatively few contraindications for usage. It is a particularly good option for women who have completed their families.

LNG-IUS

The LNG-IUS is indicated for contraceptive protection for 5 years and treatment for heavy menstrual bleeding in women who choose to use intrauterine contraception as their method of contraception. Studies have documented a reduction in menstrual blood loss of up to 94% after 3 months of use of the LNG-IUS and 80–90% after 12 months

In multiple studies, LNG-IUS has been demonstrated to be effective as treatment for pelvic pain and dyspareunia associated with endometriosis. The LNG-IUS is reportedly effective in the treatment of endometrial hyperplasia and is increasingly being studied as an adjunct to estrogen replacement therapy in menopausal women.

The package insert states that use in women over 65 has not been studied and is not approved.

Noncontraceptive benefits

Cu-IUD

The advantages of the Cu-IUD are related to its high effectiveness in preventing pregnancies, its low cost, and long useful life.

LNG-IUS

The LNG-IUS is associated with a reduction in menstrual blood loss of up to 80–90% after 12 months. It is effective in treating menorrhagia, pelvic pain, and dyspareunia associated with endometriosis.

There is an ongoing study on the use of the LNG-IUS for the prevention and treatment of endometrial hyperplasia.

Risks and adverse effects

Expulsion and removal

In the first year of use with the IUD the interval placement expulsion rate is 3% for skilled inserters and up to 10% in some studies. For postpartum placement, the expulsion rate for immediate insertion (within 10 minutes) is up to 9.5%. For insertion between 10 minutes and 48 hours postpartum, the expulsion rate is up to 37%.

For the Cu-IUD there is a 15% rate of removal for bleeding and/or pain. The incidence of these events decreases in subsequent years.

One comparative study showed that the discontinuation rate for the LNG-IUS was less than for a copper-bearing device.

> **EVIDENCE AT A GLANCE**
>
> - A large study of the **LNG-IUS** reported that the cumulative termination rates for pregnancy, bleeding and pain, and expulsion were 0.1, 7.4, and 3.4 per 100 women respectively at the end of 1 year and 0.3, 15.1, and 4.9 per 100 women respectively after 5 years.
> - A World Health Organization (WHO) study reported that the cumulative percentage discontinuation rates of the **Cu-IUD** was 1.7% for pregnancy, 35.3% for bleeding and 12.5% for expulsion at the end of 12 years.

Uterine bleeding

The majority of women discontinuing the Cu-IUD do so because of heavy, prolonged, or intermenstrual bleeding. During a normal menstrual cycle, the mean amount of menstrual blood loss (MBL) is approximately 35 mL. The Cu-IUD is associated with a 55% increase in MBL, while blood loss during LNG-IUD use is significantly reduced, declining to approximately 5 mL per cycle after 6 months of use.

Perforation

One rare but potentially serious complication of IUD insertion is partial or complete perforation of the uterus. A small partial perforation occurring at the time of IUD insertion can, over time,

Table 9.1 Medical eligibility criteria

	Cu-IUD	LNG-IUS
Nulliparous	2	2
Parous	1	1
Known thrombogenic mutations	1	2
Pelvic inflammatory disease		
Current	4 (2 for continuing)	4 (2 for continuing)
Previous, with subsequent pregnancy	1	1
Previous, without subsequent pregnancy	2	2
Vaginitis	2	2
Increased risk of STIs	2/3	2/3
HIV infected	2	2
Aids	3	3
Clinically well	2	2
Postpartum		
<48 hours	2	3
48 hours–4 weeks	3	3
>4 weeks	1	1
Past ectopic	1	1
Multiple CV risk factors	1	2
Hypertension (where blood pressure cannot be monitored)	1	2
Current heart disease/stroke	1	2
History of DVT, PE	1	2
Current DVT, PE	1	3
Current hyperlipidemia	1	2
Migraine with or without aura	1	2
Gestational trophoblastic disease		
Benign	3	3
Malignant	4	4
CIN	1	2
Breast cancer		
Current	1	4
Past, no disease in 5 yrs	1	3
Diabetes with/without vascular disease	1	2
Gallbladder disease	1	2
Hepatitis		
Active	1	3
Carrier	1	1
Anemias	2	1
Sickle cell disease	2	2

Key:
Category 1: A condition for which there is no restriction of the contraceptive method.
Category 2: A condition where the advantages of the method generally outweigh the theoretical or proven risks.
Category 3: A condition where the theoretical or proven risks usually outweigh the advantages of using the method.
Category 4: A condition which represents an unacceptable health risk if the contraceptive method is used.
Adapted from WHO 2009 (www.who.int/reproductive health/publications/en/).

become a complete perforation due to pressures exerted through uterine contractions that can force the IUD completely through the uterine wall and into the peritoneal cavity. A properly inserted IUD will not penetrate the uterine wall or wander into the peritoneal cavity.

> ☆ **TIPS & TRICKS**
>
> Perforation rates of 1–2.6 per 1000 insertions are reported for the LNG-IUS and about 1 per 3000 insertions for the Cu-IUD. Straightening the uterine axis with a tenaculum and probing the cavity with a uterine sound before IUD insertion is recommended to lessen the risk of perforation.

Complications related to pregnancy

Spontaneous abortion

If an intrauterine IUD is not removed after a diagnosis of intrauterine pregnancy is made, the incidence of spontaneous abortion is approximately 55%, about three times greater than the incidence in pregnancies with no IUD in place. In one study, the rate of spontaneous abortion for women who conceived with a Cu-IUD in place was reduced to 20% if the device was removed or spontaneously expelled. This figure is similar to the normal incidence of spontaneous abortion and significantly less than the 54% incidence of abortion reported in the same study in women retaining the device in the uterus.

> ☆ **TIPS & TRICKS**
>
> Reports indicate that while there is no increased risk of fetal death when any type of IUD is in situ, there is a significant increase in the spontaneous abortion rate and premature delivery. For these reasons, it is recommended that if the appendage is visible, removal should be attempted. A detailed informed consent should include the possibility of a wide variety of outcomes.

Some reports describe successful removal of intrauterine IUDs in the lower uterine cavity without a visible appendage using sonographic guidance during early gestation.

Septic abortion

There is no evidence that the current IUDs with monofilament tail strings increase the risk of sepsis if a spontaneous abortion occurs. However, while the IUD does not increase the risk of infection if a spontaneous abortion occurs, it does substantially increase the rate of spontaneous abortion. Since approximately 2% of all spontaneous abortions are septic, the overall incidence of septic abortion in IUD users may be increased.

Ectopic pregnancy

Because IUDs principally act by preventing fertilization through a cytotoxic effect on spermatozoa, the incidence of both ectopic and intrauterine pregnancy is decreased with their use. The estimated ectopic pregnancy rate of the Cu-IUD is only 0.2–0.4 per 1,000 women-years. This is one tenth the rate in women using no contraception, which is 3 per 1,000 women-years. In a WHO study, the cumulative ectopic pregnancy rate of the copper IUD at the end of 7 years was only 0.1 per 100 women.

> ☆ **TIPS & TRICKS**
>
> Women using a Cu-IUD have a 90% reduced risk of having an ectopic pregnancy compared with use of no contraceptive method. However, if a woman becomes pregnant with a Cu-IUD in place, the risk of the pregnancy being ectopic is increased about threefold, from 1.4% to 6% compared to women using no contraceptive method. This increased risk of ectopic pregnancy does not persist in women whose IUD has previously been removed.
>
> In a woman with an IUD and positive pregnancy test, appropriate diagnostic studies should take place early in gestation to establish the location of a pregnancy. Early diagnosis decreases the risk of tubal rupture, tubal damage, and severe blood loss.

The LNG-IUS also has a very low rate of both ectopic and intrauterine pregnancies. The 5-year ectopic pregnancy rate with the LNG-IUS is 0.1 per 100 woman.

Prematurity

If a pregnant woman has an IUD in place that can not be successfully removed and she wishes to continue her pregnancy, she should be counseled about her increased risk of prematurity, spontaneous abortion, and ectopic pregnancy. There is no evidence that there is any increased risk of other obstetric complications.

When pregnancy occurs with an IUD in place, the implantation site is usually distant to the device itself and thus the device is always extra-amniotic. Although published data is scarce, there is no evidence that infants born with a IUD in place have an increased risk of congenital abnormalities.

> ### ✋ CAUTION
>
> When an intrauterine pregnancy occurs with a Cu-IUD *in utero,* the rate of premature live births is four times greater when the Cu-IUD is left in place compared to when it is removed. *The woman should be informed to report promptly the first signs of pelvic pain, bleeding, fever, or early labor.*

Pelvic infections

In 1966, a novel research study was performed in women undergoing vaginal hysterectomy. Aerobic and anaerobic cultures were made of homogenates of endometrial tissue obtained during surgery. The surgery was timed so that cultures could be taken at various intervals after insertion of an IUD. During the first 24 hours after IUD insertion, the normally sterile endometrial cavity was consistently infected with bacteria. During the following 24 hours, the woman's natural defenses destroyed the bacteria and 80% of the samples were sterile. By 30 days, all of the cultures were sterile.

> ### ⚛ SCIENCE REVISITED
>
> • These findings indicated that development of pelvic inflammatory disease (PID) more than a month after insertion of an IUD with a monofilament tail string is due to infection with a sexually transmitted pathogen and is unrelated to the presence of the device.
>
> • A large WHO multicenter study on nearly 23,000 IUD users confirmed these findings. The PID rate was highest in the first 3 weeks after insertion and then remained low and constant (0.5 per 1000 woman-years) during the next 8 years.
>
> • One study in nulliparous women with a single sexual partner who had previously used an IUD had no increased risk of tubal infertility.
>
> • Another study found that nulliparous women who used an IUD did not have an increased risk of tubal infertility compared to women who had not used an IUD.

An IUD should not be inserted into a woman who may have recently been infected with gonorrhea or chlamydia as insertion of the device can transport these pathogens from the cervix into the upper genital tract. A large number of organisms may overcome the host defenses and cause salpingitis. If cervicitis is suspected, tests to detect pathogens should be obtained and the IUD insertion delayed until the results report no pathogenic organisms.

Administering systemic antibiotics routinely with every IUD insertion is not recommended. A randomized trial comparing treatment of azithromycin ingested just prior to IUD insertion with a placebo reported no significant differences in the subsequent rate of PID (0.1% in both study arms). In a study of the Cu-IUD, the rate of removal because of infection during the first year of use was only 0.3%.

Patient counseling

Women seeking 2–3 years or more of contraceptive protection may want to consider an IUD. Contraindications to either type of IUD are not common, but presence of uterine leiomyomas may prompt the clinician to consider whether there is distortion to the uterine cavity. Women with AIDs, unless they are stable on antiretroviral medications, are not candidates.

Women with heavy bleeding, bleeding problems, or symptomatic endometriosis and dysmenorrhea may want to consider the LNG-IUS. Women seeking 10 years or more of contraceptive protection or those with a history of breast cancer may want to consider the Cu-IUD.

Pertinent findings on physical examination include fever, tachycardia, distortions to the cervix, stenotic cervical os, purulent cervical discharge, vaginitis, enlarged or distorted uterus, position of the uterus, pelvic tenderness, or signs of pelvic infection.

Potential candidates should be counseled regarding the risks and benefits of IUDs and other contraceptive methods. Women should be aware that the risk of infection is slightly higher during the first month after insertion. They should also be aware of the change in bleeding patterns expected: use of the Cu-IUD usually results in heavier menses, whereas use of the LNG-IUS usually results in scant menses after 3–6 months of use. Women should understand that if they notice an abrupt change in bleeding patterns, or who miss a period while using the Cu-IUD, they should get a pregnancy test.

A 1–2 month check-up after insertion, especially in those with a difficult insertion, may be appropriate. Patients should be counseled to check for the string periodically (after menses).

Available options

The *Cu-IUD* (Cu T 380 A, Paragard) is currently approved in the United States for 10 years of contraceptive protection. According to a WHO study, it maintains a high level of contraceptive effectiveness for at least 12 years. At the scheduled date of removal, another device can be inserted during the same office visit.

The currently marketed *LNG-IUS* (Mirena) releases 20 µg of levonorgestrel into the endometrial cavity each day. This amount is reduced by about 50% after 5 years. This progestational action on the endometrium reduces the amount of uterine bleeding to about 5 mL per cycle. It is approved for contraception for 5 years and as treatment for heavy menstrual bleeding in women choosing an IUD for contraception.

Supplying the method
Time of insertion

> **★ TIPS & TRICKS**
>
> Although it is commonly believed that the optimal time for IUD insertion is during menses, data support that the IUD can be safely inserted on any day of the cycle as long as the woman is not pregnant. IUDs can be safely inserted immediately after a spontaneous or induced abortion or during a routine postpartum visit (after 4 weeks postpartum), even if the mother is nursing her infant. An IUD can be placed within 48 hours after a term delivery, although there is an increased expulsion rate compared with interval insertion.
> - The Cu-IUD may be placed at any time during the cycle when the clinician is reasonably certain that the patient is not pregnant.
> - The LNG-IUS is usually placed within 7 days of the onset of menses, immediately after a first-trimester abortion, or any time when it is replaced.

The method is not to be used if there are signs of puerperal infection or sepsis. Many clinics require a negative cervical gonorrhea and chlamydia test prior to insertion.

Insertion techniques are described in multiple sources including the IUD packaging and on line.

Managing problems
Pelvic inflammatory disease

It is important to assess and treat any woman who develops signs or symptoms of PID. Symptomatic PID can usually be successfully treated with antibiotics without removing the IUD until the woman becomes asymptomatic. For women with evidence of a tubo-ovarian abscess, the IUD should be removed after a therapeutic serum level of antibiotics has been reached or after a clinical response develops. An alternative method of contraception should be initiated.

Evidence exists that long-term IUD users may have an increased risk for colonization of actinomycosis in the upper genital tract. The relationship of actinomycosis to PID remains unclear, as many asymptomatic women (with and without IUDs) are noted to have colonies of actinomycosis in their vagina. If actinomycosis organisms are identified during the routine examination of cervical cytology in an asymptomatic woman, the patient should be informed but no further treatment is necessary. If there is evidence of pelvic infection, the woman should be treated with antibiotics and the IUD removed.

Cramping and pain

Treatment is with nonsteroidal anti-inflammatory medications (NSAIDs).

Excessive bleeding

Treat with NSAIDs or progestins plus iron; rule out disorders such as polyps or pregnancy.

Mefanimic acid 500 mg three times/day during the days of menstruation significantly reduces MBL in Cu-IUD users. If excessive bleeding persists despite treatment, the Cu-IUD should be removed; consideration of the LNG-IUS is appropriate.

Missing strings

Unnoticed expulsion can result in unintended pregnancy. If a patient denies an expulsion, and possible pregnancy is excluded, the cervix and uterine cavity should be probed with a uterine sound or biopsy instrument. If the IUD is properly located in the uterus, no further action is necessary. If the device is not located, a pelvic sonogram (or MRI or radiograph of pelvis and abdomen) is generally the next step.

If there is partial or total perforation of the uterine wall or cervix, the IUD may be located anywhere in the peritoneal cavity, including the subdiaphragmatic area. Removal of the IUD is indicated because of the risk of bowel injury; surgical removal with laparoscopy or laparotomy may be necessary.

Pregnancy

Women who become pregnant while using an IUD should be evaluated for ectopic pregnancy. Although users of IUDs have an overall lower risk of ectopic pregnancy than sexually active women using no method, once a pregnancy occurs in an IUD user, it is more likely to be ectopic than in a woman with a positive pregnancy test in the general population.

If an intrauterine pregnancy occurs with an IUD in place and the string is visible, the IUD should be removed if possible because the increased risk of spontaneous abortion or premature delivery. These conditions have a know risk of sepsis, septic shock, and rarely death. However, pregnancy loss may result from IUD removal.

Ovarian cysts

About 12 out of 100 women using the LNG-IUS develop a cyst on the ovary. These cysts usually disappear in 1–2 months and rarely require surgical intervention.

Amenorrhea

- About 20% of LNG-IUS users have amenorrhea 1 year after insertion; irregular and frequent bleeding often occurs during the first 6 months after insertion.
- In Cu-IUD users reporting amenorrhea, a pregnancy test should be done.

Selected references

ACOG Practice Bulletin No. 59. Intrauterine device. Obstet Gynecol 2005;105:223.

Andersson K, Odlind V, Rybo F. Levonorgestrel-releasing and copper releasing IUDs during 5 years of use: a randomized comparative trial. Contraception 1994; 49:56–72.

Daling JR, Weiss NS, Metch BJ, et al. Primary tubal infertility in relation to the use of an intrauterine device New Engl J Med 1985;313:937–41.

Farley TM, Rosenbert MJ, et al. Intrauterine devices and pelvic inflammatory disease: an international perspective. Lancet 1992; 339: 785.

Faundes A, Alvarez F, Brache V, Tejada A. The role of the levonorgestrel intrauterine device in the prefention and treatment of iron deficiency anemia during fertility regulation. Int J Gynaecol Obstet 1988;26(3);429–33.

Grimes DA, Mishell DR. Intrauterine contraception as an alternative to interval tubal sterilization. Contraception 2008;77:6.

Hildalgo M, Bahamondes L, Perrotti M, et al. Bleeding patterns and clinical performance of the levonorgestrel releasing intrauterine system up to two years. Contraception 2002; 65:129–32.

Hurskainen R, Teperi J, Rissanen P, et al. Clinical outcomes and costs with the levonorgestrel-releasing intrauterine system or hysterectomy for treatment of menorrhagia. JAMA 2004; 291:1456–63.

Lockhat FB, Emembolu JO, Konje JC. The evaluation of the effectiveness of intrauterine-administered progestogen (levonorgestrel) in the symptomatic treatment of endometriosis and in the staging of the disease. Hum Reprod 2004;19:179–84.

Mishell DR Jr, Bell JH, Good RG, Moyer DL. The intrauterine device; a bacteriologic study of the endometrial cavity. Am J Obstet Gynecol 1966;96;119.

Ortiz ME, Croxatto HB, Bardin CW. Mechanisms of action of intrauterine devices. Obstet Gynecol Surv 1996;51(12):S42–51.

Pakarinen P, Toivonen J, Luukkainen T. Randomized comparison of levonorgestrel and copper releasing intrauterine systems immediately after abortion, with 5 years' follow-up. Contraception 2003;68:31–4.

Petta C, Ferriani R, Abrao M, Hassan D, et al. Randomized clinical trial of levonorgestrel-releasing intrauterine system and a depot GnRH analogue for the treatment of chronic pelvic pain in women with endometriosis. Hum Reprod 2005;20(7):1993–8.

United Nations Development Programme/United Nations Population Fund/World Health Organization/World Bank. Special programme of research, development and research training in human reproduction. Long-term reversible contraception. Twelve years of experience with the TCU380A and TCU 220C. Contraception 1997;56:341–52.

Van Houdenhoven K, Van Kaam K, van Grootheest A, Salemans T, Dunselman G. Uterine perforation in women using a levonorgestrel-releasing intrauterine system. Contraception 2006; 73(3);257–60.

Walsh T, Grimes D, Frezieres R, et al. Randomized controlled trial of prophylactic antibiotics before insertion of intrauterine devices. Lancet 1998;351;1962–3.

WHO. Medical eligibility criteria for contraceptive use, 4th ed. Geneva: World Health Organization; 2009. Available from: http://www.who.int/reproductivehealth/publications/family_planning/9789241563888/en/index.html

Wildemeersch D, Dhont M. Treatment of non-atypical and atypical endometrial hyperplasia with a levonorgestrel-releasing intrauterine system. Am J Obstet Gynecol 2003;188: 1297–8.

10

Spermicides

DeShawn L. Taylor

Department of Obstetrics and Gynecology, Keck School of Medicine, University of Southern California, Los Angeles, CA, USA

Method of action

Spermicides are designed to prevent fertilization by killing or inactivating sperm on contact and preventing passage of sperm to the cervical canal. These agents dissolve the lipid components in the cell membrane of sperm, resulting in death or inactivation. The cytotoxic action is nonspecific and also can damage the vaginal and cervical epithelium. Spermicides act locally and are not absorbed systemically.

For most of the available spermicides, contraceptive protection commences immediately or within 10–15 minutes after insertion and lasts up to 1 hour.

Efficacy

All spermicide products have two components: a surfactant that is toxic to sperm and a carrier or base for its delivery. The most commonly used and most studied spermicidal agent is nonoxynol-9 (N-9). All spermicides available in the United States contain N-9 (Table 10.1).

Spermicides are not highly effective contraceptives when used alone and are commonly used with barrier contraceptives, such as condoms, the diaphragm, sponge, and cervical cap.

> **EVIDENCE AT A GLANCE**
>
> The failure rate of spermicides with correct and consistent use is 18%. However, with typical use the failure rate climbs to 29%.

Effectiveness is reduced if the woman does not wait long enough for the spermicide to disperse before having intercourse, if the spermicide is not placed correctly against the cervix, if intercourse is delayed for more than 1 hour after administration, or if a repeat dose is not applied before each additional act of intercourse.

Spermicides are not recommended for the purpose of preventing the spread of sexually transmitted infections (STIs). These agents should not be used by women at high risk for contacting HIV, or those who are infected with HIV or have AIDS.

Good candidates

- Any woman who wants to rely on spermicides for pregnancy prevention and is willing and able to use the product consistently and properly.
- Women who cannot or do not want to use hormonal methods or an intrauterine device (IUD).
- Women waiting to begin hormonal methods or have long-acting reversible contraceptive devices inserted.
- Couples who have intercourse infrequently.
- Couples using barrier methods of contraception.
- Couples needing a back-up method to augment other methods that may not be properly used.

Table 10.1 Commonly used spermicides in the United States

	Dosage form[a]	Brand name (manufacturer)
Vaginal contraceptive film	Supplied as 2 × 2 inch film inserts in quantities of 3, 6, or 12. Insert at least 15 min before intercourse	VCF (Apothecus)
Suppository	Supplied as individually wrapped suppositories in quantities of 12 or 18. Insert at least 10 min before intercourse	Encare (Blairex)
Gel/jelly/cream	Supplied as a tube with an applicator or prefilled applicators in quantities of 3, 6, or 10. Insert 1 applicatorful of gel/jelly/cream immediately before intercourse	Conceptrol (Ortho) Gynol II (Ortho)
Foam	Supplied as a container with an applicator. Insert 1 applicatorful of foam immediately before intercourse	Delfen (Ortho) VCF (Apothecus)

[a] All spermicides available in the United States contain N-9.

Poor candidates

- Women at risk for acquiring HIV or women diagnosed with HIV/AIDS should not use vaginal spermicides.
- Spermicides containing N-9 are not recommended for frequent daily use, so women who engage in multiple acts of intercourse daily are not good candidates for this method.
- Women who have vaginal abnormalities that interfere with the proper placement of spermicide or have frequent urinary tract infections (UTIs) are also poor candidates for spermicide use.

Medical eligibility criteria

The World Health Organization Medical Eligibility Criteria (WHO MEC) considers spermicides to be a category 3 method (risks generally outweigh the benefits) for women with positive HIV/AIDS, or those on antiretroviral therapy. Use of a spermicide and/or diaphragm with spermicide in HIV-positive woman can disrupt the cervical mucosa, leading to increased viral shedding and transmission to an uninfected partner.

Women at high risk of acquiring HIV are a category 4 (method contraindicated). Use of a spermicide in HIV-negative woman may increase the risk of a genital lesion which my increase their risk of acquiring HIV infection.

Women with cervical cancer awaiting treatment are considered category 2 (benefits generally outweigh risks).

Advantages

Spermicides can be used by a wide variety of users. They are generally less expensive than hormonal contraceptives, are widely available over the counter, are can be used with other barrier methods. They are also simple to use, easily transportable, readily available, under the control of the woman, do not require partner cooperation, and have no systemic absorption. Some women report that the spermicide provides additional lubrication for intercourse.

Disadvantages

- Due to the high risk of pregnancy with typical use, the long-term costs of using the method (primarily due to the costs of pregnancy) are very high (see Chapter 2).
- The spermicidal effect lasts only 1 hour after insertion.
- Some couples dislike the messiness, taste, delay in waiting for the suppositories to dissolve, excessive lubrication, or having to touch the genitals to insert.
- Repeated use and high-dose use of N-9 can cause vaginal and cervical irritation or abrasions. Higher rates of UTIs and vaginosis have been reported.
- Although N-9 is lethal to many organisms including chlamydia, trichomoniasis, syphilis, genital herpes, and HIV, clinical trials have reported mixed results regarding STI protec-

tion. Frequent use may be a risk factor (see "Risks and side effects," below).

Risks and side effects

Spermicides can injure vaginal and cervical epithelium. Spermicides with N-9 may increase susceptibility to HIV infection if used more than twice a day. Frequent use (twice daily or more) is associated with an increased risk of vaginal irritation, yeast infection, bacterial vaginosis, and UTIs. Allergy has been reported in up to 5% of spermicide users. There are no known general health risks.

> **✋ CAUTION!**
>
> High frequency use of N-9 products may cause epithelial damage and increase the risk of HIV infection. Women who have multiple daily acts of intercourse should be advised to choose another method of contraception.

Key history and physical elements

Identifying key points during history-taking will help determine whether a patient is an appropriate candidate to use spermicides alone for contraception. Women with multiple partners, those with a previous history of STIs, and those at risk for HIV infection, should be encouraged to use condoms for STI prevention.

Patient counseling

- Point out to the patient that spermicides can be used alone for pregnancy prevention but are most effective when used with barrier methods.
- Highlight the importance of emergency contraception use in case of incorrect or inconsistent use of spermicides (see Chapter 13).
- Address the low efficacy of spermicides compared to other contraceptive methods, particularly in women where pregnancy represents a health risk.
- Advise the patient that spermicidal agents do not protect against STIs, including HIV/AIDs.

Instructions for use vary by product. Patients should follow the instructions in the package to ensure the spermicide is used correctly. The package instructions also provide specific advice about how soon the method is effective (i.e., immediately after insertion or wait 10–15 minutes).

> **★ TIPS & TRICKS**
>
> - Tablets, suppositories, and film **need time to melt** to allow dispersal of the spermicide in the vagina prior to intercourse. Jellies, creams, and foams are dispersed upon application.
> - Patients should be advised to insert spermicides up to 15 minutes before coitus.
> - Spermicidal agents should be inserted at each coital exposure, as near to the time of coitus as possible and no longer than 1 hour prior to coitus.
> - The spermicide is placed as close to the cervix as feasible and should not be cleared from the vagina for at least 6–8 hours after intercourse.
> - Advise patients not to douche after using spermicide use as it may decrease the efficacy of the method (and some reports also indicate that it may also increase the risk of pelvic inflammatory disease and ectopic pregnancy).

Available products

All spermicide products have two components: a surfactant that is toxic to sperm and a carrier or base for its delivery. The most commonly used and most studied spermicidal agent is N-9, and all spermicides available in the United States contain N-9 (Table 10.1).

The vehicles used to deliver the spermicide include foam, gel/jelly, cream, liquid, melting and foaming suppositories, foaming tablet, and soluble film. A vaginal suppository may also be called a pessary.

Vaginal spermicides are unflavored, unscented, nonstaining, and lubricative.

New products

Other spermicidal agents available outside the United States include menfegol (available as a foaming tablet), benzalkonium chloride, and sodium docusate.

Supplying the method

Vaginal spermicides are available over the counter at drug stores. No prescription is needed.

Management of problems

If soreness, rash, or discharge develops, temporarily discontinuing use of the product may relieve the problem. Continued problems necessitate switching to another product, switching to another method, or contact with a healthcare provider.

Selected references

Farley T. WHO/CONRAD technical consultation on nonoxynol-9, World Health Organization, Geneva, 9–10 October, 2001: Summary Report. Reprod Health Matt 2002;10(20):175–81.

Grimes DA, Lopez L, Raymond EG, Halpern V, Nanda K, Schulz KF. Spermicide used alone for contraception. Cochrane Database Syst Rev 2005;19(4):CD005218.

Trussell J. Contraceptive efficacy. In: Hatcher RA, Trussell J, Nelson AL, Cates W, Stewart FH, Koweal D, eds. Contraceptive technology, 19th ed. New York: Ardent Media, Inc.; 2007.

WHO. Medical eligibility criteria for contraceptive use, 4th ed. Geneva: World Health Organization; 2009. Available from: http://www.who.int/reproductivehealth/publications/family_planning/9789241563888/en/index.html

11

Vaginal Barriers: Diaphragm, Cervical Cap, and Female Condom

Matthew F. Reeves[1] and Jill L. Schwartz[2]

[1]Medical Affairs, WomanCare Global, Chapel Hill, NC, USA
[2]CONRAD, Department of Obstetrics & Gynecology, Eastern Virginia Medical School, Arlington, VA, USA

Introduction

Female-controlled barrier methods are devices placed within the lower female genital tract to create a physical barrier to prevent sperm from ascending to the upper female genital tract. In some cases, these barriers may also prevent sexually transmitted infection (STI). This class of contraceptives includes cervical barriers and female condoms (FC). The most commonly used cervical barriers are commonly referred to as "diaphragms." The typical-use 1-year pregnancy rate is 12% for diaphragms and 21% for the FC, and the 1-year continuation rates are 57% and 41%, respectively. Barrier methods are a good method for motivated women who want an alternative to hormonal methods and desire a coitally related method for occasional use.

The use of FCs gives women the control associated with other female barriers while gaining protection against HIV and other STIs. The FC is an excellent choice for women who need STI protection but are not able to control use of male condoms.

Method of action

Cervical barriers work by physically preventing sperm from entering the cervix as they attempt to ascend the female genital tract. The addition of spermicides aids in contraceptive efficacy by killing or disabling sperm. In some cases, the barrier may function largely by holding spermicide in place to serve as a chemical barrier which aids the physical barrier. Together, the chemical and physical barriers keep sperm from ascending into the upper female genital tract, thus preventing conception. The effectiveness of this class of contraception is highly dependent upon proper use by the woman. As expected, the risk of pregnancy is greatest when the barrier device is not used with every sex act.

Good candidates

- Motivated woman with intermittent sexual activity.
- Women who want to space their pregnancies without using exogenous hormones.

Nearly all women are able to use a diaphragm safely and effectively, while essentially all women are able to use FCs.

Poor candidates

- Women with conditions that make pregnancy an unacceptable risk.
- Women who cannot use barrier methods consistently and correctly.
- Women who strongly do not want to become pregnant.

> ✋ **CAUTION**
>
> - Women who are allergic to latex should not use latex-based barrier devices.
> - Women who have a history of toxic shock syndrome should not use diaphragms, cervical caps, or sponges.
> - Women who have HIV/AIDS or are at high risk for acquiring HIV should not use diaphragms, cervical caps, or sponges (or spermicides).
> - Women who have given birth have a higher risk of cervical cap failure.
> - Women may experience an increase in urinary tract infections (UTIs) with diaphragm use, especially women with a history of UTIs.
> - Severe obesity may make diaphragm and cap placement difficult.

Medical eligibility criteria

The World Health Organization Medical Eligibility Criteria (WHO MEC) makes the following recommendations:

- Diaphragms or cervical caps are not recommended for women with a high risk of HIV acquisition (category 4) because the use of nonoxynol-9 is associated with increased HIV acquisition.
- Diaphragms or cervical caps are not recommended for women with HIV/AIDS (category 3) and for women with a history of toxic shock syndrome (category 3) unless clinical judgment determines other more appropriate methods are not possible.
- Since many diaphragms or cervical caps contain latex, caution should be used for women with allergy to latex (category 3).
- A cervical cap should not be used in women with cervical cancer awaiting treatment.

Advantages

The FC2 female condom and the Today Sponge are available over the counter and can be used without seeing a healthcare provider. The FC2 also provides protection against HIV in addition to pregnancy, based on substantial laboratory evidence for FCs and epidemiologic evidence for male condoms.

Disadvantage

Since studies have not demonstrated a protective effect of cervical barriers against HIV transmission, they cannot be recommended for HIV prevention.

> 🔬 **SCIENCE REVISITED**
>
> The MIRA study found that a diaphragm and lubricant gel did not prevent sexual acquisition of HIV infection in comparison to condoms alone. In this randomized study, condom use was high in both arms but was significantly higher in the condom-alone arm (85%) than the diaphragm arm (54%). Nonspermicidal gel was used in the MIRA study based on a prior randomized controlled trial showing that the spermicide nonoxynol-9 increased the risk of sexual acquisition of HIV is commercial sex workers.

Noncontraceptive benefits

- Vaginal barriers are controlled by the woman, have no hormonal side effects, and can be inserted ahead of time so as not to interrupt sex.
- FCs help protect against STIs, including HIV.

Risks and side effects

With barrier methods, minor irritation of the vagina or penis from the device or the spermicide is possible. With diaphragm use, an increase in UTIs and vaginal infections such as bacterial vaginosis and candidiasis can occur. Toxic shock syndrome and severe allergic reactions to the devices or spermicide are extremely rare.

Key history and physical elements

The diaphragm should not be fitted until 6 weeks after childbirth or second-trimester abortion, by which time the uterus and cervix have returned to normal size. A pelvic examination is needed before starting use of most diaphragms, so that the provider can select the size that fits properly. Single-sized devices are in development.

No fitting is needed for cervical caps or the FC.

Patient counseling

- All barrier methods require correct use with every act of sex for contraceptive effectiveness.
- The use of barrier methods requires some practice. Insertion and removal of barrier methods from the vagina becomes easier with experience.

Available options

Diaphragms

A diaphragm is composed of a latex or silicone membranous dome with a firm, flexible rim. The device is coated with gel and folded for insertion into the vagina. The diaphragm is placed deep in the vagina before sex and needs to cover the cervix for proper function. Spermicide provides additional contraceptive protection. The typical-use pregnancy rate is 12% per year when diaphragms are used with spermicidal gel.

ORTHO ALL-FLEX arcing spring diaphragm

The ALL-FLEX is a diaphragm with a shallow dome and a flexible rim containing a spring. The diaphragm is now made from silicone rather than latex rubber and is available in four sizes (65, 70, 75 and 80 mm) (Figure 11.1). The switch from latex to silicone is expected to reduce allergic adverse events experienced with latex. The ALL-FLEX is the most commonly used diaphragm in the United States.

Milex Wide Seal diaphragm

The Wide Seal is a silicone diaphragm with a shallow dome and a wide flexible rim. It has a small skirt around the rim intended to hold gel in place and improve the seal with the cervix. It is available in eight diameter sizes, from 60 to 95 mm, in 5 mm increments (Figure 11.2). The Wide Seal diaphragm is available from the manufacturer and is distributed in the United States, Canada, Europe, Asia, and the Middle East.

Cervical caps

A cervical cap is a small, firm cup designed to adhere to the cervix by suction and to hold gel close to the cervix.

FemCap

The FemCap is a clear, silicone cap with a removal strap over the dome. It has a groove between the brim and the dome that is designed to hold spermicide and trap sperm (Figure 11.3). The FemCap covers the cervix and part of the vaginal fornices. It is comes in three sizes (22, 26, and 30 mm) and is the only cervical cap currently available in the United States.

Prentif

The Prentif cervical cap is a small, flexible cup made of latex. It is thimble-shaped and fits tightly over the cervix (Figure 11.4). The Prentif cap comes in four sizes (22, 25, 28, and 31 mm).

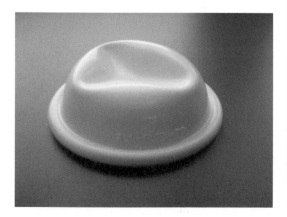

Figure 11.1 ALL-FLEX diaphragm.

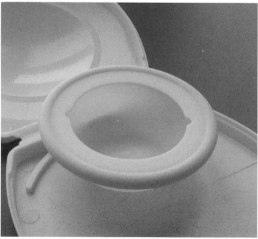

Figure 11.2 Wide Seal diaphragm.

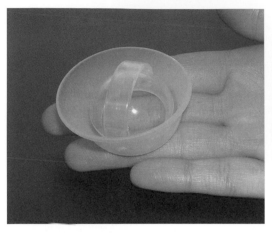

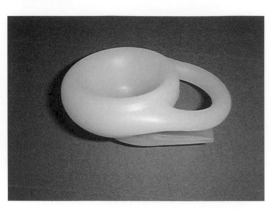

Figure 11.5 Lea's Shield.

Figure 11.3 FemCap cervical cap.

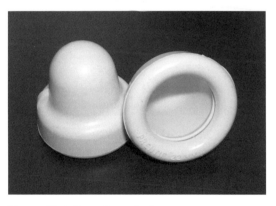

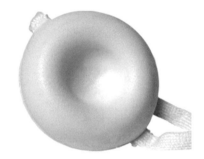

Figure 11.6 Today Sponge.

Figure 11.4 Prentif cervical cap.

Although it was the most commonly used cervical cap in the 20th century, it is no longer available in the United States.

Lea's Shield®

The Lea's Shield is a silicone barrier with a removal loop and valve for the passage of menstrual fluid and cervical secretions (Figure 11.5). It comes in one size and is approved for up to 48 hours of continuous use. Lea's Shield is now off the market but may still be in use by some women. When used with nonoxynol-9 spermicide gel, the pregnancy risk is 8.7% over 6 months of typical use.

Sponges

Today Sponge

The Today Sponge is a small, pliable, polyurethane foam sponge containing nonoxynol-9

(Figure 11.6). A concave depression is designed to fit against the cervix, and a soft loop can be grasped for removal. The sponge is designed to protect against pregnancy for 24 hours, regardless of the number of acts of intercourse, but users are counseled to leave the sponge in place for 6 hours after intercourse before removing it. The Today Sponge was removed from the U.S. market for commercial reasons in 1995, but reintroduced in 2005. In 2009 the Today Sponge was relaunched; it is now available in more than 13,000 drug stores in the United States and can also be purchased online.

Protectaid sponge

The Protectaid sponge is a barrier device made of polyurethane foam impregnated with F-5 Gel, which contains three active agents: nonoxynol-9, benzalkonium chloride, and sodium cholate

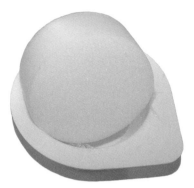

Figure 11.7 Protectaid sponge.

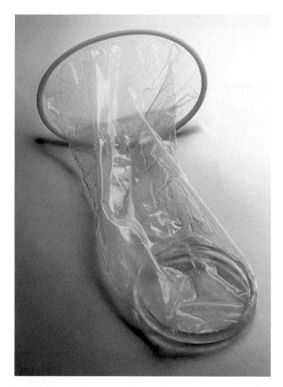

(Figure 11.7). It provides protection for a 12-hour period; a new sponge is not required if multiple acts of intercourse occur during that period. It is intended to be left in place for at least 6 hours after intercourse. In typical use, the pregnancy rate for this sponge is 23% at 12 months. The Protectaid sponge was introduced in 1996 in Canada and in 2000 in Europe, but it is not available in the United States.

Figure 11.8 FC2 female condom.

The FC2 female condom

The first FC (Figure 11.8; FC1, formerly known as Reality) was developed by the Female Health Company (FHC) and was approved by the U.S. Food and Drug Association (FDA) in 1993. FHC has recently developed the FC2, which is made of a synthetic nitrile that is formed using a dipping rather than the multistep welding process used for the FC1 condom, reducing manufacturing costs. The change in material has also decreased the amount of noise associated with use of the FC1. The FDA approved the FC2 in March 2009, and distribution within the United States has begun.

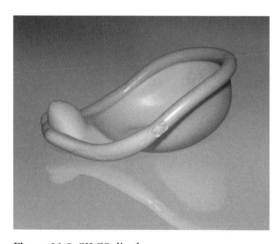

Figure 11.9 SILCS diaphragm.

New products

SILCS diaphragm

SILCS is an intravaginal barrier device currently under development (Figure 11.9). It is made of silicone with an arcing ring, and has a preshaped rim to cling high in the vaginal vault and a finger cup on one edge for easy removal. It will be a one-size-fits-most device. A contraceptive efficacy trial was completed in 2010.

BufferGel Duet

The BufferGel Duet (under development) is a reusable, one-size-fits-all, clear diaphragm made

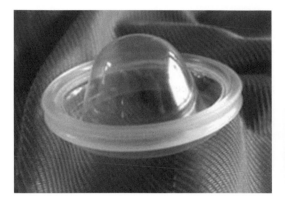

Figure 11.10 BufferGel Duet.

of dipped polyurethane (Figure 11.10). It may be marketed with pouches of BufferGel, a new contraceptive gel which has not yet been approved by the FDA.

Female condoms

The Reddy FC has received the CE mark for distribution in the European Union and is sold primarily through the private sector in several countries as the VA w.o.w. and in Brazil as the V Amour condom. It is made from highly elastic latex and is much shorter than the FC, measuring only 9 cm (3.5 inches) in length. It consists of a latex pouch with a triangular polyethylene frame at the open end and a polyurethane sponge inside the closed end to anchor the device inside the vagina.

The Natural Sensation Panty Condom is a reusable panty that serves to anchor a FC, which can be unfolded from a pouch within the panty. The FCs are replaceable. This panty condom is marketed in Latin America.

The Reddy FC and the Natural Sensation panty condom are available outside the United States but have not been approved by the FDA for contraceptive use or HIV/STI prevention.

Other designs include the Belgium FC (Mediteam, Brussels, Belgium) made of natural latex and designed to cover the entire vulva and base of the penis, and the Silk Parasol panty condom (Silk Parasol Corporation, Bodega, CA), a reusable panty that holds a replaceable FC.

PATH, a nonprofit organization, has developed the Woman's Condom (WC), a 23-cm (9-inch) pliable polyurethane pouch with a flexible soft

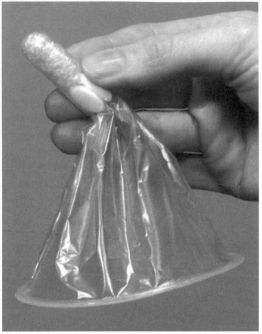

Figure 11.11 Woman's Condom.

outer ring and four foam dots on the pouch that stabilize the pouch within the vagina (Figure 11.11). To aid insertion, the distal end of the pouch and foam dots are folded and packed into a dissolving polyvinyl alcohol capsule, similar to spermicidal film. The WC performed well in a short-term acceptability study and in a comparative crossover study with the FC1. A study of the contraceptive efficacy of the WC is planned.

Supplying the method: counseling points
Female condom

★ TIPS & TRICKS

- Use a new female condom for each act of sex.
- Before any physical contact, insert the condom into the vagina.
- Ensure that the penis enters the condom and stays inside the condom.
- After the man withdraws his penis, hold the outer ring of the condom, twist to seal in fluids before removing the condom.
- Dispose of the used condom safely.

Diaphragm

- Insert diaphragm with spermicide before intercourse.
- Apply more spermicide before additional acts of intercourse.
- Leave the diaphragm in place for at least 6 hours after intercourse.
- Do not wear for more than 24 hours.

Cervical cap and FemCap

Cervical caps are approved to be worn up to 48 hours in the United States and up to 72 hours in Europe.

- Insert cap with spermicide deep in the vagina covering the cervix before intercourse.
- It is optional to apply more spermicide before additional acts of intercourse.
- Leave the cap in place for at least 8 hours after intercourse.

Management of problems

Emergency contraception should be used if the method is not used properly (see Chapter 13). For diaphragm and cervical caps, this would include dislodgement during sex or removal prior to 6 hours after sex. For FCs, incorrect usage would include invagination, misrouting of the penis around the condom, or a break in the condom.

If a woman is unable to remove a female barrier device, she should be seen in the office. Usually, the device can be easily removed by a digital or speculum examination.

Selected references

Coffey PS, Kilbourne-Brook M, Austin G, et al. Short-term acceptability of the PATH Woman's Condom among couples at three sites. Contraception 2006;73(6):588–93.

Female Health Company. 2008 Annual Report. Chicago; 2009.

Female Health Company. Female Health Company receives FDA approval for FC2 female condom. (PDF) 2009 March 11 (cited August 12, 2009). Available from: http://www.femalehealth.com/images/press_2009_03_11_FDA_FC2_Approval.pdf.

Mauck C, Glover LH, Miller E, et al. Lea's Shield: a study of the safety and efficacy of a new vaginal barrier contraceptive used with and without spermicide. Contraception 1996;53(6):329–35.

Padian NS, van der Straten A, Ramjee G, et al. Diaphragm and lubricant gel for prevention of HIV acquisition in southern African women: a randomised controlled trial. Lancet 2007;370(9583):251–61.

Schwartz JL, Barnhart K, Creinin MD, et al. Comparative crossover study of the PATH Woman's Condom and the FC female condom. Contraception 2008;78(6):465–73.

Van Damme L, Ramjee G, Alary M, et al. Effectiveness of COL-1492, a nonoxynol-9 vaginal gel, on HIV-1 transmission in female sex workers: a randomised controlled trial. Lancet 2002;360(9338):971–7.

12

Male Condoms

Anita L. Nelson

Department of Obstetrics and Gynecology, David Geffen School of Medicine at ULCA and Harbor-UCLA Medical Center, Torrance, CA, USA

Method of action and estimates of efficacy

Male condoms capture the sperm prior to entry into the woman's upper genital tract and thus prevent fertilization. Latex, polyurethane, and polyisoprene condoms also block viruses, spirochetes, and bacteria from contacting the genitalia of uninfected partners and thereby significantly reduce the spread of virtually all sexually transmitted infections (STIs).

The "natural skin" condoms manufactured from sheep cecum are reported to be more comfortable but contain pores that are up to 1.5 μm in diameter. Sperm are too large to pass through these pores, but small viruses can easily do so.

> **EVIDENCE AT A GLANCE**
>
> With correct and consistent use, the first-year pregnancy rate with male condoms should be 2%. However, in typical use, the latest estimate of first-year failure rates for male condoms is 17.4%, which is only 1% less than the pregnancy rate associated with coitus interruptus.

Estimates of nonuse of condoms are impressive; 6–9 billion condoms are used each year, but more than 24 billion are needed. One study that investigated the use patterns of 250 women who relied on male condoms for contraception and had timely access to almost unlimited numbers of condoms without any cost found that nearly half (44%) reported having had at least one act of unprotected intercourse in the last 14 days! The more acts of intercourse the couple had, the more likely they were to have had at least one episode of unprotected coitus.

Even in clinical trials where subjects are closely monitored, condom use has been suboptimal. In a review of behaviors of subjects in three large condom efficacy studies the authors noted that in one third of cycles, subjects documented in their daily diaries that they had at least one episode of unprotected intercourse.

Risk-taking behaviors can result from ambivalence about pregnancy or from an underestimation of personal risk for pregnancy or STIs. A New Zealand study of 16–18-year-olds found that only 23% of women felt they were vulnerable to acquiring an STI, even though half of them were sexually active.

Good candidates

> **★ TIPS & TRICKS**
>
> The best candidates for male condoms are couples who are familiar with and committed to the use of condoms.

Most men can be fitted with an appropriate-sized condom, and most condoms are easy to apply. The greatest challenges to success with condoms are the cost of acquisition and the need to use them with every act of intercourse.

Contraception, First Edition. Edited by Donna Shoupe.

Condoms can be used as the primary method of contraception, as a method that is used with fertility awareness methods, as a back-up method when supplies of other methods run out, or as an adjunct to any other method (except the female condom).

Poor candidates

- Men with erectile dysfunction who may have difficulty with condom slippage.
- Unmotivated couples, or those that are not aware of how to properly use condoms.
- Women who are in relationships in which they cannot negotiate for condom use and have no say in sexual practices.
- Couples who have limited access to over-the-counter condoms.

Medical eligibility criteria

The World Health Organization Medical Eligibility Criteria (WHO MEC) lists male condoms as category 1 (a condition for which there is no restriction for the use of the contraceptive method) for all conditions except latex allergy, which it lists as a category 3 (a condition where the theoretical or proven risks usually outweigh the advantages of using the method).

> **★ TIPS & TRICKS**
>
> Often, women who have serious medical problems are told to use male condoms as their method, in the belief that condoms will have no adverse impacts on the woman's health. Unfortunately, this recommendation fails to consider the impact that a pregnancy that may occur as a result of typical condom use might have on the woman's condition.

A survey of residents and fellows in internal medicine revealed that the more seriously ill a woman was, the more likely it was that her contraceptive needs would not be addressed by the primary care provider or the specialist dealing with her medical condition. Interestingly, virtually all of those surveyed reported that they felt confident in their knowledge about condoms and their ability to prescribe male condoms, but few ever recommended them to patients.

Advantages

Male condoms have many important features, which should appeal to couples:

- Condoms need to be used only at the time of intercourse. This is a particularly important consideration for couples who have infrequent coitus.
- Condoms are available without a prescription. Generally they are available over the counter, but recently some pharmacies have locked condoms up and require a staff member to open the case.
- Condoms are easily portable.
- Condoms can be used by virtually all couples.
- Condoms are relatively inexpensive on a per-unit basis. Cost is proportional to use. However, with typical use of the condom, the high costs associated with unintended pregnancies make the method quite costly over time (see Chapter 2).

Noncontraceptive benefits

Condoms have several noncontraceptive benefits. The most important is their dramatic potential for reducing the risk of acquisition and/or transmission of STIs. Other potential benefits derive from the special features that have been developed for some types of condoms. These include helping men with premature ejaculation maintain an erection. Enhancing coital pleasure has been the goals for newer condoms with ribbing, flavors, and lubrication. Condoms may be packaged with accessories, which are designed to more explicitly increase arousal or the intensity of stimulation.

Reducing the risk of sexually transmitted infections

The use of latex condoms has been recognized by both the United Nations and WHO as the best defense in preventing STIs. This protection has been validated for a wide variety of STIs. In a community-based randomized controlled investigation of antibiotic use in rural Uganda in the mid 1990s, consistent condom use was associated with a significant reduction in acquisition of many STIs compared to nonuse; the relative risk was 0.37 for HIV, 0.71 for syphilis, and 0.5 for gonorrhea/chlamydia/infection.

Because the of transmission risk of a sexually transmitted infection (STI) is generally higher than pregnancy risk, consistent and correct use of condoms is even more important to the success of condoms in reducing the spread of STIs than it is for pregnancy protection. For example, one episode of intercourse mid cycle carries about 20% risk of pregnancy, but if the man has gonorrhea, his female partner faces a 50% chance of acquiring that infection from one coital exposure at any time in the cycle.

The evidence of risk reduction with condom use is clear for several STIs.

HIV

Evidence from discordant couples where the male partner acquired his infection from blood transfusion shows that seroconversion of the female partner was reduced by 80% in condom using couples compared to condom nonusers.

The use of condoms reduces the risk of ulcerative STIs, such as herpes simplex virus (HSV), chancroid, and syphilis, which increase both the susceptibility of the uninfected partner and the infectiousness (active shedding) of the HIV-infected partner.

In addition to reducing horizontal transmission of HIV, condoms also reduce vertical transmission from mother to child. Condoms have been shown to have the potential to avert the 28.6% more births of HIV-positive babies than the use of nevirapine by the women during delivery and by the newborn for the first 72 hours of life.

Gonorrhea and chlamydia

In a systematic review of all studies published in 1966–2004, condom use was associated with reduced risk of gonorrhea and chlamydia in most studies. In the studies that distinguished between consistent and inconsistent use and/or between new and pre-existing infection in one at-risk population, condoms were shown to reduce the risk of these two infections by 80%.

In a subsequent study of sexually active teenagers aged 14–18 followed for 6 months, 17.8% of those who reported consistent condom use were found to have a positive test for gonorrhea, chlamydia, or trichomoniasis whereas 30% of those who did not consistently use condoms had a positive test.

Herpes simplex virus

Because HSV is spread by skin-to-skin contact, there was a theoretical concern that the male condom would not cover all the susceptible areas on the genitalia, and women would, therefore, not be provided risk reduction. However, epidemiologic data confirmed that condom use can reduce the spread of HSV-2. Information about condom efficacy from a failed vaccine trial found that those who frequently used condoms had a 25% reduction in the risk of acquiring HSV-2 infection, but condom use did not significantly impact on seroconversion for HSV-1.

In an 18 month study, use of condoms more than 25% of the time reduced women's risk of acquiring HSV-2 by 92%. Since shedding occurs when the infected partner is asymptomatic, consistent condom use should be the rule for discordant couples not trying to conceive.

Human papillomavirus

The human papillomavirus (HPV) is also acquired by cutaneous contact, but can spread throughout the external genitalia and vagina and cervix. Continuous condom use was associated with more rapid regression of the cervical dysplasia. Men with penile lesions who used condoms also had more rapid regression of their lesions.

Condoms help reduce the spread of HPV. In an 8 month study of college coeds following their sexual debut, those whose partners consistently used condoms had an incidence of genital HPV infection that was 70% lower than that found among women whose partners only infrequently used condoms.

Syphilis

In a recent systematic review of epidemiologic studies assessing condom use and the risk of syphilis, the two most rigorously designed studies suggested a reduction risk of syphilis with consistent condom use.

Reducing the risk of cancer

By reducing the spread of hepatitis B and HPV, condoms reduce the risk of two of the most important virally induced cancers—hepatocellular carcinoma and the full array of genital cancers that are HPV linked: squamous and adenocarcinoma of the cervix, squamous cell cancer of the vagina and the vulva in reproductive-age women, anal cancer, and penile carcinoma. If condoms or dental dams are used with oral–genital sex, the risk of laryngeal papillomatosis and some head and neck squamous cell cancers may also be reduced.

Until more vaccines can be developed and given to all sexually active people, safer sex practices (with an emphasis on condom use and careful partner selection) may provide the only lines of defense for sexually active individuals.

Risks and side effects

The greatest single risk associated with condom use is *pregnancy*. However, only a very small portion of condom failure derives from breakage or slippage of condoms. The vast majority of failure results from inconsistent condom use. In the United States, the quality of condoms has been very significantly improved. Breakage rates for latex condoms in recent clinical studies were 3–4/1000.

Surveys of men with personal condom breakage rates in excess of 20% reveal curious practices, such as stretching the condom prior to placing it, inflating the condom prior to application, or neglecting to unroll it.

Latex condoms can cause problems for those with *latex allergies*. It has been estimated that 1–2% of the general population, 2–4% of those in the medical profession, and nearly 15% of latex workers have latex allergies. Generally the allergy presents as a delayed contact dermatitis—an irritation that develops shortly after exposure and resolves within 24–48 hours. Women with this allergy often misinterpret the symptoms as being due to a yeast infection and inappropriately treat themselves with other-the-counter antifungal agents. For couples with latex allergies, condoms made of polyurethane (eg. Avanti, Trojan Supra) or polyisoprene (Skyn) are good choices. Breakage and slippage rates of the polyurethane condoms are higher (0.6–7.2%) than for latex condoms (0.4–2.3%), but pregnancy rates are not different.

On a different level, the request for a partner to use a condom *may convey a sense of mistrust* (or may be anticipated to convey such a message). Many teenage women report they are afraid to ask their partners to use condoms. Many men do not like conventional condoms. Asking them to use condoms can create friction in a relationship.

Commercial sex workers in many areas have to reduce their fees if they make the customers use a condom. In an interesting study of the legalized ranches in Reno, Nevada, a measurable number of potential customers had to be escorted out by security guards because, despite the clever persuasions of the women, they refused to use a condom. *Ordinary women do not have security guards protecting them from unsheathed partners.*

Key history and physical examination elements

When prescribing male condoms for women, it is important to learn if the woman believes that her partner is willing to use condoms correctly and consistently. As mentioned, some women may find it difficult to raise the issue and persuade their partner to use them.

Women whose partners have already tried to use condoms should be asked about any past problems:

- Postcoital irritation in either partner could suggest a latex allergy.
- Higher slippage rates suggest either incorrect sizing (see below) or incorrect placement/removal techniques.
- High breakage rates require more detailed analysis.
- Dislike of condoms may relate to inadequate lubrication, sizing, or need for a more stimulating condom.

Patient counseling

There are two important aspects of patient counseling. First is the message that it is necessary to use condom with *every* act of intercourse. Con-

Table 12.1 Instructions for correct condom use

Open the condom package with care. Do not use sharp instruments, such as scissors or teeth to open it.
Apply the condom before any penetration (e.g., vaginal, rectal, or oral) for contraception and before any genital contact for STI risk reduction.
Use a fresh new condom on the tip of the penis where it can be rolled down completely over the shaft. Leave a space at the tip of the flat-topped condom to allow for movement to prevent breakage. Do not leave extra space in the reservoir-tipped condom; only the reservoir needs to be left empty.
Immediately following ejaculation, hold the condom at the base of the penis and withdraw from the partner. If the penis loses its erection before withdrawal, the semen may spill from the condom.
Inspect the condom for damage, such as tears or holes. Wrap it in a tissue and put in the trash. Do not flush down the toilet.
If the condom breaks or slips off during the sex act, remove the penis immediately. The woman should use emergency contraception to prevent pregnancy, and each partner should consider the need for sexually transmitted infection prophylaxis if at risk.
Do not turn the condom inside out and reuse; discard after one use. Use a new condom with each sexual act.
If lubrication is needed, use commercial water-based lubricants.
Do not use oil-based lubricants, because they can degrade latex (e.g., avoid using cooking oil, mineral oil, cold cream, petroleum jelly, vaginal medication for yeast infection).
Use good-quality condoms, not those purchased at novelty shops; those have not been tested by the standards set by the FDA.
Do not use condoms that have passed their expiration date.
Store condoms at room temperature.

Modified from Nelson AL, Woodward J. Sexually transmitted diseases. Humana Press. Totowa, NJ; 2006, p. 314.

sistent use requires that potential barriers be identified in advance and eliminated. Second is the need to provide detailed, hands-on experience with every aspect of condom use.

Education about condoms is certainly important to their success. By failing to provide young people information about condom use, abstinence-only education resulted in increased vulnerability of young people to STIs when they became sexually active. This was a lesson our country should have learned from our experience during World War I, when U.S. doughboys were refused condoms by the military who were under pressure from groups that advocated that if men were to engage in immoral acts, they should pay the price. The result of that decision was a generation of women and children who contracted the deadly disease from returning veterans. Before a cure was found for syphilis, the infection had spread so rapidly that the Surgeon General predicted that within a generation, 10% of all U.S. citizens would be infected.

Internationally, mistrust of condoms abounds. Rumors that newer condoms are coated with HIV block adoption of their use, while use of old condoms is characterized as "farming with your hoe in a sack".

Education is needed for every aspect of condom use (Table 12.1). First, patients need to learn how to open the condom packet. This is not always easy to do in a moment of passion. However, use of sharp objects, such as teeth, should be avoided. Potential threats to condom integrity—such as sharp edges of long nails, or jewelry (rings) as well as tongue rings or labial rings should be avoided.

Users must also be able to easily recognize which way the condom should be placed on the tip of the penis for unrolling to avoid wastage, frustration, and the cost of replacement units.

For condoms without a reservoir tip, a little extra space must be maintained at the top of the unit to allow room to collect the ejaculate. The user needs to pinch that space between the thumb and forefinger of one hand while unrolling the condom with the other hand.

If there has been any loss of erection during condom placement (30% of men experience this problem), the base of the condom should be grasped and held against the base of the penis during intercourse to prevent slippage until a full erection is re-established.

To prevent terminal spillage after ejaculation, the ring at the base of the condom should be promptly grasped and again held against the base of the penis while the condom-covered penis is removed from the vagina. Once the penis is away from the woman's genital area, the penis can be removed from the condom. The condom should then be inspected for any defects, tied off at its open end, and disposed of in the solid waste container. If there is any suspicion of breakage or spillage, women should be told so she can use emergency contraception promptly.

Available options

Many different types of male condoms are now available. The quality of U.S. condoms today is quite impressive. In a recent evaluation of 20 condoms by a leading consumer product testing group, 7 condoms all achieved perfect scores (100%), and 6 more scored 90% or more. Only one condom did not meet the criteria, which were very stringent. For example, a condom under test had to able to be inflated to hold 25 L or more without bursting and must show no defects in submersion tests.

Male condoms are now available in latex, polyurethane (Avanti, Trojan Supra), polyisoprene (Skyn), and "lambskin". Latex condoms are very stretchable, but the polyurethane condoms are more stiff. On the other hand, latex can feel cold, while polyurethane transmits body heat. The polyurethane condoms prevent passage, even of small viruses, as effectively as their latex counterparts. The so-called "natural" condoms provide contraception, but cannot offer comprehensive STI protection.

The most remarkable new developments in condom design have arisen from the manufac-turers' realization that while potential customers recognized that they *should* use condoms; most did not *want* to use them. User complaints included the facts that condom placement interrupted love-making and could be awkward. The condom created a cold, unlubricated sensation and could be messy for the man. The standard condoms can fall off some men or uncomfortably constrict others. Latex allergies created problems for other users. As a result, condoms have just not been used reliably.

> ### ☆ TIPS & TRICKS
>
> In response to all these complaints, manufacturers have developed new condoms and created condom accessories that are designed not only to minimize the negative aspects of condom use, but also to add pleasure with condom use and incentivize people to make them want to use condoms.

Different condom sizes

Condoms now can be sized to fit more men. There are "snugger fit" condoms for developing young men, and for adult men who are less well endowed. There are extra large condoms for some men who cannot comfortably fit into a standard size condom. There are two different models of larger condoms from which to choose—those that have a standard condom for the shaft of the penis but provide extra capacity at the glands, and those that increase the condom diameter along the full length of the condom.

Different condom designs

Condoms are made with ribbing, swirling patterns, or studdings, to enhance sensation with condom use. There are condoms "scented" (a.k.a. flavored) with strawberry, cherry, and mint for a wider range of sexual pleasuring activity. To simplify condom placement, some condoms can be unrolled in either direction.

Marketing to women

Time and motion studies show that women can feel intimidated when buying condoms in stores, and spend only a few seconds to quickly pick up a particular brand without doing any comparison shopping. In stores, 20–30% of condoms are purchased by women. In a more private online purchasing environment, over half of condoms are sold to women. In order to allow women more time to explore new options, companies have packaged male condoms into boxes which appeal to women and, they have placed those boxes in areas of the stores where women may feel more secure—next to the sanitary napkins.

Condom accessories

Not only have condoms been redesigned to enhance sensations themselves, but they are now packaged with, or comarketed with, pleasure-enhancing products, such as refreshing wipes and an array of vaginal lubricants designed to increase female arousal.

The penultimate development in this arena was a slender ring that fit over the condom-covered penis to rest at the base. Attached to this ring was a single battery-operated vibrating unit. This vibrator was so popular that it was soon replaced by a slender ring with two battery-operated vibrating rings (his and hers).

For men with premature ejaculation (or those going for the Guinness book of erection records), condoms are available with an internal coating of benzocaine.

New products

Research continues to test new nonlatex materials for traditional male condoms. New ways to incentivize condom use by providing accessories or features to enhance sexual pleasure are also being explored. Some vaginal gels are being characterized as "invisible condoms" under female control. For true male condoms, another approach has been to try to develop so-called "spray on" condoms to be used after full erection.

Supplying the methods

When discussing condoms, suggest that the patient obtain an ample supply to have ready at all times.

- For men, storing the condom in their wallet is a reasonable option. Women can carry a condom discreetly between pictures in their wallets.

- Young women have more challenges since they have tiny purses.
- Condoms can be placed in all areas where sex might take place.

Management of problems

As discussed above, there are only a limited number of problems that can arise during condom use.

- *Latex allergy* can be dealt with by recommending polyurethane or polyisoprene condoms.
- *Slippage*: Immediately, have the women use EC. If repeated slippage occurs, investigate if the couple is using the correct size condom and if they are using correct techniques, especially for condom removal after ejaculation.
- *Breakage*: Immediately, have the women use EC. If breakage occurs more than rarely, consider other condom sizes or materials. Ask about the possibility of sharp objects. See if the couple is trying to reuse condoms.
- *Inconsistent use*: Incentivize with pleasure enhancement designs and accessories. Remind patient about the risks of intermittent use (carrot and stick appearance). Consider other contraceptive methods if the couple is unable to effectively use condoms.

★ TIPS & TRICKS

- Have an array of condoms for the woman to evaluate. Tell her how to shop for male condoms in stores and also online.
- Show her some of the different accessories to help her incentivize her partner to use condom with every act of intercourse.
- Always offer/provide emergency contraception to all condom users. With a prescription, the insurance company may cover the cost. Advise her to buy EC in advance to have it ready in her medicine cabinet when she needs it.

✋ CAUTION

- Do not assume **anyone** knows how to use a condom.

- There are numerous pitfalls in opening the packet, placing the condom correctly, and removing it without spillage.
- Have lifelike practice models. Teach the women how to place the condom if the man is not available to teach.
- Watch out for sharp objects that can tear the condom.

Conclusions

Clearly, many of the technical issues about condom design have been very successfully dealt with in the last 20 years. However, the most fundamental barrier to condom success is inconsistent use. The answers to that challenge may be beyond technical condom designs and rest with behavioral interventions, which have to date only been marginally effective. The more basic problems underlying inconsistent condom use require massive societal changes. Women's abilities to protect themselves with male condom use are clearly related to larger issues of the status of women in any given society. For example, in Nigeria it is food insecurity that drives most female commercial sex workers into the profession and discourages the use of condoms.

There have been encouraging new developments and insights. Just as network analysis has proven a useful tool in understanding the spread of STIs, it may also have a potential for increasing condom use. Studies have shown that when a woman is in a group of friends who discuss condom use, she is more likely to become a user; social marketing of condoms (especially free condoms) increases use. Programs targeted to encourage condom use among commercial sex workers have demonstrated some success, especially when condoms are provided and licensing rules require STI testing and condom use.

Providing education in schools about condom use has been convincingly shown to be associated with lower rates of future STIs. Condom promotion programs, along with other prevention strategies targeted to different age groups, life stages, epidemic levels, and settings, should be included in STI and HIV prevention programs.

As these and other tools and messages are spread both within clinical settings and in larger public forums, it is to be hoped that condom use will increase and the male condom will more fully achieve its potential for providing protection both against pregnancy and the spread of STIs.

Selected references

Ahmed S, Lutalo T, Wawer M, Serwadda D, et al. HIV incidence and sexually transmitted disease prevalence associated with condom use: a population study in Rakai, Uganda. AIDS 2001;15(16):2171–9.

Albert AE, Warner DL, Hatcher RA, Trussell J, Bennett C. Condom use among female commercial sex workers in Nevada's legal brothels. Am J Public Health 1995;85(11):1514–20.

Bosage P. Barrier methods to prevent STIs in sexually transmitted diseases: a practical guide for primary care. Totowa, NJ: Humana Press; 2006, p. 313.

Bleeker MC, Hogewoning CJ, Voorhorst FJ, et al. Condom use promotes regression of human papillomavirus-associated penile lesions in male sexual partners of women with cervical intraepithelial neoplasia. Int J Cancer 2003; 107(5):804–10.

Brückner H, Bearman P. After the promise: the STD consequences of adolescent virginity pledges. J Adolesc Health 2005;36(4):271–8.

Choi KH, Gregorich SE. Social network influences on male and female condom use among women attending family planning clinics in the United States. Sex Transm Dis 2009;36(12): 757–62.

Consumer Reports. Most reliable condoms. Consumer Reports 2009 (December):52.

Crosby RA, DiClemente RJ, Wingood GM, Lang D, Harrington KF. Value of consistent condom use: a study of sexually transmitted disease prevention among African American adolescent females. Am J Public Health 2003;93(6): 901–2.

Dodge B, Reece M, Herbenick D. School-based condom education and its relations with diagnoses of and testing for sexually transmitted infections among men in the United States. Am J Public Health 2009;99(12):2180–2.

Hogewoning CJ, Bleeker MC, van den Brule AJ, et al. Condom use promotes regression of cervical intraepithelial neoplasia and clearance of human papillomavirus: a randomized clinical trial. Int J Cancer 2003;107(5):811–16.

Holmes KK, Levine R, Weaver M. Effectiveness of condoms in preventing sexually transmitted infections. Bull World Health Organ 2004; 82(6):454–61.

Koss CA, Dunne EF, Warner L. A systematic review of epidemiologic studies assessing condom use and risk of syphilis. Sex Transm Dis 2009; 36(7):401–5.

Kost K, Singh S, Vaughan B, Trussell J, Bankole A. Estimates of contraceptive failure from the 2002 National Survey of Family Growth. Contraception 2008;77(1):10–21.

Oyefara JL. Food insecurity, HIV/AIDS pandemic and sexual behaviour of female commercial sex workers in Lagos metropolis, Nigeria. Sahara J 2007;4(2):626–35.

Plummer ML, Wight D, Wamoyi J, Mshana G, Hayes RJ, Ross DA. Farming with your hoe in a sack: condom attitudes, access, and use in rural Tanzania. Stud Fam Plann 2006;37(1): 29–40.

Renaud TC, Bocour A, Irvine MK, et al. The free condom initiative: promoting condom availability and use in New York City. Public Health Rep 2009;124(4):481–9.

Reynolds HW, Janowitz B, Homan R, Johnson L. The value of contraception to prevent perinatal HIV transmission. Sex Transm Dis 2006;33(6): 350–6.

Trussel J. Choosing a contraceptive: efficacy, safety and personal consideration. In: Hatcher RA, Trussell J, Nelson AL, Cates W, Stewart FH, Koweal D, eds. Contraceptive technology, 19th ed. New York: Ardent Media, Inc.; 2007, p. 24.

Warner L, Stone KM, Macaluso M, Buehler JW, Austin HD. Condom use and risk of gonorrhea and Chlamydia: a systematic review of design and measurement factors assessed in epidemiologic studies. Sex Transm Dis 2006;33(1): 36–51.

Wald A, Langenberg AG, Link K, et al. Effect of condoms on reducing the transmission of herpes simplex virus type 2 from men to women. JAMA 2001 27;285(24):3100–6.

Wald A, Langenberg AG, Krantz E, et al. The relationship between condom use and herpes simplex virus acquisition. Ann Intern Med 2005;143(10):707–13.

Weller S, Davis K. Condom effectiveness in reducing heterosexual HIV transmission. Cochrane Database Syst Rev 2002;(1):CD003255. Review.

Winer RL, Hughes JP, Feng Q, et al. Condom use and the risk of genital human papillomavirus infection in young women. N Engl J Med 2006;354(25):2645–54.

13

Emergency Contraception

Ronna Jurow

Department of Obstetrics and Gynecology, Keck School of Medicine, University of Southern California, USA

Introduction

In 1995, international organizations from seven countries, convened by the Rockefeller Foundation, established the International Consortium for Emergency Contraception (EC). Their purpose was "to promote EC as a part of mainstream reproductive health care worldwide". Dedicated products for this purpose were "virtually unknown" and there was little awareness of EC as an option. The consortium developed a product called Postinor-2 (equivalent to Plan B and Next Choice) for distribution and then began marketing and educational programs throughout the world. Plan B was approved by the U.S. Food and Drug Authority (FDA) in 1999, and since then three other dedicated pill options, the copper intrauterine device (Cu-IUD), and Yupze regimens (regimens of particular combination oral contracptives) have been approved. Although the social awareness of these products and their availability in the United States has increased substantially, further educational programs are needed.

> ### 🔬 SCIENCE REVISITED
>
> The most commonly quoted statistics from the Guttenmacher Institute are that in the United States unwanted pregnancies approach 3.1 million, or the often-stated fact that 50% of the pregnancies in the United States are unintended.

A national study conducted by the Kaiser Foundation in 2003 reported that while two thirds of women aged 18–44 had knowledge about EC, only 6% had ever used it. It has been estimated that widespread use of EC could cut the abortion rate in the United States by 50%.

EC provides women with another choice, particularly the 4.6 million women at risk for pregnancy who are not using a regular method. It provides the 6.8 million women using condoms a concrete alternative if they have used a condom that has slipped, broken, or fallen off during intercourse. It can also be a young woman's introduction to contraception, by serving as the bridge to be continued in the same or just slightly altered form as her first birth control method.

There are excellent products, a wide variety of choices, evidence-based literature on the products, and FDA approval for four methods. Of these four methods, three are pills and one is an intrauterine contraceptive, commonly called a Cu-IUD, the copper containing Paragard Intrauterine System.

Relationship to high-risk sex and pregnancy terminations

In December 2005, an ACOG Practice Bulletin on Emergency Contraception stated "A prominent concern among both women and health care providers is that making emergency contraception more readily available could encourage irresponsible sexual behavior, which would increase the risks of both unintended pregnancy and sexually transmitted diseases. *However, numerous studies have shown that this concern in unfounded.*"

Contraception, First Edition. Edited by Donna Shoupe.
© 2011 Blackwell Publishing Ltd. Published 2011 by Blackwell Publishing Ltd.

A review by contraceptive experts in 2007 provided further support for these findings. "Reported evidence demonstrates that making EC more widely available does not increase risk taking and that women who are the most diligent about ongoing contraceptive use are those most likely to seek emergency treatment." (Trussell and Raymond).

There is controversy regarding the impact of EC on lowering the rate of abortions in the United States or abroad. Multiple studies have been unable to document a lowering of abortion rates in countries with either prescription access to older Yupze-regimen EC, over-the-counter access to progestin-only EC, or advanced distribution of free EC supplies. A large study in China confirmed that in a randomized trial, advance access to EC compared to women with no access did not have an effect on pregnancy rates. On the other hand, researchers note that increased use of EC as a back-up method may have accounted for up to 43% of the total reduction in abortion rates between 1994 and 2000.

Effectiveness

Progestin-only EC pill

> **EVIDENCE AT A GLANCE**
>
> The FDA reports that progestin-only emergency contraception reduces the expected pregnancy rate by 89% if taken within 72 hours of unprotected intercourse.

The effectiveness of ECs is usually expressed as the percentage reduction in pregnancy rate for a single use of EC. The package insert for Plan B explains its effectiveness with the following statement: "*Seven out of every eight women who would have gotten pregnant will not become pregnant.*"

Effectiveness is highly dependent on the duration between unprotected intercourse and ingestion of the first dose of EC. (Figure 13.1)

Yupze regimens

The effectiveness of Yupze regimens (Tables 13.1 and 13.2) is reported as ranging from a high of 74% to a low of 50%. These regimens, as well as the progestin-only EC pills, have a higher rate of effectiveness if taken within 12 hours of intercourse. A study by the WHO in 2002 reported some reasonable degree of effectiveness for EC pills taken for up to 5 days after intercourse.

Cu-IUD used for EC

> **EVIDENCE AT A GLANCE**
>
> If the Cu-IUD is inserted within 5 days of unprotected sex, it reduces the risk of pregnancy by more than 99%.

The WHO guidelines state that if ovulation can be estimated, the insertion can be extended beyond 5 days after intercourse but not more than 5 days after ovulation.

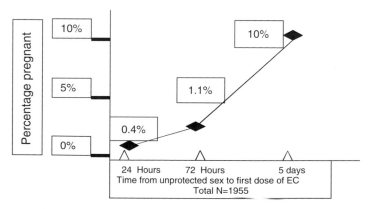

Figure 13.1 Large randomized trials document that the sooner the first dose of EC is taken after intercourse, the greater the effectiveness. Adapted from Piaggio et al. (1999) and Guillebaud (1998).

Table 13.1 Equivalents of common oral contraceptives for use as emergency contraception (equivalent generics can be substituted)

Agent	Pills per dose[a]	Ethinyl estradiol (µg/dose)	Norgestrel (mg/dose)[b]
Yupze options			
Ovral	2 white	100	1
Alesse	5 pink	100	0.50
Levlite	5 pink	100	0.50
Nordette	4 light orange	120	0.60
Levlen	4 light orange	120	0.60
Levora	4 white	120	0.60
Lo/Ovral	4 white	120	1.2
Triphasil	4 yellow	120	0.50
Tri-Levlen	4 yellow	120	0.50
Trivora	4 pink	120	0.50
Ogestrel	2 white	100	1
Low-Ogestrel	4 white	120	1.2
Progestin only			
Ovrette	20 yellow	0	1.5

[a]The amount of norgestrel/tablet is twice the amount of levonorgestrel.
[b]Treatment consists of two doses taken 12 hours apart.

Mechanism of action

Progestin-only ECs

> **SCIENCE REVISITED**
>
> The FDA states that *progestin-only emergency contraception works by preventing ovulation.* The FDA adds that "it is possible" that progestin-only emergency contraceptive pills (ECPs) may interfere with the blastocyst implanting in the uterine lining, but that they have no effect on pregnancies if taken after implantation.

Several studies have shown that the rate of ovulation suppression is approximately equal to the effectiveness of EC, suggesting that this is the dominant mechanism involved. Thickening of cervical mucus, alterations in tubal transport or direct inhibition of fertilization may play a secondary role. Several studies indicate that progestin-only EC may cause secondary changes within the endometrium that may interfere with implantion.

The overwhelming agreement is that there is reduced efficacy when treatment is delayed. Leading experts in the field continue to point out that if ECPs cause direct interference with implantation, then delays in use would not reduce their efficacy, as long as they were used before implantation. However, there is a continuing controversy and it cannot be easily concluded that EC never prevents pregnancy after fertilization.

Cu-IUDs

The Cu-IUD is a very effective method of contraception when used as a regular method. It acts primarily through spermicidal actions of the copper ions and inflammatory changes in the endometrium. It is not known whether these toxic effects, or the insertion of the IUD and further disruption of the endometrium, may have a harmful effect on embryos. This may be a consideration for some women when considering an IUD for EC.

Table 13.2 Available Yupze options in the United States

Agent	Manufacturer	Pills per dose
Alesse	Wyeth-Ayerst	5 pink
Aviane	Duramed	5 orange
Cryselle	Barr	4 white
Enpresse	Barr	4 orange
Lessina	Barr	5 pink
Levlen	Berlex	4 light orange
Levlite	Berlex	5 pink
Levora	Watson	4 white
Lo/Ovral	Wyeth-Ayerst	4 white
Low-Ogestrel	Watson	4 white
Lutera	Watson	5 white
Nordette	Wyeth-Ayerst	4 light orange
Ogestrel	Watson	2 white
Ovral	Wyeth-Ayerst	2 white
Portia	Barr	4 pink
Seasonale	Barr	4 pink
Tri-Levlen	Berlex	4 yellow
Triphasil	Wyeth-Ayerst	4 yellow
Trivora	Watson	4 pink

Regimen: First dose taken as early as possible and not later than 72 hours after unprotected sex and a 2nd dose taken 12 hours later.

Good candidates

EC pills

Treatment within 72 hours of unprotected sex for the following conditions:

- Unplanned, unprotected sexual relationship at any time during cycle
- Late in starting new patch, new oral contraceptive (OC) pack or vaginal ring
- Missed 2 or 3 OCs (especially during the first week of OCs)
- 3 or more hours late taking a progestin-only pill
- Condom breakage, slippage, or improper use
- Cap, diaphragm, or shield improper usage
- Late getting depot medroxyprogesterone acetate (DMPA, Depo-Provera) injection
- Mistake in calculating "safe days" when practicing natural family planning
- Rape victims

Cu-IUD

Insertion within 5 days of unprotected sex is an especially good option for women following unprotected sex who would like to use an IUD as a routine contraceptive method

According to the World Health Organization Medical Eligibility Criteria (WHO MEC), if the time of ovulation can be estimated, insertion can occur later than 5 days after unprotected sex as long as the insertion occurs not more than 5 days after ovulation.

> ⚡ **TIPS & TRICKS**
>
> Cu-IUD insertion is indicated for candidates as listed above for EC pills, except that special precautions and clinical judgment should be used for **rape victims**, because of the risk of sexually transmitted infections (STIs), and for other women at **high risk for STIs** (see Chapter 8). The Cu-IUD for emergency contraception in rape victims can also be used in a woman with a low risk of STIs.

Women who have unprotected sex with infected partners, those who use intravenous (IV) drugs, or who have a partner that uses IV drugs, are *not* good candidates for a Cu-IUD.

WHO has specified two STIs, chlamydia and gonorrhea, as organisms that increase the risk of pelvic inflammatory disease (PID). WHO feels there is increased risk of PID with placement of intrauterine contraception if these organisms are present.

Many family planning clinics and hospital-based emergency facilities caring for assaulted woman give appropriate STI treatment following guidelines from the U.S. Centers for Disease Control and Prevention (CDC). Following treatment and attainment of appropriate antibiotic levels, a Cu-IUD can be safely placed.

Medical eligibility criteria (WHO MEC)

EC pills

The attractiveness of EC pills lies in the fact that there are very few "poor candidates". There are few contraindications to its use because of the small dosage of hormone and short time of exposure.

> ★ TIPS & TRICKS
>
> According to the WHO Medical Eligibility Criteria for Emergency Contraceptive Pills(WHO MEC), there are no medical conditions where the risks outweigh the benefits of using either the progestin-only emergency contraceptive pills or combination oral contraceptive regimens.

Even in conditions that exclude the use combination OCs for routine contraceptive protection (including history of severe cardiovascular disease, stroke, angina, migraine, or severe liver disease including jaundice), the advantages of using EC pills generally outweigh the theoretical or proven risks (category 2). In these situations, the progestin-only EC pill is preferable. The progestin-only EC pill is also preferred in a woman with idiopathic thrombosis.

- EC pills do not protect against STIs.
- EC pills are not indicated in women who are pregnant. (Existing pregnancy is not a contraindication in terms of safety, as there is no known harm to the fetus if EC pills are inadvertently taken, but the medication will be ineffective.)
- EC pills should not be used in a woman with a known hypersensitivity of any component of the product or those with undiagnosed vaginal bleeding.

Cu-IUD

> ★ TIPS & TRICKS
>
> The eligibility criteria for inserting a **Cu-IUD** as a routine contraceptive method also apply for insertion of the Cu-IUD as emergency contraception (see Chapter 8).

Note particularly:

- Pregnancy is category 4—a condition which represents an unacceptable health risk if the contraceptive method is used.

- High risk of STI is a category 3 condition—theoretical or proven risks usually outweigh the advantages of using the method.
- For *rape victims*, good clinical judgment should be used to assess the STI risk, treatment options, and use of a Cu-IUD for EC protection.

Advantages of emergency contraceptive methods

Advantages of EC pills

- EC pills are safe for almost all women.
- No serious side effects or reported deaths have been linked to EC pills.
- EC pills can be bought in advance and kept on hand for use in an emergency.
- In the event of failure, no teratogenic or other adverse outcomes are reported after exposure to EC pills.
- The FDA allows women 17 or older to purchase EC pills over the counter. Women under 17 can obtain EC pills with prescription.

Advantages of Cu-IUD

- The IUD provides an ongoing highly effective method of contraception lasting 10 years.
- The IUD can be inserted up to 5 days after unprotected sex. WHO states that insertion can be done later than 5 days after intercourse but not later than 5 days after the estimated day of ovulation.

Risks and side effects

Progestin-only EC pills

Possible side effects include nausea (23%), abdominal pain (19%), fatigue (17%), headache (17%), heavier menstrual bleeding (14%), lighter menstrual bleeding (12%), dizziness (11%), breast tenderness (11%), vomiting (7%), and diarrhea (5%). These side effects are short lived and usually resolve within 24 hours.

Progestin-only EC pills have a lower rate of side effects than the estrogen–progestin (Yupze) EC pill regimens. One comparative study reported nausea 23% and vomiting 6% on progestin-only EC pill compared with 50% and 19% on estrogen–progestin EC pills.

After taking progestin-only EC pills, some women may have spotting for a few days. About

75% of the time, users will have a normal menses within 3 days of their expected time, and 87% will have their next menses within 7 days of their expected time; 13% will have heavier bleeding and 12% will have less. If there is a delay in menses of more than 1 week, testing for pregnancy is indicated.

A previous ectopic pregnancy is not a contraindication to the use of progestin–only EC pills.

Progestin-only ECs may be associated with the same metabolic effects seen with progestin-only OCs (see Chapter 4), although these changes are only short term and are quickly normalized.

> ### ✋ CAUTION
>
> Progestin-only EC pills are not recommended for routine use as a contraceptive and are not effective in terminating an existing pregnancy.

Noncontraceptive benefits

Use of EC pills, even the combination OC (Yupze) regimens, is not associated with the noncontraceptive benefits appreciated with use of OCs for contraception (see Chapters 3 and 4).

The noncontraceptive benefits of EC appear to be:

- the chance to educate all women on all contraceptive options
- the opportunity to form better relationships with the very large population of underserved women
- the initiation of relationships with very young woman for whom the subject of contraception has not been discussed.

The anticipated benefit of EC to decrease unplanned pregnancy rates and abortion rates has not been seen. Despite availability in more than 140 countries, 50 of them where EC is available without a doctor's prescription, there has not been a decrease in the rates of abortion or unintended pregnancy.

Even the push to assure advance availability of EC pills has not been shown to be effective. In the major studies where women were given either the medication itself for future use or a prescription to be used in the event of an unprotected event, the trials reported that a large percentage of women failed to use the medication as they did not consider all unprotected acts of intercourse to be emergencies. A large study in San Francisco using advance provision of EC pills reported that 45% did not use them. In the Nevada/North Carolina trial, 33% of women in the advance provision group admitted to at least one uncovered act.

Patient counseling

If taken properly, EC has very few disadvantages. The importance of healthcare providers providing accurate information to their patients about availability and proper use of contraceptive options, including EC, cannot be emphasized enough.

Progestin-only EC pills are available over the counter for women 17 and older. However, many sexually active women are unaware of this possibility, or poorly informed regarding use of EC pills. A timely telephone call or clinic visit can provide access to a healthcare provider for women seeking information or access to EC. *There is great advantage in early use of EC pills.*

For the healthcare provider, the most important questions to ask are *when* the unprotected sexual activity occurred and *during which part of the woman's cycle* (the risk of pregnancy is significantly higher for unprotected sex during the 3–4 days before and after mid-cycle). Other important information includes establishment of the dates of the two prior menstrual periods, regularity of the patient's cycles, contraceptive methods, health status, medications, and any symptoms of bleeding or cramping.

If patients are within 72 hours of unprotected sex, they are candidates for EC and can be directed to a pharmacy for Plan B, Plan B One-Step, or Next Choice without a prescription if they are 17 or older.

Counseling regarding the side effects of EC pills includes possible nausea, cramping, bleeding and alterations of next menses. Offering a prescription for an antiemetic is recommended. Users should be advised they need to return if they have heavy bleeding, severe cramps, persistent bleeding, or a positive pregnancy test. If the next menses if more than 1 week late, a pregnancy test should be done.

Finally, counseling regarding contraceptive options, and timing of initiation of a chosen contraceptive method are an important parts of this visit (see "Bridging to routine contraceptive method," below)

Good clinical judgment should be used to determine the use of a pelvic examination and pregnancy test. A urine pregnancy test (the resolution of urinary hCGs is now 100–150 milli-IU/mL) is usually positive during or just after a missed menses.

Patients who are within 72 hours of an unprotected act of sexual intercourse, are interested in a Cu-IUD for continuing contraception, and have a negative pregnancy test are candidates for EC using the Cu-IUD.

Where progestin-only OCs are not available/preferred and the patient is within 72 hours of unprotected sex, the Yupze regimens (see Tables 13.1 and 13.2) are appropriate. The more frequent and more severe side effects with these regimens can be lessened by pretreatment with antiemetics. (see "Management of problems," below).

Bridging to routine contraceptive method

One of the more recent family planning advances has been in "Quick Start" or "bridging" methods. Bridging from EC pills to combination OCs, discussion of the Cu-IUD for EC and for long-term contraception, or discussion and selection of one of the other contraceptive methods is an important part of this visit.

The fact that EC provides no protection for STIs makes the visit for EC an opportunity to discuss risk factors, screening, and ways to lower the risk of acquiring STIs.

★ TIPS & TRICKS

It is important to counsel women that emergency contraception is not 100% effective. If a normal menses does not occur within a week of the expected time, a pregnancy test should be done.

Available options

- *Plan B* contains two 0.75 mg levonogestrel tablets. The first pill is to be taken as soon as possible within the 72 hour window of unprotected intercourse and the second is taken 12 hours later.
- *Plan B One-Step:* The package contains one 1.5 mg levonorgestrel tablet. The single tablet is taken as soon as possible after unprotected sex and within 72 hours. It has been found to be just as well tolerated and effective as the two-pill regimen.
- *Next Choice* is the generic equivalent of Plan B. It is less expensive than Plan B, and it is often covered by state and federally funded programs.
- Yupze regimen: Combination OCs containing levonorgestrel/norgestrel with ethinyl estradiol, as shown in Tables 13.1 and 13.2. In 1997 the FDA issued a statement, placed in the Federal Register, that certain combination OCs are safe and effective for use as postcoital EC.
- Copper intrauterine contraception (ParaGard): Insertion of the Cu-IUD is the most effective EC available today and it is approved for use up to 5 days after unprotected intercourse.
- A new emergency contraceptive pill, called Ella (ulipristal acetate) has been approved in tablet form by the US FDA. It is available by prescription only, and prevents pregnancy if taken within five days after unprotected sexual intercourse or contraceptive failure. [see below under New Products]

New products

A second-generation progesterone receptor antagonist, ulipristal acetate, is already being marketed in Europe by HRA Pharma, and looks very promising as an effective alternative; it has fewer side effects than other FDA-approved agents and can be safely used up to 5 days after unprotected sexual intercourse. It is given in a single dose of 30 mg and has been shown to be highly selective and to effectively suppress ovulation. It has only one notable side effect, a delay in menstruation, but appears to be better tolerated than the other oral EC agents. Data comparing the progestin-only EC pill and combined EC pills with ulipistal acetate indicate that ulipistal has a higher efficacy than both other options. Ulipristal is effective for up to 120 hours. In May, 2009, ulipristal acetate was approved by the European Medicines Agency for use up to 5 days after unprotected intercourse. It was clinically tested in more than 4,000 women both in the United States (several in Planned Parenthood sites) and Europe. No adverse events have been reported. It is currently awaiting clearance from the FDA.

Supplying the method

- Women 17 and older can purchase progestin-only EC pills over the counter.
- Some insurance companies will cover the medication only if a prescription is obtained.
- Women under 17 can only purchase the medication when they have a prescription.
- Combination OC pill regimens (Yupze regimens) are available by prescription.
- The Cu-IUD is inserted by a healthcare provider.
- Ella (ulipristal acetate) is available by prescription only.

Management of problems

Method failure

The most poignant problem is a failure after use of EC, meaning conception has occurred. A timely discussion with the woman about options and potential referrals is recommended. Appropriate options should be clearly discussed without prejudice. Appropriate referral is to a clinician or clinic that is comfortable and knowledgeable about her particular issues.

There is no data linking teratogenicity of the EC to the fetus or known harm to the pregnant woman. Most of the reassuring data comes from use of OCs during early pregnancy, where no adverse events are reported.

Nausea

- Meclizine has been shown to reduce nausea risk, but other options (including sublingual options) are now available, e.g. ondansetron (Zofran), metoclopramide (Reglan).
- Antiemetics should be given as a premedication, prior to beginning the ECP; if vomiting still occurs, a second dose should be considered.

- Taking EC pills during meals may reduce nausea, but some studies have found it ineffective.
- Simethicone (Gas-X), trimethobenzamide (Tigan) suppositories, vitamin B_6, and diphenhydramine (Bendectin) are also used.

Selected references

AAP Committee on Adolescence. Emergency contraception (PDF). Pediatrics 2005;116(4): 1026–35.

ACOG Practice Bulletin No. 69. Emergency contraception. Obstet Gynecol 2005;106(6):1443–52.

Belzer M, Sanchez K, Olson J, Jacobs AM, Tucker D. Advance supply of emergency contraception: a randomized trial in adolescent mothers. J Pediatr Adolesc Gynecol. 2005;18(5):347–54.

Cheng L, Gulmezoglu AM, Oel CJ, Piaggio G, Ezcurra E, Look PF. Interventions for emergency contraception. Cochrane Database Syst Rev 2004;(3):CD001324.

Croxatto HB, Brache V, Pavez M, et al. Pituitary-ovarian function following the standard levonorgestrel emergency contraceptive dose or a single 0.75-mg dose given on the days preceding ovulation. Contraception 2004;70(6): 442–50.

Demers L. The morning-after pill. N Engl J Med 1971;284(18):1034–6.

FDA. Plan B Rx to OTC switch medical reviews (August 22, 2006) (PDF) pp. 32–7, 133–77.

FDA. Certain combined oral contraceptives for use as postcoital emergency contraception. Fed Regist 1997;62(37):8610–2.

Gainer E, Kenfack B, Mboudou E, Doh A, Bouyer J. Menstrual bleeding patterns following levonorgestrel emergency contraception. Contraception 2006;74(2):118–24.

Glasier A. Emergency contraception: Is it worth all the fuss? BMJ 2006;333(7568):560–1.

Glasier A, Baird D. The effects of self-administering emergency contraception. N Engl J Med 1998; 339(1):1–4.

Glasier A, Fairhurst K, Wyke S, Zieblad S, Seaman P, Walker J, Lakha F. Advanced provision of emergency contraception does not reduce abortion rates. Contraception 2004;69(5):361.

Gold MA, Wolford JE, Smith KA, Parker AM. The effects of advance provision of emergency contraception on adolescent women's sexual and contraceptive behaviors. J Pediatr Adolesc Gynecol 2004;17(2):87–96.

Gottardi G, Spreafico A, de Orchi L (). The post-coital IUD as an effective continuing contraceptive method. Contraception 1986;34(6): 549–58.

Grimes DA, Raymond EG. Emergency contraception. Ann Intern Med 2002;137(3):180–9.

Guillebaud J. Time for emergency contraception with levonorgestrel alone. Lancet 1998;352: 416–17.

Hatcher RA, Stewart GK, Stewart F, Guest F, Josephs N, Dale J. Contraceptive technology 1982–1983, 11th ed. New York: Irvington Publishers; 1982, pp. 152–7.

Hu X, Cheng L, Hua X, Glasier A. Advanced provision of emergency contraception to postnatal women in China makes no difference in abortion rates: a randomized controlled trial. Contraception 2005;72(2): 111–16.

Jackson RA, Schwarz EB, Freedman L, Darney P (2003). "Advance supply of emergency contraception: effect on use and usual contraception—a randomized trial". Obstet Gynecol 102 (1): 8–16.

Lo SS, Fan SYS, Ho PC, Glasier AF. Effect of advanced provision of emergency contraception on women's contraceptive behavior: a randomized controlled trial. Hum Reprod 2004;19(10):2404–10.

Piaggio G, von Hertzen H, Grimes DA, Van Look PF. Timing of emergency contraception with levonorgestrel or the Yuzpe regimen. Task Force on Postovulatory Methods of Fertility Regulation. Lancet 1999;353:721.

Polis CB, Schaffer K, Blanchard K, Glasier A, Harper CC, Grimes DA. Advance provision of emergency contraception for pregnancy prevention: a meta-analysis. Obstet Gynecol 2007;110(6):1379–88.

Raine T, Harper C, Leon K, Darney P. Emergency contraception: advance provision in a young, high-risk clinic population. Obstet Gynecol 2000;96(1):1–7.

Raine TR, Harper CC, Rocca CH, et al. Direct access to emergency contraception through pharmacies and effect on unintended pregnancy and STIs: a randomized controlled trial. JAMA 2005;293(1):54–62.

Raymond E, Goldberg A, Trussell J, Hays M, Roach E, Taylor D. Bleeding patterns after use of levonorgestrel emergency contraceptive pills. Contraception 2006;73(4):376–81.

Raymond EG, Stewart F, Weaver M, Monteith C, Van Der Pol B. Impact of increased access to emergency contraceptive pills: a randomized controlled trial. Obstet Gynecol 2006;108(5): 1098–106.

Stewart FH, Trussell J. Prevention of pregnancy resulting from rape: A neglected preventive health measure. Am J Preventive Med 2000; 19(4):228.

Task Force on Postovulatory Methods of Fertility Regulation. Randomised controlled trial of levonorgestrel versus the Yuzpe regimen of combined oral contraception for emergency contraception. Lancet 1998;352(9126):428–33.

Trussell J, Ellertson C, Stewart F. The effectiveness of the Yuzpe regimen of emergency contraception. Fam Plann Perspect 1996;28(2):58–64, 87.

Trussell J, Ellertson C, von Hertzen H, et al. Estimating the effectiveness of emergency contraceptive pills. Contraception 2003;67(4): 259–65.

Trussell J, Hedley A, Raymond E. Ectopic pregnancy following use of progestin-only ECPs. J Fam Plann Reprod Health Care 2003; 29(4):249.

Trussell J, Raymond EG. Emergency contraception: a cost-effective approach to preventing unintended pregnancy. In Kruger TF, van der Spuy ZM, Kempers RD, eds. Advances in Fertility Studies and Reproductive Medicine. Cape Town, SA: Juta & Co; 2007, pp. 252–66.

Trussell J, Rodriguez G, Ellertson C. Updated estimates of the effectiveness of the Yuzpe regimen of emergency contraception. Contraception 1999;59(3):147–51.

Walsh TL, Frezieres RG. Patterns of emergency contraception use by age and ethnicity from a randomized trial comparing advance provision and information only. Contraception 2006;74(2):110–17.

WHO. Question 20. What can a woman do to prevent nausea and vomiting when taking emergency contraceptive pills (ECPs)? In: Selected practice recommendations for contraceptive use, 2nd ed. Geneva: World Health Organization; 2005.

WHO. Question 21. What can a woman do if she vomits after taking emergency contraceptive pills (ECPs)? Selected practice recommendations for contraceptive use, 2nd ed. Geneva: World Health Organization; 2005.

WHO Task Force on Postovulatory Methods of Fertility Regulation. Randomised controlled trial of levonorgestrel versus the Yuzpe regimen of combined oral contraceptives for emergency contraception. Lancet 1998;352(9126): 428–33.

WHO/HRP. Levonorgestrel is more effective, has fewer side-effects, than Yuzpe regimen. Prog Hum Reprod Res 1999;51:3–5.

Yuzpe A, Thurlow H, Ramzy I, Leyshon J. Post coital contraception—A pilot study. J Reprod Med 1974;13(2):53–8.

Zhang L, Chen J, Wang Y, Ren F, Yu W, Cheng L. Pregnancy outcome after levonorgestrel-only emergency contraception failure: a prospective cohort study. Hum Reprod 2009;24(7): 1605–11.

14

Tubal Sterilization

Charles M. March

California Fertility Partners and the Department of Obstetrics and Gynecology, Keck School of Medicine, University of Southern California, USA

Worldwide, tubal sterilization is used by 33% of married women using contraception, making it the most common contraceptive option. Although vasectomy is as efficacious as methods available to women—as well as being faster, safer, less complex, and less costly—more women than men undergo sterilization, the current ratio being approximately 3:2. Features of the "ideal method" of sterilization are listed in Table 14.1.

EVIDENCE AT A GLANCE

In the United States, rates of tubal sterilization have been as high as almost 50% in women aged 40–44, but recently, the rates have been declining. *This decline is thought to be due to the improved access to a variety of highly effective reversible methods including IUDs and the implant.*

Failure rates

Long-term failure rates of tubal sterilization are 1–2%, and vary considerably according to the method used (Table 14.2). During the first year failure rates are between 0.1 and 0.8%. The 10-year cumulative probability of pregnancy was 18.5 per 1,000 procedures (95% confidence interval (CI) 15.1–21.8) among the 10,685 women enrolled in the U.S. Collaborative Review of Sterilization study.

In that study luteal-phase pregnancies (estimated to be 2–3 per 1,000) were not reported as failures Curettage at the time of sterilization will reduce the risk that a procedure done in the luteal phase will not "fail" because of a pre-existing pregnancy. Limiting surgery to the follicular phase reduces the risk of a "luteal pregnancy" and also reduces the risk of traumatizing a fresh corpus luteum.

For unipolar tubal coagulation the rate was only 7.5 per 1,000 procedures, compared to 36.5 per 1,000 procedures after clip application. Failures occurred more commonly among younger women because of their higher fertility which is maintained for a longer time. For bipolar coagulation, the failure rate may be reduced by coagulating three or more sites.

Good candidates

- Sexually active reproductive-aged women who have completed their families
- Women with medical problems that make pregnancy undesirable.

Medical eligibility criteria

The World Health Organization Medical Eligibility Criteria (WHO MEC) classifies over 60 medical conditions in categories according to the risk that tubal ligation procedure would have in that particular condition. Each medical condition is assigned to one of four categories: A, accept; D, delay; C, caution; S, special circumstances. The assignment to these categories follows the guidelines for general standard of care for surgical candidates (see Table 14.3).

Contraception, First Edition. Edited by Donna Shoupe.
© 2011 Blackwell Publishing Ltd. Published 2011 by Blackwell Publishing Ltd.

Table 14.1 Attributes of the ideal method of sterilization

Minimal skill and training required
Performed by paramedical personnel
One-time procedure
Highly effective
Effective immediately
Office procedure
Local or no anesthesia
Minimal pain
Minimal morbidity
No mortality
Little equipment required
Reusable equipment
Equipment maintenance minimal
No visible scar
Performed during pregnancy, postpartum, or postabortion
Inexpensive
Reduces/prevents STIs
Reversible

STI, sexually transmitted infection.

Table 14.2 Cumulative 10-year failure rates of tubal sterilization by method

Method	Failure rate (%)
Postpartum partial salpingectomy	0.75
Unipolar coagulation	0.75
Silastic ring	1.77
Interval partial salpingectomy	2.01
Bipolar coagulation	2.48
Hulka clip	3.65

Noncontraceptive benefits

One prospective study of 396,000 women demonstrated that the risk of ovarian cancer was 30% less in the group who had undergone tubal ligation. Some have suggested that exposure to carcinogens which may ascend in the reproductive tract is reduced or that damage to the tube plays a role. Tubal closure also reduces the frequency of salpingitis and pelvic peritonitis.

> **⚠ CAUTION**
>
> Sterilization does not protect against sexually transmitted infections (STIs) or HIV, and the correct and consistent use of condoms is recommended for women at risk, either alone or with another contraceptive method. Male latex condoms are proven to protect against STI/HIV.

Advantages

- Sterilization is a permanent, not coitally related, nonhormonal, highly effective method of contracpetion.
- Inexpensive methods are available: hysteroscopic methods are the most cost-effective (see Chapter 2).
- It is a good option for women who are poor candidates for other methods: those with multiple risk factors for cardiovascular disease, or poor compliance with other methods.

Risks and side effects

The likelihood that a pregnancy will be extrauterine is greater if it occurs after a sterilizing operation than otherwise. The proportion of ectopics increases over time, being three times higher in years 4–10 than in the first 3 years following tubal sterilization. Ectopics are most common after bipolar coagulation (65%) and interval partial salpingectomy (43%). Unipolar coagulation (17%) and spring clip application (15%) are associated with the lowest proportion.

The morbidity and mortality of laparoscopy are low. In 1993 the American Association of Gynecologic Laparoscopists reported a death rate of 1 in 22,966 procedures. In another report, the mortality rate was 1.5 in 100,000. Many of these deaths occurred in patients with medical conditions and most are attributed to anesthetic complications or vascular or intestinal injuries.

The complication rate is reported to be twice as high in those who undergo a laparotomy compared to those who have laparoscopic surgery. Laparotomy is associated with longer operating and convalescence times, higher rates of wound

Table 14.3 WHO Medical Eligibility Criteria (WHO MEC)

Category	Condition	Comments
A	Postpartum <7 days or >42 days Mild pre-eclampsia Postabortion (uncomplicated) Thrombogenic mutation STIs (excluding HIV and hepatitis) Hypertension during pregnancy, currently normal Benign gestational trophoblastic disease History of DVT/PE Viral hepatitis carrier or chronic Mild compensated cirrhosis Benign focal nodular hyperplasia/ liver tumor Sterilization at time of cesarean section	
D	Pregnancy Postpartum 7–42 days Severe pre-eclampsia or eclampsia Prolonged rupture of membranes ≥24 hours Puerperal sepsis, intrapartum or puerperal fever Severe antepartum or postpartum hemorrhage Severe trauma to the genital tract: cervical or vaginal tear at time of delivery or abortion Postabortion sepsis or fever Severe post-abortion hemorrhage Acute hematometra Unexplained vaginal bleeding (before evaluation) Current ischemic heart disease Malignant gestational trophoblastic disease Local infection	
		Clarification: there is an increased risk of postoperative infection
	Infection or gonorrhea Current PID Current purulent cervicitis or chlamydia or gonorrhea infection Acute bronchitis, pneumonia	
		Clarification: The procedure should be delayed until the condition is corrected. There are increases in anesthesia-related and other perioperative risks
	Systemic infection or gastroenteritis Viral hepatitis (acute or flare) Current symptomatic gallbladder disease Iron deficiency anemia (Hb <7g/dL) Acute DVT/PE Gestational trophoblastic disease with persistently elevated β-HCG Cervical or endometrial cancer Current breast cancer	

(Continued)

Table 14.3 *Continued*

Category	Condition	Comments
C	Young age	Young women should be counseled regarding the permanency of the method and the availability of alternative, long-term, highly effective methods
	Depressive disorders	
	Current breast cancer	
	Obesity (BMI >30)	Clarification: the procedure may be more difficult. There is an increased risk of wound infection and disruption. Obese women may have limited respiratory function and more likely to require general anesthesia
	Uterine fibroids	
	Previous abdominal or pelvic surgery	
	Endometriosis	
	Uterine fibroids	
	Diaphragmatic hernia	
	Previous abdominal or pelvic surgery	
	Hypertension (adequately controlled)	Elevated blood pressure levels (properly taken measurements) systolic 140–159 or diastolic 90–99
	History of ischemic heart disease or cerebrovascular accident	
	Uncomplicated valvular heart disease	
	Hypothyroid	
	Diabetes (type 1 or 2) but no vascular disease	
	PID without subsequent pregnancy	
	Liver hepatocellular adenoma or malignant hepatoma	
	Hemoglobin ≥ 7 to $<10\,g/dL$	
	Thalassemia	
	Fibrosis of liver	
	Kidney disease	
	Severe nutritional deficiencies	
	SLE (without clotting problems or on immunosuppressive medication)	
	Epilepsy	
S	Postpartum or postabortion uterine rupture or perforation	Clarification: If exploratory surgery or laparoscopy is conducted and the patient is stable, repair of the problem and tubal sterilization may be performed concurrently if no additional risk is involved
	Hypertension: systolic >160 or diastolic >100	Clarification: Elevated blood pressure should be controlled before surgery. There are increased anesthesia-related risks and an increased risk of cardiac arrhythmia with uncontrolled hypertension. Careful monitoring of blood pressure intraoperatively is necessary

Table 14.3 *Continued*

Category	Condition	Comments
	Vascular disease or multiple risk factors for arterial cardiovascular disease	
	Asthma, bronchitis, emphysema, lung infection	
	Complicated valvular heart disease (pulmonary hypertension, risk of atrial fibrillation)	
	Diabetes with nephropathy/retinopathy/ neuropathy or other vascular disease or diabetes >20 years	
	Severe decompensated cirrhosis	
	DVT/PE on anticoagulant therapy	
	Positive of antiphospholipid antibodies, severe thrombocytopenia	
	Coagulation disorders	
	Immunosuppressive therapy	
	AIDS	
	Hyperthyroid	
	Pelvic tuberculosis	
	Fixed uterus due to previous surgery or infection	
	Abdominal wall or umbilical hernia	Clarification: Hernia repair and tubal sterilization should be performed concurrently, if possible
	Endometriosis	

BMI, body mass index; DVT/PE, deep venous thrombosis/pulmonary embolism; HCG, human chorionic gonadotropin; PID, pelvic inflammatory disease; SLE, systemic lupus erythematosus.
Key:
Category A: Accept. There is no medical reason to deny sterilization
Category D: Delay. The procedure is delayed until the condition is evaluated and/or corrected. Alternative temporary methods of contraception should be provided.
Category C: Caution. The procedure is normally conducted in a routine setting, but with extra preparation and precautions
Category S: Special circumstances. The procedure should be undertaken in a setting with an experienced surgeon and other back-up medical support. The capacity to decide on the most appropriate procedure and anesthesia regimen is also needed. Alternative temporary methods of contraception should be provided, if referral or other delay is anticipated.
Adapted from WHO Medical Eligibility Criteria: http://whqlibdoc.who.int/publications/2004/9241562668.pdf

infections and greater postoperative pain. Mini-laparotomy reduces the risks associated with laparotomy.

Laparoscopic complications are rare but include vascular and bowel injuries. Patient selection, intra- and postoperative vigilance, and operator experience and judgment influence complication rates. Another complication of laparoscopy is the inability to complete the procedure laparoscopically because of adhesions, poor visualization, or other distortions to the normal anatomy.

Sterilization does not affect ovarian function or alter the age of menopause, sexual function or desire, or increase the risk of hysterectomy or psychological problems. Although irregular menses and dysmenorrhea are reported to occur more often after tubal sterilization, most of these reports are in women who previously used oral contraceptives, often to relieve these same problems.

Patient counseling

Tubal sterilization should be considered permanent and the decision to have the procedure should not be made when the patient is under unusual conditions or in a stressful situation.

Avoiding and managing regret

Regret is a serious concern. Does the request for sterilization emanate from a reaction to a difficult pregnancy? The desire for sterilization often rests on the assumption that the newly delivered infant is and will remain healthy. The delivery of an infant whose health status is uncertain is cause for concern. Would a neonatal or infant death cause the couple to desire another pregnancy? Because the delivery of a very ill infant might not have been suspected, re-evaluation of the couple's wishes in the delivery room is mandatory.

In a study of 7,000 women followed for at least 5 years after sterilization, the frequency of regret was reported to be 6%. The frequency of regret within 14 years after surgery was 20.3% for women who were below 30 years at the time of surgery, and 5.9% in those older. Those under 30 attributed regret to the desire to have for more children, whereas those over 30 attributed various disorders to the sterilization, a claim that is not supported by data. Parous women and those in unstable relationships are more likely to have regret than are nulliparas.

Careful counseling prior to sterilization is critical. Those who request a method that "may be reversible" are obviously going down the wrong path.

The method selected should be that with which the surgeon has the most experience. Most patients who undergo sterilization will not regret their decision, and to penalize them by performing a procedure with lower efficacy is inappropriate.

Available options

Sterilization may be performed in close proximity to a pregnancy or it may be an interval procedure. Each should be evaluated against the backdrop of the "ideal method".

Postpartum sterilization

The ready access to the oviducts at the time of cesarean section makes sterilization convenient. Postpartum sterilization allows recovery from both the delivery and the procedure to occur simultaneously, obviating the need for a subsequent surgery. Although sterilization after delivery carries more risks than interval sterilization (because the pelvic viscera are more vascular), extra bleeding is usually recognized and controlled immediately.

Although there are different methods of sterilization after delivery, some modification of the Pomeroy partial salpingectomy is most common. The Uchida and Irving procedures take longer to perform and have a slightly higher morbidity. Clips or bands are not used postpartum because they are more difficult to apply at this time and are associated with a higher failure rate compared to application during interval sterilizations.

Fimbriectomy is not more effective and has important disadvantages. Hydrosalpinges may develop and become quite large, causing pain, undergoing torsion, becoming infected, or being interpreted as neoplasms leading to another surgery. The intrauterine pregnancy rate after reversal of a fimbriectomy is significantly lower than that following reversal of midtubal sterilization.

On occasion, significant tubal pathology will be discovered and sterilization should be by salpingectomy.

Interval methods

Interval methods allow the patient to make her decision without the stress of a recent or current pregnancy. The surgery is done in the follicular phase in order to avoid the possibility that the woman may be pregnant.

Laparotomy

In addition to the same operations performed at the time of cesarean section, rings or clips can be applied. Laparotomy performed exclusively for sterilization is rarely performed but may occasionally be done if there are contraindications to laparoscopy. These women are best served by a hysteroscopic approach. However, if a laparotomy is required for other reasons, tubal sterilization adds little cost or morbidity.

Minilaparotomy

Minilaparotomy via a 2–5 cm suprapubic incision is performed in the lithotomy position on an outpatient basis. A uterine elevator facilitates access to the oviducts. Except in very obese women, access is easy. A paracervical block significantly reduces the discomfort for those who elect local anesthesia.

Tubal occlusion may be by partial salpingectomy, ring, or clip. If significant pelvic adhesions are present, the incision may be enlarged and general anesthesia utilized.

Laparoscopy

Laparoscopy is faster, safer, cheaper and has a shorter recovery period and superior cosmetic result. An operating laparoscope permits the operation to be performed more rapidly and may allow surgery under local anesthesia with less Trendelenberg positioning and minimal pneumoperitoneum. For those with pelvic adhesions, pelvic pain, or other pathology, the use of a secondary trocar permits a full diagnostic laparoscopy to be performed with treatment of any pathology.

Electrical methods

Monopolar coagulation is the original method of tubal fulguration. The procedure is done by grasping the midportion of the oviduct and coagulating and dividing it. Although this is highly effective, three potential problems were recognized:

- The occurrence of bowel injuries: If thermal injury to the intestine is detected, its extent will probably be far greater than that seen initially and immediate repair with bowel resection or at least close observation is mandatory.
- Tuboperitoneal fistulae and pregnancies, especially ectopics: These occurred because the electrical energy spread laterally towards both the uterus and fimbriae, damaging more tissue that was apparent at the time of surgery. The frequency of ectopic pregnancies is not

high but the proportion tends to rise as the interval from surgery increases. This suggests that late failures are related to tubal recanalization rather than method failure.

- Often little residual fallopian tubes remained because of excessive tubal damage, making reversals very difficult.

Bipolar coagulation is the method of choice for many today. Because the energy is confined between the jaws of the forceps, bowel burns have been reduced markedly. Tubal damage is also less extensive, and reversal of sterilization is usually possible if only one area is coagulated.

If a single-burn technique is used, many surgeons divide the tube in its center. Neither the coagulation nor the incision should be carried into the mesosalpinx because the former may compromise ovarian blood supply and the latter may lead to immediate or delayed hemorrhage. If the oviduct is divided, the proximal and distal stumps are coagulated again so as to reduce the risk of fistula formation. Double- and triple-burn techniques also are employed and, although the failure rate is reduced, the chance of reversal is mostly eliminated.

To insure complete coagulation it is advisable to use a generator with an ammeter which provides audible signals when the coagulation is complete. Using an endocoagulator is another way to reduce the risk of damaging other structures: heat is applied directly to the tubes, increasing safety. However, few surgeons use an endocoagulator for other procedures and thus this instrument has not gained widespread use.

Mechanical methods

Tubal occlusion by mechanical means obviates the safety concerns of electrosurgery; however, these methods are not suitable for use postpartum or in the presence of dilated tubes. Surgeons should select the method they believe to be the best and use it exclusively, with electrosurgery as back-up. Efficacy is greatest when the nuances of each instrument are learned through prolonged experience.

Silastic rings: Yoon band or Falope ring

A 3.6 mm silastic band (impregnated with 5% barium sulfate to provide radio-opacity) is mounted on an applicator that is inserted through an accessory trocar. Immediately before application, the band is advanced over the outer cylinder of the applicator. The tube is grasped at the junction of its proximal and middle thirds, a 2.5 cm portion of tube is drawn into the inner cylinder, and the ring is advanced over this segment. It is important to confirm that the ring is "seated" properly over the knuckle of tube without incorporating any mesosalpingeal vessels. Application of a local anesthetic to the site reduces postoperative pain. If one or both oviducts are large, if bleeding occurs, or if adhesions are present, conversion to an electrosurgical method is advised. The failure rate is approximately 1% after 2 years. The lack of an excessive inflammatory reaction or adhesion formation and the small amount of tubal damage makes this method reversible in most cases.

Clips

These devices are associated with the least amount of tubal damage and thus are most amenable to reversal.

- The *Hulka spring-loaded clip* has two plastic jaws with multiple teeth. It is placed perpendicular to the long axis of the tubal isthmus. The jaws are closed and a gold-plated stainless steel spring is advanced over the jaws, sealing the tube. The teeth of the clip must extend into the mesosalpinx, ensuring complete tubal closure.
- The *titanium Filshie clip* is lined with silicone rubber and has a concavity on its antimesenteric side which conforms to the shape of the oviduct. Application of the clip must be perpendicular to the tubal isthmus. Initially, the clip occludes the tube by the pressure applied during application. However, as tubal necrosis ensues, the silicone rubber expands and maintains luminal obstruction.

Salpingectomy

Salpingectomy has a limited but important role. Patients with hydrosalpinges or extensive tubal damage may be candidates for salpingectomy.

For those who undergo laparoscopic sterilization in conjunction with endometrial ablation, the small isthmic segment of oviduct may fill with blood and secretory products from uterine cornua, causing the "postablation–tubal sterilization syndrome". Salpingectomy, including entry into the lateral intramural segment (as well as leaving the lateral troughs of the endometrial cavity intact during the ablation), avoids this complication.

During salpingectomy, clamps should be placed immediately below the oviduct in order to spare collateral ovarian blood supply.

Vaginal approach

Sterilization via *colpotomy* is performed very infrequently. After colpotomy and identification of the fallopian tubes, fimbriectomy or partial salpingectomy is performed, often with an Endo-Loop type device.

Factors that have reduced the frequency of this approach include adhesions of the tubes and/or ovaries to the site of incision, vaginal scarring causing dyspareunia, and fewer training opportunities.

Transcervical approach

Transcervical sterilization has many advantages and disadvantages (Table 14.4).

The intramural oviduct is tortuous, often preventing long, rigid devices from remaining intraluminal. The myometrium around this portion of the tube can contract and expel rigid plugs. It is also somewhat compliant and may dilate after a device is placed, preventing complete occlusion. Its secretory capability can prevent the adherence and tissue ingrowth needed for some devices to be effective. Healing and regeneration may also lead to failures.

Transcervical sterilization must be performed early in the proliferative phase and at a time well removed from a pregnancy. No currently available method is effective immediately.

Essure

The 4 cm insert consists of a flexible stainless steel inner coil; a very elastic, expandable outer coil of a nickel titanium alloy; and a layer of polyethylene terephthalate (PET) running along and through the inner coil (Figure 14.1). Hysteroscopy is performed under local anesthesia. Using a narrow-diameter release catheter, the device is maintained in a "wound-down" configuration

Table 14.4 Advantages and disadvantages of transcervical sterilization

Advantages	Disadvantages
Office procedure	Complex delivery systems
Less invasive	Expensive disposables
Local/no anesthesia	Long learning curve?
No incision	Possible intraperitoneal injury
Safe	Not possible postpartum
Effective	Not possible postabortion
Inexpensive	Follicular phase timing required
Rapid recovery	Normal anatomy required
Ideal for high-risk patient	Delayed efficacy
	Long-term effectiveness unknown?
	Long-term risks uncertain?
	Insurance coverage variable

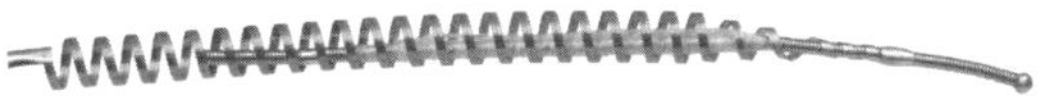

Figure 14.1 Essure microinsert.

(0.8 mm) in order to facilitate placement. After the ostium has been identified, the insert is advanced into the intramural portion until only 5–10 mm remains visible. The device is released and the outer coil expands to up to 2.0 mm, anchoring it and spanning the distance between the ostium and proximal isthmus.

EVIDENCE AT A GLANCE

Successful placement of the Essure device can be achieved in 90% or more of women.

The PET fibers induce a foreign body reaction which peaks 2–3 weeks later. Over 3 months, tissue ingrowth occludes the tube. This ingrowth affects 5 cm of tube. The reaction spares both the serosa and the tubal epithelium distal to the device. Contraception is utilized until a hysterosalpingogram (HSG) demonstrates tubal obstruction. Safety, efficacy, and patient satisfaction were demonstrated in prospective multicenter trials of more than 700 patients. Adverse events were reported in 7%. Three months after surgery, proper placement and bilateral tubal occlusion was demonstrated in 96%. Almost all others had occlusion 3 months later. In summary, after placement by very experienced hysteroscopists, 87% relied on the method for permanent contraception.

After 9,620 women-months of exposure, no pregnancies were reported. Of 643 women followed for up to 5 years, there were no pregnancies in 29,357 women-months of follow-up. Levy et al. reviewed 64 pregnancies and found that patient or physician noncompliance (30) or a misread radiograph (18) were the most common problems. Eight patients were pregnant at the time of placement.

EVIDENCE AT A GLANCE

The efficacy of the Essure device approaches that of monopolar laparoscopic tubal sterilization. Insertion under local anesthesia together with a mild oral sedative and an NSAID is acceptable to most patients.

In a recent report, 118 different physicians, all members of a large multispecialty group, attempted to place Essure in 884 women during 897 procedures (13 had 2 attempts). Each physician performed between 1 and 54 procedures. The initial attempt was successful in 850 (96.2%), failed in 31 (3.1%), and unknown in 3. Bilateral tubal occlusion was reported in 687 (93.0%) of the 739 who had an HSG. There was no correlation between efficacy and increasing physician experience. These results may reflect the willingness of physicians to attempt more difficult procedures as their experience grows, or may be related to the procedure being "user friendly".

This procedure costs one third less than laparoscopic sterilization. This fact, coupled with its ease and effectiveness, has caused the Detroit Medical Center to use Essure for more than half of their sterilizations.

Optical marker   Radiofrequency electrode array

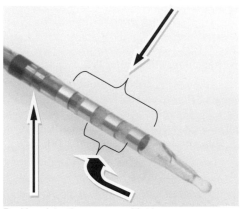

Position detection array   Matrix

Figure 14.2 Adiana device.

Adiana

In July, 2009, the U.S. Food and Drug Authority (FDA) approved the Adiana system (Figure 14.2). The Adiana protocol is similar to that used in the Essure trials but this device uses a considerably different two-step procedure.

Under hysteroscopic guidance a catheter is placed into the intramural portion of the tube. An electrode delivers low level (<5W) radiofrequency energy, causing superficial epithelial destruction. The generator maintains a desired tissue temperature during lesion formation, thereby limiting the amount of damage and individualizing treatment to compensate for variations in anatomy. Exact placement of the catheter in the center of ostium is critical and assured via a unique monitoring device. After the lesion has been created, a porous nonbiodegradable matrix implant of medical-grade silicone is deposited into the area. This matrix induces tissue ingrowth and complete occlusion. Proper placement is documented visually and by ultrasound immediate after surgery. An HSG and follow-up ultrasound are performed 3 months later.

In a prospective multicenter trial of 770 women, bilateral placement was achieved in 611 of 645 women (95%). Bilateral occlusion was confirmed in 570 of 645 (88.4%). The 1-year pregnancy prevention rate by life-table methods was 98.9%.

Palmer and Greenberg compared the Essure and Adiana procedures. They reported that after

7 years Essure has proven to be safe, effective, and well-tolerated versus only 12 months for the Adiana system. Results from the pivotal study documented that as with Essure, the Adiana system is well tolerated with few side effects. The bilateral placement rates for both are similar (94% vs 95%), as are the rates of tubal occlusion by HSG.

Although Essure has been used successfully to treat women with hydrosalpinges prior to in-vitro fertilization (IVF), the presence of a portion of the device in the uterus may make the Adiana device (which is wholly intratubal) a better choice for these patients.

Hysteroscopic sterilization may be performed with a Mirena intrauterine device (IUD) in place. Timing is more flexible in these patients, the endometrium is thinner, and contraception is assured during the 3 month interval prior to HSG. These procedures, as well most of those mentioned below, can be combined with one of the global methods of endometrial ablation. This combination should obviate the risk of the postablation–tubal sterilization syndrome.

Endometrial ablation

Ablation alone is not a method of sterilization. Although pregnancy after ablation is rare, perhaps 1 in 400, these data are difficult to interpret. Most women who undergo ablation are older and relatively infertile, have been sterilized, or use contraception. Thus, their risk of pregnancy is low. Because there have been serious complications in some pregnancies that have occurred after ablation, simultaneous hysteroscopic sterilization should be considered. NovaSure ablation combined with Essure sterilization has been demonstrated to be effective.

Reversal of sterilization

Factors affecting the success of reversing tubal sterilization are listed in Table 14.5. The chance of success is inversely related to the amount of tubal damage caused by the procedure. The most damage occurs after monopolar coagulation, followed by fimbriectomy, multiple-burn bipolar coagulation, single-burn bipolar coagulation, partial salpingectomy, Falope rings, and clips. Very little data are available to assess the likelihood of reversing hysteroscopic sterilization.

If reversal is requested, referral should be to a reproductive surgeon experienced in tubal microsurgery who will review the prior surgical and pathology reports. If these reports do not reveal a contraindication to reversal (e.g., a bilateral salpingectomy), a semen analysis, evaluation of ovulatory function, and HSG should be performed. The HSG can evaluate the uterus and proximal oviducts.

A discussion of the alternatives (IVF and reconstructive surgery) for restoring fertility can follow. Factors to consider are live birth rate per cycle, the cumulative live birth rate after a specific number of cycles, the risk of multiple pregnancy, abortion and extrauterine pregnancy, and the additional successes based on transfer of any frozen embryos.

IVF avoids major surgery, has a very low rate of ectopic pregnancy, and is successful in the presence of male factor infertility. However, it is expensive and usually not covered by health insurance. It is also associated with a high rate of multiple pregnancies and an increase in the rate of spontaneous abortion, and may have to be performed multiple times especially in those who may wish to have more than one child.

Reconstructive surgery offers a basically endless number of cycles in which the couple can achieve one or more pregnancies and the risk of

abortion is not increased. The risk of an ectopic pregnancy following mid-tubal reanastomosis is very low. However, as with IVF, tubal surgery is usually not covered by insurance and usually involves a laparotomy. Morbidity occurs more often after surgery than after IVF.

The types of procedures are multiple and their outcomes vary considerably (Table 14.6). If the patient fails to become pregnant following surgery, a repeat operation is almost never justified and the patient should consider IVF.

Investigational procedures

The worldwide need for "easy", affordable sterilization will continue to stimulate research efforts.

Quinacrine

Quinacrine has been used in a solution, in quinacrine-impregnated IUDs, and as pellets. It is the safest, most effective, and most widely used nonsurgical method. In solution form, bilateral closure rates of 55%, 80%, and 95% were achieved after one, two and three instillations, respectively.

Quinacrine-impregnated IUDs, which prevent peritoneal spillage and intravascular administration, deliver quinacrine close to the tubal ostia, eliminate the need for multiple applications, and provide contraception while tubal closure is progressing. However, they do not improve efficacy.

Seven 36 mg quinacrine pellets are delivered to the top of the fundus via an IUD introducer monthly for 2 months. They dissolve within 30 minutes and scar tissue forms within 12 weeks. The bilateral tubal closure rate of 73% rose to 84% after a third insertion. The failure rate was 3.7%.

A more practical approach is the delivery of quinacrine rods to the intramural oviducts under hysteroscopic guidance. The ease of

Table 14.5 Factors influencing the success of tubal sterilization reversal

| Method of sterilization |
| Amount of tubal damage |
| Patient age |
| Presence of other infertility factors |
| Surgeon experience |

Table 14.6 Outcome of tubal reconstructive surgery

Procedure	IUP (%)	Live birth (%)	Ectopic (%)
Salpingostomy by laparotomy	20–40	18–35	10–40
Salpingostomy by laparoscopy	10–40	10–30	10–35
Reanastomosis by laparotomy	45–80	30–80	2–10
Reanastomosis by laparoscopy	50–75	50–60	3–30
Tubocornual anastomosis	50–60	30–50	5–15

IUP, intrauterine pregnancy.

administration and very low cost of quinacrine are likely to maintain ongoing interest in this method.

Tissue adhesives

Gelatin–resorcinol–formaldehyde was highly efficacious, but peritoneal spillage occurred. Bilateral closure rates were 66% after one instillation and 89% after two instillations. As methyl-cyanoacrylate flows from the proximal to distal oviduct it changes from a monomer to a polymer. The polymerized form on the outside of the advancing stream protects the peritoneum from injury should spillage occur. Cell necrosis begins within 24 hours and proceeds rapidly. By 12 weeks the tubes are scarred. Bilateral closure rates were 74–80% after one application but rose to 90–98% after a second one. The cumulative pregnancy rate is reported to be 3.7% after 24 months.

Microwave sterilization

The same approach to endometrial destruction by means of microwaves may be applied to the intramural oviduct. If trials demonstrate safety, studies may begin, perhaps with delivery under ultrasound guidance.

Other methods

Other research methods include hysteroscopic tubal coagulation, neodymium:yttrium aluminum garnet (Nd:YAG) laser, Brundin P-block, Hosseinian uterotubal junction device (UTJD), Hamou intratubal thread, rigid plugs, formed-in-place silicone plugs, intratubal ligation device, and reversible tubal occlusion devices.

Conclusion

Table 14.7 compares various methods of sterilization available today. Although the ideal

Table 14.7 Today's methods of sterilization versus the ideal method

	Ideal	PS	LTC	LTB	BTC	HSC
Skill/training	Minimal					+
Paramedic procedure	Yes				+	
One treatment	Yes	+	+	+		+
Effectiveness	High	+	+	+		+
Effective immediately	Yes	+	+	+		
Office procedure	Yes				+	+
No anesthesia	Yes				+	±
Pain	Minimal		+	+	+	+
Morbidity	Minimal	+	+	+	+	+
Mortality	None	±	±	±	−	−
Equipment needed	Little	+				+
Reusable equipment	Yes	+	+	±		
Equipment maintenance	Minimal	+			+	
Visible scar	None				+	+
Possible during pregnancy	Yes	+				
Possible postpartum or abortion	Yes	+	+		±	
Inexpensive	Yes					+
Reduce/prevent STIs	Yes					
Reversible	Yes	+	±		+	

BTC, blind transcervical; HSC, hysteroscopic; LTB, laparoscopic application of band or clip; LTC, laparoscopic tubal coagulation, monopolar or bipolar; PS, partial salpingectomy (at cesarean section, interval, abdominal or vaginal).

sterilization option has not been developed, the hysteroscopic approaches remain the most attractive interval procedures.

Selected references

Centers for Disease Control and Prevention. Deaths following female sterilization with unipolar electrocoagulation. MMWR 1980; 30:150.

Cooper JM, Carignan CS, Cher D, et al. Microinsert nonincisional hysteroscopic sterilization. Obstet Gynecol 2003;102:59–67.

Donnadieu AC, Fernandez H. The role of Essure sterilization performed simultaneously with endometrial ablation. Curr Opin Obstet Gynecol 2008;20:359–63.

Feldblum P, Hays M, Zipper J, et al. Pregnancy rates among Chilean women who had non-surgical sterilization with quinacrine pellets between 1977 and 1989. Contraception 2000; 61:379–84.

Goldhaber MK, Armstrong MA, Golditch IM, et al. Long term risk of hysterectomy among 80,007 sterilized and comparison women at Kaiser Permanente, 1971–1987. Am J Epidemiol 1993;138:508–21.

Hillis SD, Marchbanks PA, Tylor LR, et al. Post-sterilization regret: findings from the United States Collaborative Review of Sterilization. Obstet Gynecol 1999;93:889–95.

Kerin JF, Carignan CS, Cher D. The safety and effectiveness of a new hysteroscopic method for permanent birth control: results of the first Essure pbc clinical study. Aust N Z J Obstet Gynaecol 2001;41:364–70.

Kerin JF, Cattanach S. Successful pregnancy outcome with the use of in vitro fertilization after Essure hysteroscopic sterilization. Fertil Steril 2007;87:1212.

Kraemer DF, Yen PY, Nichols M. An economic comparison of female sterilization of hysteroscopic tubal occlusion with laparoscopic bilat-eral tubal ligation. Contraception 2009;80: 254–60.

Levy B, Levie MD, Childers ME. A summary of reported pregnancies after hysteroscopic sterilization. J Minim Invas Gynecol 2007;14: 271–4.

March CM, Israel R. A critical appraisal of hysteroscopic tubal fulguration for sterilization. Contraception 1975;11:261–9.

Miracle-McMahill HE, Calle EE, Kosinski AS, et al. Tubal ligation and fatal ovarian cancer in a large prospective cohort study. Am J Epidemiol 1997;145:349–57.

Palmer SN, Greenberg JA. Transcervical sterilization: A comparison of Essure(r) permanent birth control system and Adiana(r) permanent contraception system. Rev Obstet Gynecol 2009;2(2):84–92.

Peterson HB, Xia Z, Hughes JM, et al. The risk of ectopic pregnancy after tubal sterilization. New Engl J Med 1997;336:762–7.

Peterson HB, Xia Z, Hughes JM, et al. for the U.S. Collaborative Review of Sterilization Working Group: The risk of pregnancy after tubal sterilization from the U.S. Collaborative Review of Sterilization. Am J Obstet Gynecol 1996;174: 1161–70.

Savage UK, Masters SJ, Smid MC, et al: Hysteroscopic sterilization in a large group practice. Experience and effectiveness. Obstet Gynecol 2009; 114:1227–1231.

Shavell VI, Abdallah ME, Shade GH Jr, et al. Trends in sterilization since the introduction of Essure hysteroscopic sterilization. J Minim Invasive Gynecol 2009;16:22–7.

Townsend DE, McCausland V, McCausland A, et al. Post-ablation-tubal sterilization syndrome. Obstet Gynecol 1993;82:422–4.

Vancaillie TG, Anderson TL, Johns DA. A 12-month prospective evaluation of transcervical sterilization using implantable polymer matrices. Obstet Gynecol 2008;112(6):1270–7.

Section 3

Guidelines for Use in Selected Populations

15

Postpartum Contraception

Stephanie B. Teal

Department of Obstetrics and Gynecology, University of Colorado Denver School of Medicine, Aurora, CO, USA

Introduction

The postpartum period is one of intense emotional, physical, and social change for a woman and her family. A patient may have been satisfied with her prepregnancy contraceptive method and a stable user of it over many years. Postpartum, however, she is facing changes in physiology, body image, fertility risk, sexual behavior, desire for future fertility, and tolerance for an unintended pregnancy. Any of these factors may change the appropriateness of her prior contraceptive choice. Further, these factors vary over the first 6–12 postpartum months, especially for women who choose to breast-feed.

The postpartum visit

For the postpartum woman, resumption of contraceptive use after an extended break may not be a top priority. While many healthcare providers see patients in the office for a 6-week postpartum check-up, this interval is arbitrary and does not take into account many health needs which arise prior to 6 weeks.

Health concerns that should be addressed prior to this interval include successful initiation of breast-feeding and any impending disorders related to it; mental health and emotional wellbeing; and contraception. Although many prenatal care providers address postpartum contraceptive plans during the third trimester, it is rare for these plans to be put into action before the standard 6-week check-up.

Even at that visit, many women delay contraceptive initiation if sexual intercourse has not resumed. When the woman does resume intercourse some weeks or months later, it is not uncommon for the main concerns to be avoidance of pain or disruption of repaired tissue, as well as re-establishment of her relationship with her partner, with prevention of pregnancy receiving only secondary and reduced attention.

In studies across multiple societies, approximately half of postpartum women resumed sexual intercourse within 6 weeks of delivery, regardless of mode of delivery or lactation.

SCIENCE REVISITED

Non-breast-feeding women begin to ovulate around 4 weeks postpartum, and most ovulate before the first menses occurs. Thus, a significant number of women are at risk for rapid repeat pregnancy in the immediate postpartum period.

Lactation and contraception

Because of its well-documented health benefits to both mother and child, breast-feeding should be encouraged for virtually all postpartum women. Over two thirds of new mothers initiate breastfeeding, but by 12 weeks postpartum only half continue to breastfeed at all, and only about 40% are breastfeeding exclusively. By 6 months, these numbers drop to 35% and 13% respectively. Lactation should not be seen as oppositional to effective contraception. However, contraceptive needs and risks will change with changes in the continuation, frequency, and intensity of nursing. Careful consideration of the changing

Contraception, First Edition. Edited by Donna Shoupe.

contraceptive needs of the patient from delivery through the initial 6–12 months postpartum will allow the woman to achieve both her breastfeeding and family planning goals.

Contraceptive efficacy of lactation: using LAM

⚙ SCIENCE REVISITED

Endocrinology of lactation

Lactation can effectively suppress ovulation, and has been one of the most important mechanisms for birth spacing throughout human history.

- At 7–8 weeks gestation, estrogen levels begin to increase, initially by conversion of maternal androgens in the placental compartment, and by 20 weeks, almost exclusively by conversion of fetal adrenal androgens.
- The increased level of estrogen suppresses hypothalamic dopamine (prolactin inhibiting factor) and directly stimulates prolactin gene transcription in the pituitary.
- Although prolactin levels are very high through most of pregnancy, lactation is inhibited by placental progesterone, which interferes with activation of the prolactin receptor in breast alveolar cells, antagonizing the positive action of prolactin on its own receptor and reducing prolactin binding.
- The rapid disappearance of estrogen and progesterone from the maternal circulation after delivery triggers milk production within the alveolar cell and its secretion into the alveolar lumen. Milk secretion begins 3–4 days postpartum when estrogen and progesterone have been sufficiently cleared. Prolactin levels drop more slowly, and can be maintained by suckling.
- If breastfeeding does not occur, prolactin declines to the nonpregnant levels by approximately 7 days postpartum. If the woman does breastfeed, the baseline prolactin level remains at 2–4 times nonpregnant levels, but increases 10–20-fold each time she nurses.

The effectiveness of lactation as a contraceptive method depends on several important criteria being met. If the woman is less than 6 months postpartum, has not resumed menses, is exclusively nursing without supplementation, and is nursing at least every 4 hours, she is considered to be using the lactational amenorrhea method (LAM, see Figure 15.1). While the effectiveness rate of LAM is considered to be over 97%, it depends on both the intensity and frequency of infant suckling. Breast pumping is not equivalent to suckling for maintenance of LAM, because it does not stimulate the maternal neuroendocrine response to the same extent.

If a patient plans to use LAM as her birth control method in the initial postpartum period, it is very important to review these criteria with her. If all is going well otherwise, she may not call her doctor, or her baby's doctor, to report that she has started supplemental feeds, or decided to stop nursing. Any patient who uses LAM should have a clear plan in place and supplies available for when this method is no longer reliable for her.

Considerations for use of hormonal contraception in lactation

★ TIPS & TRICKS

Once menses returns, lactation intensity diminishes, or 6 months has passed, the breastfeeding mother cannot rely on LAM for high-level contraceptive efficacy.

If she chooses to use a hormonal contraceptive while continuing to nurse, considerations include contraceptive effectiveness, effect on the quality or quantity of milk available to the infant, and transfer of exogenous hormone to the infant. During pregnancy, both estrogen and progesterone block the effect of prolactin on breast tissue.

Full milk production does not begin until a few days after delivery, when the high estrogen and progesterone levels of pregnancy have dropped. Thus, concern has long existed that giving estrogen- and progestin-containing contraceptives during lactation would diminish milk production. The American Congress of Obstetricians and Gynecologists (ACOG), the International

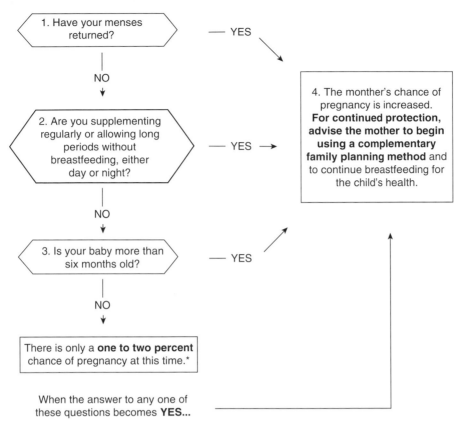

Figure 15.1 Criteria for effectiveness of lactational amenorrhea as a contraceptive method. Source: Labbok M, Cooney K, Coly S. Guidelines: Breastfeeding, family planning, and the lactational amenorrhea method—LAM. Washington, DC: Institute for Reproductive Health/ Georgetown University, 1994.

Planned Parenthood Federation (IPPF), and the World Health Organization (WHO) all advise against the use of combined hormonal contraceptives (CHCs) in lactating women, mostly based on this theoretical concern of decreased milk production.

The actual effect of hormonal contraceptives on lactation has been difficult to study. A systematic review of all randomized controlled trials on this topic found only five trials that compared a hormonal contraceptive to another hormonal contraceptive, a nonhormonal contraceptive, or placebo in lactating women. The authors concluded that even these studies were of limited quality and did not have the ability to demonstrate an effect of hormonal contraceptives on milk quality and quantity. The high loss to follow-up rates, selection and confounding biases, and probably inadequate methods for measuring milk production led the authors of this review to conclude that no recommendation could be supported or refuted by the studies that exist to date.

⚙ SCIENCE REVISITED

Given the lack of good scientific evidence, many practitioners suggest waiting until the milk supply and feeding pattern is well established before starting a contraceptive, and using a nonhormonal or progestin-only contraceptive until weaning. Even women with well-established lactation patterns may experience a decrease in milk production with CHCs.

Non-randomized studies with progestin-only contraceptives started immediately postpartum have been reassuring regarding effect on maternal health parameters, milk production, and infant growth.

- Depot medroxyprogesterone acetate (DMPA, Depo-Provera) has been studied extensively in the postpartum period and has been found to have minimal or even positive effect on milk quality and infant growth. A small study in Thailand found no evidence of DMPA metabolites in infant urine, or changes in infant hormonal parameters.
- The etonogestrel subdermal implant (Implanon) has also been studied in the immediate postpartum period and found to have minimal effect on breastfeeding parameters and infant growth.
- While WHO recommends waiting 6 weeks to initiate progestin-only contraception, studies on progestin-only pills, injectables, and implants initiated as soon as 2 days postpartum have found reassuring results on breastfeeding continuation, milk quality and infant growth.

The risk of deep venous thromboembolism (DVT) is increased in the postpartum period, even above the risk during gestation. Exogenous progestins are not associated with increased risk of venous thromboembolism (VTE).

★ TIPS & TRICKS

Taking into account the increased risk of VTE in the early postpartum period, and the need for early contraception in the non-breast-feeding woman, many providers recommend using progestin-only contraception until 6–7 weeks postpartum, after which combined hormonal methods may be resumed.

✋ CAUTION

Estrogens and venous thromboembolism
The risk of deep venous thromboembolism (DVT) is increased approximately fourfold throughout pregnancy compared to the nonpregnant state, due to increased concentrations of several hepatic clotting factors. In the postpartum period, the risk is even greater, rising by another factor of 5–20-fold above baseline risk, and the risk of pulmonary embolism is about 15 times higher in the postpartum period than during gestation. This risk is especially dramatic, given that the postpartum time period is much shorter: 12 weeks compared to 40 weeks of gestation. Half of postpartum DVTs occur in the first 2 weeks postpartum. DVTs are uncommon after 6 weeks. The already high risk of venous thrombosis in the postpartum woman makes estrogen-containing contraceptives less attractive, even in non-breast-feeding women. Non-breast-feeding women should resume contraception by the third postpartum week, but estrogen-containing methods are probably best begun after the sixth postpartum week. Progestin-only pills may be used as a bridge method for the woman who desires initiation of combined hormonal contraceptives.

Intrauterine contraception

The use of the copper-bearing intrauterine device (Cu-IUD) or the levonorgestrel-releasing intrauterine system (LNG-IUS) provides effective contraception that is virtually maintenance free. In lactating women, Cu-IUDs do not increase breast milk copper concentration. The systemic dose of levonorgestrel from the LNG-IUS is lower than that of progestin-only contraceptive pills. A randomized trial of over 300 women that compared breastfeeding performance, infant growth, and infant development over 1 year in women assigned to the Cu-IUD versus the LNG-IUS found no differences in any of these parameters.

Other potential concerns regarding postpartum intrauterine contraception include possible higher risks of expulsion or uterine perforation for placements in the earlier postpartum period (less than 8 weeks) compared to IUD placement later. Most data supports a low rate of expulsion, similar to interval IUD placement, when the IUD is placed 6–12 weeks postpartum and uterine involution is confirmed.

A possible increased risk of perforation remains controversial. A case-control study conducted over 25 years ago found that perforated IUDs were 10 times as likely to have been placed postpartum. However, another study from the same time compared 411 IUD placements between 4 and 8 weeks postpartum to 1,197 placements after 8 weeks, and found no difference in perforation, pregnancy, expulsion, or removals for pain or bleeding. A more recent 6-year prospective study examined 8,343 women by ultrasound 1 year after IUD placement. Only 18 perforations were found (0.22%). However, IUD placement either 0–3 months or 3–6 months postpartum increased the relative risk of perforation compared to placement at least 6 months postpartum.

Best practices dictate that IUD placement in the postpartum woman follows a careful pelvic examination to ascertain whether uterine involution is complete. If involution is not complete, indicated by an enlarged, soft uterus beyond what one would expect at an interval examination, IUD placement should be delayed until involution has been achieved. If available, placement under ultrasound guidance can be considered. Finally, care should be given to the depth of sounding. If the uterus sounds beyond 10 cm, IUD placement should not occur at that time.

Postplacental IUD placement

Immediate postplacental IUD placement has been gaining in popularity in the United States in recent years. Several advantages include early contraceptive protection, no interference with breastfeeding, and an opportunity to achieve contraception for women with little access to follow-up medical care.

☆ TIPS & TRICKS

Postplacental IUD placement after vaginal delivery
The Cu-IUD may be placed either manually or with ring forceps, the LNG-IUS either manually or with its usual inserter.

Manual IUD placement
- After uterine massage, but before perineal repair, change into new sterile gloves.
- Pitocin may be administered per routine.
- Prophylactic antibiotics are not routinely administered.
- Special or additional anesthesia is not needed.
- Remove IUD from the inserter.
- Place IUD between the index and middle fingers.
- Place the opposite hand on the abdomen to externally stabilize the uterus.
- Within 10 minutes of delivery of the placenta, insert the IUD to the top of the uterine fundus.
- To ensure fundal placement, the operator should feel the impact of the device against the fundus both internally and through the abdominal wall. Placing the device too low in the uterus may lead to expulsion.
- As the internal hand is removed, rotate it about 15° to avoid dislodging the IUD.
- Cu-T380 IUD strings are 12 cm long and should not be visualized after insertion; if the strings are visible, the IUD may be too low and reinsertion should be considered. The strings usually descend spontaneously through the cervix and can be trimmed at a follow-up visit. If fundal placement is confirmed and strings are seen, trim to the level of the cervix. LNG-IUS strings should also be trimmed to the level of the cervix.

Manual insertion requires no instruments; however, it may be more painful than insertion with ring forceps or the IUD applicator in the absence of anesthesia.

Insertion with ring forceps or LNG-IUS applicator
- Prepare the LNG-IUS applicator as usual or grasp the IUD with the ring forceps at a slight angle so that the ball of the stem and the strings are parallel to the forceps.

- If using ring forceps, the top of the IUD should be even with the tip end of the forceps.
- Using a hand or retractor, expose and visualize the anterior cervix.
- Grasp the cervix with another ring forceps.
- While retracting gently on the cervix and under direct visualization, introduce the IUD through the cervix into the lower uterus.
- Release the hand that was retracting the cervix and place it on the abdomen.
- Stabilize the uterus with this hand.
- Advance the IUD to the uterine fundus.
- Confirm fundal placement with both the abdominal hand and the inserting hand.
- Release the IUD from the ring forceps or Mirena IUD applicator.
- Rotate the ring forceps about 45° and move it laterally to avoid dislodging the IUD. If a Mirena IUD applicator is used, it can be removed in the typical fashion.

Ultrasound guidance may be used at the provider's discretion to assure fundal placement.

Immediate IUD placement has not been associated with increased infection, uterine perforation, abnormal postpartum bleeding, or uterine subinvolution. Some providers stress the importance of placement within 10 minutes of placental delivery, while others advocate placement within the first 48 hours postpartum.

Six studies have directly compared the safety and effectiveness of immediate postpartum insertion (within 10 minutes of placental delivery) to delayed postpartum placement. Comparisons of these methods have generally found similar rates of complications (most frequently expulsion), although some studies have found lower expulsion rates in women receiving their IUDs within 10 minutes after placental delivery. Four other studies have examined immediate or delayed postpartum placement compared to placement at 6 weeks or greater postpartum. All these studies found higher rates of expulsion in postpartum placements (typically ranging from 9% to 16%) compared to interval placements, with typical expulsion rates of around 3%.

Nonhormonal methods

Natural family planning (NFP), sometimes called periodic abstinence or the rhythm method, can be difficult to practice during the postpartum period. For most women, the first postpartum menses is preceded by ovulation, and thus women are at risk for unintended conception before being able to use a calendar day-based method.

Postpartum lochia and irregular ovulation can make cervical mucus evaluation less reliable. If a woman is using LAM, and menses has not returned at 6 months, she should be advised that she can no longer rely on LAM for high-level efficacy, but she probably cannot rely on NFP prior to return of menses. Such women who do not want to start a hormonal method should be encouraged to use other nonhormonal methods, such as condoms, a diaphragm, and/or spermicide to provide a higher level of contraceptive protection.

A woman who has used a diaphragm previously should be refitted after delivery. Even if the patient did not undergo labor or a vaginal delivery, changes in the pelvis and changes in body weight distribution can affect correct diaphragm sizing.

Sterilization

For the woman desiring no future childbearing, *immediate postpartum sterilization* has some advantages:

- The uterus is still an abdominal organ, and the fallopian tubes can be easily accessed through a small infraumbilical incision. The procedure should be performed within the first 48 hours postpartum, as later procedures are technically more difficult and carry a higher risk of infection.
- Postpartum tubal ligation is simpler than interval laparoscopic sterilization. The patient

is already in the hospital, and does not have to find additional childcare or take additional time off work. She may have qualified for publicly funded insurance based on her pregnancy status, and may lose her opportunity to have a desired sterilization with the impending loss of that insurance coverage. Further, postpartum sterilization is more cost-effective than interval sterilization, and seems to have the lowest risk of failure.

Conversely, immediate postpartum sterilization is a demonstrated risk factor for regret regarding the loss of fertility, so the motivation for this option should be carefully explored with the patient during the antepartum period. Care should be taken to keep the separation of mother and infant as short as possible, to minimize disruption of bonding and breast-feeding. The patient should be encouraged to nurse just prior to the procedure, and regional or local anesthesia is preferred to minimize delay in breastfeeding postoperatively.

Hysteroscopic sterilization is not possible immediately postpartum. Because hysteroscopic sterilization relies on adequate visualization of the tubal ostia, this procedure can occur in the fully breast-feeding woman after complete uterine involution and cessation of bleeding, with the assumption that estrogen production and endometrial proliferation will be adequately suppressed to allow adequate visualization.

In partially or non-breast-feeding women, additional hormonal manipulation may be necessary to ensure a successful procedure. This may consist of one cycle of a combined hormonal contraceptive with the procedure occurring around the fifth day of the withdrawal bleed, or use of DMPA. Waiting for a spontaneous menses puts the patient at risk of

Table 15.1 Time frames for resumption of contraceptive methods in postpartum nonlactating women

Method	Time frame	Comments
Combined oral contraceptive	>21 days	Immediately after a first- or second- trimester abortion or ectopic pregnancy
Progestin-only contraceptives	<21 days	Immediately after a first- or second- trimester abortion or ectopic pregnancy
Intrauterine devices	<48 hours >4 weeks (category 2—benefits outweigh risks)	Immediately post first trimester Immediately post second trimester (category 2—benefits outweigh risks) Puerperal sepsis—do not place
Barrier methods	Any time, no restrictions	
Fertility awareness methods	<4 weeks >4 weeks Postabortion	D A C
Female surgical sterilization	<7 days 7–42 days >42 days Severe pre-eclampsia; sepsis; prolonged rupture of membranes; severe trauma Postabortion Postabortion: severe trauma, hemorrhage, sepsis, hematometra Postabortion: perforation	A D A D A D S

Key:
A, accept; D, delay; C, caution; S, special circumstances.

pregnancy and makes scheduling of the procedure difficult.

Postpartum contraception in nonlactating women

> ☆ **TIPS & TRICKS**
>
> Women who do not breastfeed their infants may resume combined hormonal contraception. Since ovulation can resume as soon as 26 days after delivery, contraception should resume in the third postpartum week.

Postpartum nonlactating women may resume the following contraceptive methods in the time frames shown in Table 15.1 providing they do not have any of the medical contraindications for a particular method as described in Chapters 3–14.

Summary

Thoughtful decision-making regarding postpartum contraception will help women achieve their desires regarding successful lactation, the health of the infant, their own well-being, and desired birth spacing and family size.

> ☆ **TIPS & TRICKS**
>
> Postpartum changes in physiology, fertility risk, and desire for future fertility may make the patient's prior contraceptive method less appropriate during this time, and for the future. Counseling should begin during pregnancy, so an appropriate plan is in place before fertility returns.

Selected references

Brito MB, Ferriani RA, Quintana SM, et al. Safety of the etonogestrel-releasing implant during the immediate postpartum period: a pilot study. Contraception 2009;80:519–26.

Caliskan E, Ozturk N, Dilbaz BO, Dilbaz S. Analysis of risk factors associated with uterine perforation by intrauterine devices. Eur J Contracept Reprod Health Care 2003;8:150–5.

Grimes D, Schulz K, Van Vliet H, Stanwood N. Immediate post-partum insertion of intrauterine devices. Cochrane Database Syst Rev 2003:CD003036.

Heartwell SF, Schlesselman S. Risk of uterine perforation among users of intrauterine devices. Obstet Gynecol 1983;61:31–36.

Heit JA, Kobbervig CE, James AH, et al. Trends in the incidence of venous thromboembolism during pregnancy or postpartum: a 30-year population-based study. Ann Intern Med 2005;143.697–706.

Labbok M, Cooney K, Coly S. Guidelines: breastfeeding, family planning, and the lactational amenorrhea method—LAM. Washington, DC: Institute for Reproductive Health; 1994.

Li R, Darling N, Maurice E, Barker L, Grummer-Strawn LM. Breastfeeding rates in the United States by characteristics of the child, mother, or family: the 2002 National Immunization Survey. Pediatrics 2005;115:e31–7.

McCann MF, Moggia AV, Higgins JE, Potts M, Becker C. The effects of a progestin-only oral contraceptive (levonorgestrel 0.03 mg) on breast-feeding. Contraception 1989;40:635–48.

Mishell DR, Jr., Roy S. Copper intrauterine contraceptive device event rates following insertion 4 to 8 weeks post partum. Am J Obstet Gynecol 1982;143:29–35.

Moggia AV, Harris GS, Dunson TR, et al. A comparative study of a progestin-only oral contraceptive versus non-hormonal methods in lactating women in Buenos Aires, Argentina. Contraception 1991;44:31–43.

Rodriguez MI, Kaunitz AM. An evidence-based approach to postpartum use of depot medroxyprogesterone acetate in breastfeeding women. Contraception 2009;80:4–6.

Shaamash AH, Sayed GH, Hussien MM, Shaaban MM. A comparative study of the levonorgestrel-releasing intrauterine system Mirena versus the Copper T380A intrauterine device during lactation: breast-feeding performance, infant growth and infant development. Contraception 2005;72:346–51.

Speroff L, Mishell DR, Jr. The postpartum visit: it's time for a change in order to optimally initiate contraception. Contraception 2008; 78:90–8.

Speroff L, Fritz M. Clinical gynecologic endocrinology and infertility, 7th ed. Philadelphia: Lippincott Williams & Wilkins; 2005.

Taneepanichskul S, Reinprayoon D, Thaithumyanon P, et al. Effects of the etonogestrel-releasing implant Implanon and a nonmedicated intrauterine device on the growth of breast-fed infants. Contraception 2006;73:368–71.

Truitt ST, Fraser AB, Grimes DA, Gallo MF, Schulz KF. Hormonal contraception during lactation. systematic review of randomized controlled trials. Contraception 2003;68:233–8.

16

Adolescents: Compliance, Ethical Issues, and Sexually Transmitted Infections

Melanie E. Ochalski and Joseph S. Sanfilippo

Department of Obstetrics and Gynecology and Reproductive Sciences, Center for Fertility and Reproductive Endocrinology, University of Pittsburgh Physicians, Magee-Womens Hospital, Pittsburgh, PA, USA

Introduction

Providing contraception to adolescents requires an understanding of the unique needs of this population, with particular emphasis on discretion and ease of use. The adolescent reproductive health visit represents a unique opportunity to engage the patient in important reproductive health decisions, and can set the stage for a lifetime of healthy, informed decisions. Many teens do not seek out contraception until months after their sexual debut, so inquiring about sexual activity at the adolescent's initial health care evaluation is essential. The American College of Obstetricians and Gynecologists (ACOG) recommends that this visit occur between 13 and 15 years, with a pelvic examination reserved for specific indications. At this visit, risks of pregnancy and sexually transmitted infections (STIs) should be discussed, and contraceptive counseling should be offered. In addition, sexually active teens require STI screening, as discussed below.

Teenage pregnancy continues to be a national health problem, despite recent declines in adolescent pregnancy rates. Each year in the United States, approximately 1 million adolescents become pregnant. Children born to teenage mothers are more likely to be born preterm, have low birth weight, suffer from child abuse, neglect, poverty, and death, and have behavioral disorders and difficulties in school. There is therefore a need to develop better strategies for preventing unintended pregnancies in this age group. The healthcare provider can make a big impact on this important health problem.

EVIDENCE AT A GLANCE

- ~60% of young women have had sexual intercourse by age 18.
- Within a relatively short time after becoming sexually active, 58% of adolescent females have had sex with two or more partners.
- Half of sexually active teenagers do not use condoms, placing them at increased risk for STIs.

When to initiate

The onset of fertility following menarche varies among individuals; therefore any sexually active teenager is at risk for pregnancy and STIs. Studies have repeatedly documented that adolescents do not seek contraception for many months to a year or more after initiating sexual activity. However, once teenagers begin using contraception, many are consistent users. It is preferable to delay use of a hormonal agent—the oral contraceptive pill (OCP)—until linear growth ceases, usually approximately 2 years after menarche.

Estrogen induces closure of the epiphyseal plate. To avoid stunting growth, it is recommended to not start oral contraceptives containing estrogen until 2 years after menarche.

Table 16.1 Common indications for a pelvic examination at the initial visit

History of vaginal intercourse
Abnormal pubertal development
Abnormal vaginal bleeding
Pelvic pain
Pathologic vaginal discharge

Barriers to access

Most adolescents do not seek contraceptive services until they have been sexually active for at least 6 months. Two significant reasons why teens delay accessing contraception are fear of the pelvic examination and confidentiality concerns. Deferring the physical examination until after contraception is provided is appropriate in many situations. Table 16.1 lists several common indications for performing a pelvic examination at the initial visit. However, the external genitalia should be inspected in all patients, if allowed. Discussing the patient's privacy rights at the start of the visit will encourage open communication and promote trust. Many states allow minors to consent to contraceptive services, without their parent's involvement. Clinicians should know their state laws regarding consent by minors for reproductive health services. The Guttmacher Institute's "State policies in brief: minors' access to contraceptive services" outlines the laws by state and can be accessed freely through the internet (www.guttmacher.org).

EVIDENCE AT A GLANCE

The 2007 Youth Risk Behavior Surveillance System found that:
- 47% of high-school students have had sexual intercourse.
- 7% of high- school students had sex before they were 13 years old.
- 15% of high-school students reported having sex with four or more partners.

In order to effectively communicate about sexual activity, it is essential for the healthcare professional to understand the unique perspective and pressures of the adolescent patient. Adolescents 17 years and younger often think in concrete terms, and are less able to connect present action with future consequence. Simply put, the teenager who admits to some noncoital sexual experimentation may not be able to recognize the likelihood of sexual intercourse in the near future in the same way that an adult may be able to. Indeed, when a group of teenagers was surveyed about the top reason for unprotected intercourse, lack of forethought was the most frequently cited reason. Furthermore, television and movies, often the main source of examples of sexual relationships for teenagers, disconnect sex from pregnancy and STIs.

It is therefore important to describe definitive adverse consequences of sexual activity and encourage the use of contraceptive methods that do not require future planning or intercourse-related use.

★ TIPS & TRICKS

Many misperceptions about sexual activity exist among teenagers (and others). Be sure to address these:
- Pregnancy can occur with each sexual encounter, even during "the first time". A sexually active teen has a 90% chance of becoming pregnant the first year.
- Many noncoital activities can spread STIs. Any contact with mucous membranes should be protected with a barrier contraceptive.
- Many STIs are asymptomatic, but can cause significant health problems in the future. Always use a barrier method of protection.
- Douching is not a protective means of contraception or STI prevention.

Education

Early, exploitative, or risky sexual activity may lead to health and social problems, such as unin-

Table 16.2 Internet contraception resources for adolescents

Association of Reproductive Health Professionals, Adolescent Health	http://www.arhp.org/Topics/Adolescent-Health
Planned Parenthood of America	www.plannedparenthood.org
Our Bodies, Ourselves	http://www.ourbodiesourselves.org
Reproductive Health Access Project	http://reproductiveaccess.org

tended pregnancy and STIs. Adolescents should be encouraged to communicate with their parents about sexual matters, as studies have demonstrated the favorable influence that such open dialogue has on sexual behaviors. However, for many patients, their healthcare provider is their sole access to accurate information about sexuality and contraception. The confidential and longitudinal relationship formed with a teenager can make a lasting impact on her reproductive and psychological health.

Adolescents need formal, comprehensive sex education that covers everything from abstinence to various contraceptive methods. One strategy for opening up the line of communication with your adolescent patient is to inquire about her level of understanding of risks associated with sexual activity. Specific points to cover include the actual risk of pregnancy with unprotected coital activity, the risk of STI acquisition and the need for annual screening, and the variety of contraceptive options available. Even patients in the precontemplative stage will benefit from this information, and studies support the benefits of this comprehensive approach, while not encouraging sexual activity.

To help patients become informed about their choices, providers can direct them to educational internet sites for material that is understandable and accurate (Table 16.2). The healthcare provider can play an important role in implementing strategies that endorse responsible sexual behavior. The adolescent health visit represents a unique opportunity to cover a variety of reproductive health maintenance items; Table 16.3 lists several key elements to be covered at each adolescent visit.

The ACOG recommends that sexually active women aged 25 years or younger should be screened annually for *Chlamydia trachomatis*, and all sexually active adolescents should be

Table 16.3 Strategies for promoting responsible sexual behavior

Review menstrual cycle and risks for getting pregnant
Review contraceptive options; encourage her to commit to a method that day
Review emergency contraception instructions, indications; give a prescription that day
Review the transmission of STIs and the importance of condom use with each sexual encounter. If already sexually active, screen for gonorrhea and chlamydia
Offer the HPV vaccine

★ TIPS & TRICKS

STI screening and counseling

- Patients should be informed that any form of sexual contact—vaginal, anal, or oral—may transmit a sexually transmitted infection (STI).
- With few exceptions, all adolescents in the United States can legally consent to the confidential diagnosis and treatment of STIs. STI screening should be obtained with each new sexual partner (Table 16.4).
- Screening has become much easier with the availability of urine and vaginal swab testing, without the need for pelvic examination.
- Teenagers should be aware that use of a barrier method is effective at preventing STIs, including the human papillomavirus (HPV).

screened for *Neisseria gonorrhoeae*. Urine-based screening without a speculum examination is sufficient. In addition, all adolescents who are sexually active should be screened for HIV. The U.S. Centers for Disease Control (CDC) estimates

Table 16.4 Screening for sexually transmitted infections

Chlamydia trachomatis
Neisseria gonorrhea
Trichomonas vaginalis
HIV
Syphilis
Hepatitis B and C

All women presenting for STI screening should be offered the HPV vaccine and the hepatitis B vaccine, if not already immunized.

that half of all HIV infections in the United States occur among young people under the age of 25, and HIV infection is the sixth leading cause of death among 15–24-year-olds in the United States.

The HPV vaccine should be offered to all teenagers, ideally before initiation of sexual activity. Cervical cancer screening should begin at age 21 years, regardless of sexual history.

EVIDENCE AT A GLANCE

In November 2009, ACOG issued revised guidelines for cervical cancer screening. Based on this, screening before age 21 should be avoided, because women less than 21 years old are at very low risk of cancer, and screening these women may lead to unnecessary and harmful evaluation and treatment.

EVIDENCE AT A GLANCE

Half of all HIV infections in the United States occur among young people under the age of 25, and HIV infection is the sixth leading cause of death among 15–24-year-olds in the United States (www.cdc.gov/std).

Contraceptive counseling

Most teenagers are interested in discussing contraception, especially by age 15. However, most will not initiate the dialogue. Trust is an essential component of the clinician–adolescent interaction. The teenager must be reassured of the con-

fidentiality of the interaction. Research has confirmed that requiring parental notification deters young people from using contraception and protecting against STIs. Therefore, privacy and confidentiality should be stressed. However, all teenagers should be encouraged to develop an open communication with their parents, as this also has been shown to improve contraceptive use.

Contraceptive counseling should be provided to all adolescents, including those who are not currently sexually active and those who have taken abstinence or virginity pledges. A recent comparison of sexual behaviors between virginity pledgers and nonpledgers showed no difference in premarital sex, STIs, lifetime sexual partners, and age of first sexual encounter. That said, a pledge of abstinence by a teenage patient should be praised, and the emotional and reproductive health benefits reviewed.

Effective contraceptive counseling provides an overview of the breadth of choices, while highlighting two or three "best fit" options based on the patient's individualized needs. When surveyed about the characteristics that were most important to their contraceptive choice, adolescent women prioritized safety, convenience, privacy, and efficacy. There are many resources available online to help patients make an informed decision (Table 16.2). Adolescents should be encouraged to seek out this information, and be proactive about their reproductive health.

Over half of the unintended pregnancies in the United States are due to contraceptive failures. Once teenagers access contraception, compliance issues can diminish contraceptive efficacy. Instructions on correct use are as important as writing the prescription. Many teens have never filled a prescription before, so discussing the cost and explaining how to obtain it is helpful.

There are a variety of contraceptive methods available to the adolescent (Table 16.5). Contraceptive failure is nearly twice as likely to occur in teenagers as in women age 30 years or older. When discussing contraceptive failure rates, it is less confusing to report the "usual experience" with a method. Therefore, the failure rates reported in this chapter are the "typical" failure

Table 16.5 Contraceptive options for adolescents

Method	Failure rate (Typical use)	Dosing regimen	Potential side effects	Caution	Advantages
No method	85%	—	—	—	—
Withdrawal	23.6%	—	—	—	—
Male latex condom	15%	With each sexual intercourse	If latex allergy: use polyurethane condom	—	Protects against HIV and other STIs Easy accessibility
Spermicides	25.7%	With each sexual intercourse	Vaginal or penile irritation	Nonoxynol-9 may raise the risk of HIV	Easy accessibility
Female latex condom	21%	With each sexual intercourse	Vaginal or penile irritation	May slip out of place during intercourse	Protects against HIV and other STIs
Combination OCP	8%	Daily	May cause nausea, vomiting, weight gain, headaches, decreased libido May cause spotting for the first month	Contraindicated with known thrombogenic mutations Efficacy may be decreased if used with medications that alter liver enzymes (ie anticonvulsants)	May alleviate dysmenorrhea and menorrhagia May improve acne Lowers risk of ovarian cancer after 4 years of use
Progestin-only OCP	3%	Every 24 hours	Irregular bleeding w/in the first 3 months	Must take within 27 hours of the previous pill	

Method	Efficacy	Directions	Side effects	Contraindications	Advantages
Combination contraceptive patch (Ortho Evra)	8%	Apply a new patch once a week for 3 weeks. No patch in week 4	May irritate skin under patch	Known thrombogenic mutations (contraindicated) BMI >30 kg/m² as efficacy may be diminished	Private; Does not require daily dosing
Combined hormonal vaginal ring (Nuva Ring)	8%	Insert a new ring vaginally for 3 weeks. No ring in week 4	May increase vaginal discharge	Known thrombogenic mutations (contraindicated)	
Progestin-only injection (Depo-Provera)	0.3%	Single intramuscular shot of 150 mg is administered every 3 months	Irregular bleeding may occur in the first 3 months of use. Average weight gain of 5.5 lbs, 8 lbs, and 14 lbs the first, second and third year, respectively	May worsen depression, acne and facial hair	Minimal intervention; At 1 year, 60% of users will be amenorrheic.
Intrauterine device and system (Copper-ParaGard and Levonorgestrel-Mirena)	<1%	Copper-ParaGard may be left in place for up to 10 years; Levonorgestrel-Mirena for 5 years	Cu-IUD may worsen cramps and heavy menses. May cause irregular spotting	Active cervicitis or current PID	Nothing to take/place before sex
Single-rod contraceptive implant (Implanon)	<1%	3-year contraceptive duration	Menstrual irregularities are common		High continuation rate in the adolescent population

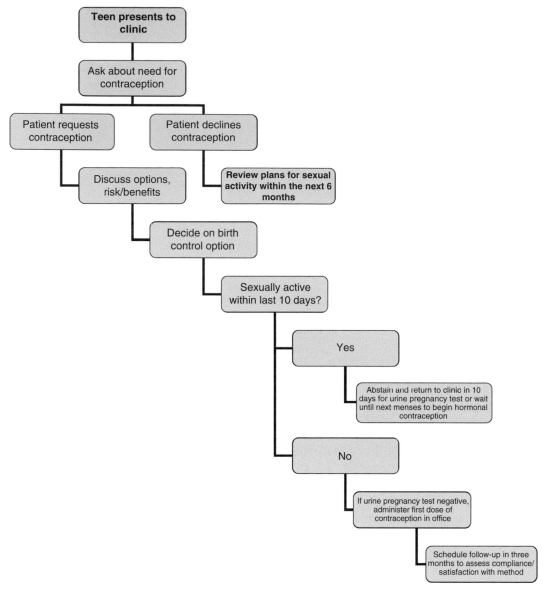

Figure 16.1 Algorithm for supplying contraception to the adolescent.

rates during the first year of use. Figure 16.1 provides a simple algorithm for supplying contraception to the adolescent.

Abstinence

The most reliable way to avoid pregnancy and transmission of STIs is to abstain from sex. Counseling that encourages abstinence from sexual intercourse is a crucial part of any comprehensive contraceptive counseling. This method should be promoted among adolescents who are not yet capable of coping with sex and its consequences. Adolescents who have been sexually active previously should also be counseled regarding the benefits of postponing future sexual relationships, and the consequences of multiple partners with future sexual interactions.

Barrier methods

Barrier methods should be encouraged to prevent STIs, even when the teen is on another form of contraception. The most common form of barrier method used by adolescents is the male condom. Barrier methods have several drawbacks particular to the adolescent, including cost, accessibility, and need for planning ahead. However, because the male condom is the most effective method of preventing STI acquisition, after abstinence, this method should be encouraged. Studies have shown that condom use increases only when discussions occur before the initial sexual encounter. In addition, it is important to review instructions on proper use. Key points include:

- Consistency: A condom should be used with *every* sexual activity.
- Timeliness: A condom should be placed prior to any mucous membrane contact.
- Hygiene:A condom should be changed between anal and vaginal contact in order to prevent the spread of disease.

The female condom is a less popular method of contraception, but with correct use can prevent STIs and pregnancy. The advantage of this method is that it can be used if the male refuses to use a condom, thus making this option worth mentioning. A less expensive version of the female condom made of synthetic latex (nitrile), called FC2, has been approved by the U.S. Food and Drug Authority (FDA).

Spermicides can be used alone or with other forms of barrier methods, and should be included in the adolescent's contraceptive repertoire.

Combination estrogen/progestin contraceptives

Combined oral contraceptive pills

Over 50% of sexually active adolescent women use the OCP to prevent pregnancy, making it the most commonly used method in this age group. OCPs also have a number of noncontraceptive benefits that make them particularly appealing to young women. Acne, premenstrual dysphoric disorder (PMDD), dysmenorrhea, and menorrhagia are among some of the indications for OCPs. A low-dose formulation containing ethinyl estradiol (20 μg) and drospirenone (3 mg) in a 24–4 regimen has proven efficacy against acne and PMDD.

It is important that patients are educated about the importance of compliance, particularly with the low-dose formulations. One-third of patients 17 years old and younger reported missing two or more pills in their most recent cycle. Patients should be instructed to use a back-up method if they miss more than three pills in a row, and emergency contraception offered. In addition, a pregnancy test should be taken if the next menses is missed.

Extended regimens of OCPs, such as the 84–7 package of ethinyl estradiol 30 μg/levonorgestrel 150 μg have not been well studied in the adolescent population, but have clear benefits of four menses/year with only a mild increase in breakthrough bleeding. This option should be offered to adolescents, particularly those who desire less frequent menses, such as athletes or those with dysmenorrhea.

A "quick start" initiation on the day that the prescription is given can help improve compliance. Having the patient take the first pill in the office is ideal. The improvement in compliance with this type of initiation as compared to the traditional Sunday start outweighs the risks.

Transdermal patch/vaginal ring

The transdermal patch and vaginal ring have the advantage of maintaining a constant level of hormones, with a weekly or monthly dosing regimen. Compliance rates have been greater than with OCPs. This may be a good alternative for adolescents who have compliance problems with the pill.

> **✋ CAUTION**
>
> Two absolute contraindications for contraception use:
> - Thromboembolic mutations and the use of estrogen-containing methods.
> - Current pelvic inflammatory disease or mucopurulent vaginal discharge and initial placement of an intrauterine device (IUD).

Progestin-only contraception

Progestin-only contraception includes the progestin-only pill (POP), depot medroxyprogesterone acetate (DMPA), levonorgestrel-releasing intrauterine system (LGS-IUD, Mirena) and the Etonogestrel implant (Implanon). As a class, they have excellent contraceptive efficacy and are ideal for patients for whom exogenous estrogen is contraindicated. There are a number of non-contraceptive health benefits of progestin-only agents, including amelioration of endometriosis pain; treatment of specific menstrual disorders, such as dysfunctional uterine bleeding or menorrhagia; protection against uterine fibroids and cancer; treatment of anemia associated with sickle cell disease; and reduction in seizure frequency in patients with epilepsy.

Adverse events include irregular bleeding, weight gain, acne, mood changes, loss of libido, and breast tenderness. The hypoestrogenic state created by long-term use of DMPA has been associated with decreased bone mineral density (BMD) in adolescents, especially those who use the method for over 2 years. However, BMD has been shown to recover to the level of nonusers once DMPA is discontinued, and the benefits of the regimen are though to outweigh the theoretic fracture risks in the adolescent population (this is the World Health Organization (WHO) position). The following recommendations should be stressed to all adolescent women: appropriate calcium intake (1500 mg/day), tobacco cessation, and active lifestyle. Monitoring of BMD should be considered in adolescents on DMPA for more than 2 years.

⚙ SCIENCE REVISITED

Progestin-only contraceptives (POCs) act in a number of ways to prevent pregnancy, including:
- Thickening the cervical mucus to hinder migration of sperm
- Inhibiting the egg's ability to travel through the fallopian tubes
- Suppressing ovulation
- Partially suppressing the ability of sperm to penetrate and fertilize the egg
- Altering the uterine lining to prevent implantation of a fertilized egg.

Intrauterine devices and systems

Intrauterine devices and other systems are an excellent method for the adolescent, one that is underutilized for pregnancy prevention. STI acquisition and ascending infection can be easily avoided with proper condom use and screening for STIs prior to insertion. Many misperceptions persist about the association of intrauterine contraception with pelvic inflammatory disease (PID) and its reproductive sequelae. However, studies have shown no increase in infertility or STI incidence, and use of this method is advocated by both WHO and the Adolescent Healthcare Committee of ACOG.

☆ TIPS & TRICKS

Placing the IUD/IUS in the nulliparous patient is facilitated by pretreating her with misoprostol 50 μg per vagina, 1 hour before insertion.

The high prevalence of *Chlamydia trachomatis* and gonococcal infection in adolescents warrants screening for these two infections prior to IUD/IUS placement.

Emergency contraception

The use of hormonal medications to prevent an unwanted pregnancy after unprotected coitus has utility in the adolescent population, yet is underutilized in this setting. It is our practice to counsel all adolescents about the availability of emergency contraception (ECP), and provide a prescription with their birth control method. Educating the patient about the mechanism of action is key to improving the likelihood of use, and promoting correct usage. ECP is most effective when used within 24 hours of the event, but has efficacy up to 72 hours.

- The most commonly used method, "Plan B–OneStep" consists of levonorgestrel 1.5 mg, taken as a single dose.
- Patients who vomit within 2 hours of taking their dose should repeat the dose.
- Misconceptions about the dispensing of ECP being related to risk-taking behavior and increase in sexual activity have been unfounded.

- "Plan B" is available over-the-counter for adolescents 17 years or older, and by prescription only for those younger than 17.

Summary

- Adolescents have a wide variety of contraceptive options available, and treatment should be tailored to their specific needs.
- Effective counseling focuses on the importance of compliance and instructions dealing with missed pills or lost vaginal rings or patches.
- An adolescent-friendly environment that fosters open communication is vital.
- Clinicians who care for adolescents are obligated to help these individuals realistically assess their sexual futures, and plan accordingly.
- Empowering the adolescent patient to take charge and responsibility of her reproductive life can have lasting benefits.

Selected references

Lara-Torre, E. Update in adolescent contraception. Obstet Gynecol Clin North Am 2009;36: 119–28.

Rosenbaum JE. Patient teenagers? A comparison of the sexual behavior of virginity pledgers and matched nonpledgers. Pediatrics 2009; 123(1):e110–20.

Sanfilippo J, Lara-Torre E. Adolescent gynecology. Am J Obstet Gynecol 2009;113:935–47.

Speroff L, Darney P. A clinical guide for contraception, 4th ed. Philadelphia, PA: Lippincott, Williams & Wilkins; 2005.

Whitaker A, Gilliam M. Contraceptive care for adolescents. Clin Obstet Gynecol 2008;51: 268–80.

Yen S, Saah T, Hillard PJ. IUDs and adolescents—an under-utilized opportunity for pregnancy prevention. J Pediatr Adolesc Gynecol 2010; 23(3):123–8.

Websites

Centers for Disease Control and Prevention—sexually transmitted disease: http://www.cdc.gov/std/default.htm.

This website contains vital statistics about STIs, as well as treatment guidelines and patient handouts.

Guttmacher Institute: www.guttmacher.org.

A website with important resources about sexual and reproductive health policy, research and education.

World Health Organization: family planning: http://www.who.int/topics/family_planning/en/

Provides information on safety and use of contraceptive methods.

17

Women 35 Years and Older: Safety Issues

Catherine Cansino[1] and Mitchell Creinin[2]

[1]Department of Obstetrics and Gynecology, The Ohio State University, Columbus, OH, USA
[2]Department of Obstetrics, Gynecology and Reproductive Sciences, University of Pittsburgh School of Medicine and Magee-Womens Research Institute, Pittsburgh, PA, USA

Introduction

The contraceptive needs of women 35 years of age and older can be simple, but require careful consideration. Advanced age is an independent risk factor for many conditions that influence contraceptive choices. For all women in their reproductive years, healthcare providers should account for any pre-existing comorbidities that may be more prevalent among older women. Providers should consider these factors when identifying appropriate contraceptive options to women in the latter part of their reproductive years.

Special considerations regarding symptomatology and safety issues in perimenopause are discussed in Chapter 18.

Contraceptive choices

Factors that influence contraceptive choices do not differ among older women: effectiveness, ease of use, safety, reversibility, side effects, and cost. For all women with comorbidities, especially older women who may be at higher risk for these conditions, healthcare providers must balance the woman's need for effective contraception and the risks associated with each method.

Use of spermicide, withdrawal, fertility awareness-based, and barrier methods eliminate the risk of adverse events associated with hormonal contraception. However, decreased compliance and the relatively higher failure rate associated with these methods classify them as less than ideal. Surgical risks associated with female sterilization can also limit contraceptive options for women with comorbidities. Women with significant health problems, among whom pregnancy may pose even greater medical risks compared to hormonal contraception, should be offered effective contraception, including hormonal contraceptives.

Although risks are commonly a focus of individualized contraceptive counseling, healthcare providers should also include information for patients about the medical benefits that *hormonal contraception* offer. These benefits are often of interest to women with advancing age, and their associated risks are often either misinterpreted or overemphasized.

- *Combined hormonal contraceptives* (CHCs) offer many noncontraceptive benefits as well as improved bleeding control and are a good option in healthy women over 35 with no contraindications. (Tables 17.1–17.3; see Chapters 3 and 6).
- *Progestin injectable contraceptive* (DMPA) may decrease heavy or abnormal bleeding that is especially common in perimenopausal women (see Chapter 21).

Table 17.1 US CDC MEC for contraceptive use: classification

Category	With clinical judgment	With limited clinical judgment
1	Use the method in any circumstances	Yes (Use the method)
2	Generally use the method	
3	Use of method not usually recommended unless other more appropriate methods are not available or not acceptable	No (Do not use the method)
4	Method not to be used	

Table 17.2 US CDC MEC for contraceptive use: conditions that require special consideration among older women[a]

Age ≥40 years	Category 2 for CHCs such as COCs, contraceptive patch, contraceptive vaginal ring
Age >45 years	Category 2 for CHCs and DMPA
Age ≥35 years and Smoking <15 cigarettes/day	Category 3 for CHCs
Age ≥35 years and Smoking ≥15 cigarettes/day	Category 4 for CHCs
Migraine headaches without aura, age ≥35 years	Category 2 for initiation or continuation of DMPA, contraceptive implant, LNG-IUS, and POPs. Category 3 for initiation of CHCs. Category 4 for continuation of CHCs

CHC, combined hormonal contraceptive; COC, combined oral contraceptive; DMPA, depot medroxyprogesterone acetate; IUD, intrauterine device; POP, progestin-only pill.
[a]Unless otherwise specified, contraceptive options are considered category 1.

- *Progestin implant or the progestin-only pill* (POP) are safe for the majority of women over 35.
- In addition to hormonal methods, the long-term effectiveness and relatively few contraindications of the copper or levonorgestrel-releasing *intrauterine devices* (Cu-IUD or LNG-IUS) make them an excellent choice for older women (see Chapter 9).

- *Tubal sterilization* is appropriate for those women who have completed their families.
- *Barrier methods* are a safe contraceptive option for motivated couples.

Benefits of hormonal contraceptives in older women

Combined hormonal contraceptives, specifically combined oral contraceptives (COCs) offer several health benefits that are particularly applicable to older women. For women in the later reproductive years, use of low-dose COCs (formulations with <50 µg of ethinyl estradiol (EE)) and other CHCs can provide increased bone mineral density and benefit in relation to cycle control and reduction of vasomotor symptoms:

- Decreased menstrual blood loss, especially among women with heavy bleeding (menorrhagia)
- Decreased breakthrough bleeding (metrorrhagia).

Current and previous COC users also benefit from a reduction in risk of epithelial ovarian cancer and endometrial cancer. Risk reduction is noted even among women who use newer COC formulations with less than 50 µg of estrogen. Since the postulated physiologic mechanism is related to decreased ovulation and endometrial proliferation, other combined hormonal contraceptives may also reduce the risk of these gynecologic cancers. Since the risk reduction of ovarian cancer among carriers of the *BRCA1* and *BRCA2* mutations is inconclusive, CHC use for cancer prevention in these women is not recommended regardless of age.

Table 17.3 US CDC MEC for contraceptive use: selected medical conditions that are more prevalent among older women[a]

Cardiovascular disease	
Multiple risk factors for arterial cardiovascular disease (such as older age, smoking, diabetes, and hypertension)	Category 2 for POPs, contraceptive implant and LNG-IUS Category 3 for DMPA Category 3/4 for CHCs
Hypertension	
(a) Adequately controlled hypertension, where blood pressure CAN be evaluated	Category 2 for DMPA Category 3 for CHCs
(b) Elevated blood pressure levels (properly taken measurements), systolic 140–159 or diastolic 90–99	Category 2 for DMPA Category 3 for CHCs
(c) Elevated blood pressure levels (properly taken measurements), systolic > 160 or diastolic > 100	Category 2 for POPs, contraceptive implant and LNG-IUS Category 3 for DMPA Category 4 for CHCs
(d) Vascular disease	Category 2 for POPs, contraceptive implant and LNG-IUS Category 3 for DMPA Category 4 for CHCs
History of high blood pressure during pregnancy (where current blood pressure is measurable and normal)	Category 2 for CHCs
DVT/PE	
(a) History of DVT/PE, not on anticoagulant therapy with higher risk of recurrent DVT/PE [≥1 risk factors such as (1) history of estrogen-associated DVT/PE, (2) pregnancy-associated DVT/PE, (3) idiopathic DVT/PE, (4) known thrombophilia, including antiphospholipid syndrome, (5) active cancer, metastatic, on therapy or within 6 months after clinical remission, excluding non-melanoma skin cancer, (6) history of recurrent DVT/PE]	Category 2 for POCs Category 4 for CHCs
(b) History of DVT/PE, not on anticoagulant therapy with lower risk for recurrent DVT/PE (no risk factors)	Category 2 for POCs Category 3 for CHCs
(c) Acute DVT/PE	Category 2 for POCs and Cu-IUD Category 4 for CHCs
(d) DVT/PE and established on anticoagulant therapy for at least 3 months with higher risk for recurrent DVT/PE [≥1 risk factors such as known thrombophilia, including antiphospholipid syndrome, (2) active cancer, metastatic, on therapy or within 6 months after clinical remission, excluding non-melanoma skin cancer, (3) history of recurrent DVT/PE]	Category 2 for POCs and Cu-IUD Category 4 for CHCs

Table 17.3 *Continued*

(e) DVT/PE and established on anticoagulant therapy for at least 3 months with lower risk for recurrent DVT/PE (no risk factors)	Category 2 for POCs and Cu-IUD Category 3 for CHCs
Current and history of ischemic heart disease	Category 2 for initiation of POPs, contraceptive implant and LNG-IUS Category 2 for initiation of POPs, contraceptive implant and LNG-IUS Category 3 for DMPA and continuation of other POCs Category 4 for CHCs
History of stroke	Category 2 for LNG-IUS and initiation of POPs and contraceptive implant Category 3 for DMPA and continuation of POPs and contraceptive implant Category 4 for CHCs
Known hyperlipidemia	Category 2 for POCs Category 2/3 for CHCs
Uncomplicated valvular heart disease	Category 2 for CHCs
Complicated valvular heart disease (pulmonary hypertension, risk for atrial fibrillation, history of subacute bacterial endocarditis)	Category 4 for CHCs

Reproductive system disorders

Irregular bleeding pattern without heavy bleeding	Category 2 for POPs, DMPA, and contraceptive implant
Heavy or prolonged bleeding (includes regular and irregular patterns)	Category 2 for POPs, DMPA, contraceptive implant, Cu-IUD, and continuation of LNG-IUS
Unexplained vaginal bleeding (suspicious for serious condition, before evaluation)	Category 2 for CIICs, POP, and continuation of both levonorgestrel and Cu-IUDs Category 3 for DMPA and contraceptive implant Category 4 for initiation of both levonorgestrel and Cu-IUDs
Cervical cancer (awaiting treatment)	Category 2 for CHCs, DMPA, contraceptive implant and continuation of both levonorgestrel and Cu-IUDs Category 4 for initiation of both levonorgestrel and Cu-IUDs
Breast disease—undiagnosed mass	Category 2 for all hormonal contraception
Current breast cancer	Category 4 for all hormonal contraception
Personal history of breast cancer and no evidence of current disease for 5 years	Category 3 for all hormonal contraception
Endometrial cancer	Category 2 for continuation of both levonorgestrel and Cu-IUDs Category 4 for initiation of both levonorgestrel and Cu-IUDs
Ovarian cancer	Category 12 for all contraception

Table 17.3 *Continued*

Endocrine conditions	
Diabetes	
(a) Both insulin dependent and non-insulin dependent	Category 2 for all hormonal contraception
(b) Nephropathy/retinopathy/neuropathy or other vascular disease, or diabetes of > 20 years' duration	Category 2 for POPs, contraceptive implant, and LNG-IUS Category 3 for DMPA Category 3/4 for CHCs
Gastrointestinal conditions	
Gallbladder disease	
(a) asymptomatic or treated by cholecystectomy	Category 2 for all hormonal contraception
(b) Current disease	Category 2 for POCs Category 3 for CHCs

CHC, combined hormonal contraceptive; COC, combined oral contraceptive; Cu-IUD, copper-containing intrauterine device; DMPA, depot medroxyprogesterone acetate; DVT/PE, deep venous thrombosis/pulmonary embolism; IUD, intrauterine device; LNG-IUS, levonogestrol intrauterine system; POP, progestin-only pill.

Endometrial suppression from the LNG-IUS improves altered bleeding patterns during the perimenopause. Use of the LNG-IUS, associated with relatively high progestin levels within the endometrial cavity, has been investigated in the treatment of endometrial hyperplasia or early endometrial cancer among select women. At this time, there are no conclusive data supporting routine use. The potential for progression of disease remains a cause for concern and researchers emphasize the need for continued endometrial surveillance.

Progestin-only methods (progestin-injectable, POPs, implant) protect the endometrium from unopposed estrogen and hyperplasia. The progestin injectable often reduces blood loss after 6–12 months of use.

Risks

Hormonal contraception and arterial cardiovascular disease

The relationship between hormonal contraception and arterial disease is complex. Estrogen and certain progestins can have a negative impact on specific serum lipid levels. Such surrogate markers, however, do not necessarily translate to clinically significant effects.

Currently available low-dose COC formulations can cause a slight increased risk of hypertension. However, COCs, when used in appropriate candidates, are not associated with an increased risk of myocardial infarction or stroke, even after adjusting for age. Among women with a history of hypertension, oral and injectable progestin-only contraceptives may predispose women to a higher risk of cardiovascular events.

EVIDENCE AT A GLANCE

- Smoking is an independent risk factor for myocardial infarction. Smoking increases the risk of myocardial infarction associated with CHCs among women 35 years and older.
- Beginning at age 35, the age-related mortality risk from cardiovascular events among smokers is greater among women who use combined hormonal contraception compared to pregnant women.
- Generally, older women who smoke should be counseled against CHCs.
- CHCs offer safe, reliable contraception to healthy, nonsmoking women older than 35 years.

Hormonal contraception and venous thromboembolism

While the absolute risk of venous thromboembolic disease (VTE) among reproductive-age women remains low, the relative risk of VTE increases with age. COCs appear to augment the effect of age on the risk of VTE. The higher exposure to exogenous estrogen associated with the contraceptive patch compared to other CHCs has also raised concern regarding the potentially greater risk of VTE among patch users. However, there is no conclusive evidence of a difference in VTE risk among such women. The age-related VTE risk among patch users may be similar to the risk among users of other combined hormonal methods.

> ### ✋ CAUTION
>
> When counseling women about VTE risk and hormonal contraception, you should note that pregnancy is associated with greater risk of VTE than CHC use. In addition, the higher risk of VTE appears to decrease after CHC discontinuation.

Similarly, women who use progestin-only contraceptives (POCs) do not appear to be at greater risk of developing VTE.

Hormonal contraception and gynecologic cancer

Among women 35–64 years of age, current or past COC users do not have an increased risk of breast cancer. Current and previous COC users have a reduced risk of epithelial ovarian cancer and endometrial cancer. Use of the LNG-IUS has been investigated in the treatment of endometrial hyperplasia or early endometrial cancer among some women.

Progestins and bone mineral density

There is limited data on the relationship between POCs and bone mineral density (BMD) among older women. Use of the progestin injectable (depot medroxyprogesterone acetate, DMPA)) for more than 2 years may be associated with decreased BMD among postmenopausal women. However, long-term DMPA users are noted to have a slower rate of decline in BMD during early menopause compared to nonusers. The attributable risk of nontraumatic fracture among older women who use POCs is unknown.

Advanced age as an independent risk factor, and pre-existing comorbidities

The US Centers for Disease Control and Prevention Medical Eligibility Criteria for Contraceptive Use (US CDC MEC) provides guidelines with regard to medical conditions that affect contraceptive choices. The document was adapted from the World Health Organization Medical Eligibility Criteria for Contraceptive Use, 4th edition. It uses a classification scheme that serves as a practical tool for assessing patient eligibility for contraceptives by summarizing relative and absolute contraindications (see Table 17.1).

There are certain conditions that require special consideration with regard to women with advancing age. Table 17.2 focuses on contraceptive eligibility that takes into account age as an independent risk factor for specific medical conditions. These recommendations are based on evidence for the combined effect of age and smoking on a woman's risk for cardiovascular events, as well as the combined effect of age and history of migraines with or without aura on the risk for stroke.

> ### ✶ TIPS & TRICKS
>
> Careful history-taking and appropriate health screening can help identify women who may be predisposed to medical conditions that are more prevalent among women at 35 years and older compared to younger women. Contraceptive eligibility for women with pre-existing comorbidities that are more prevalent among older women is presented in Table 17.3. These conditions are discussed in greater detail in Chapter 19.

Selected references

ACOG Practice Bulletin No. 73. Use of hormonal contraception in women with coexisting medical conditions. Obstet Gynecol 2006;107: 1453–72.

ACOG Practice Bulletin No. 110. Noncontraceptive uses of hormonal contraceptives. Obstet Gynecol 2010;115:206–18.

Centers for Disease Control and Prevention. U.S. Medical Eligibility Criteria for Contraceptive Use, 2010. MMWR 2010:59(No. RR-4).

Chasan-Taber L, Willett WC, Manson JE, et al. Prospective study of oral contraceptives and hypertension among women in the United States. Circulation 1996;94(3):483–9.

Cundy T, Cornish J, Roberts H, Reid IR. Menopausal bone loss in long-term users of depot medroxyprogesterone acetate contraception. Am J Obstet Gynecol 2002;186:978–83.

Marchbanks PA, McDonald JA, Wilson HG, et al. Oral contraceptives and the risk of breast cancer. N Engl J Med 2002;346(26):2025–32.

Montz FJ, Bristow RE, Bovicelli A, Tomacruz R, Kurman R. Intrauterine progesterone treatment of early endometrial cancer. Am J Obstet Gynecol 2002;186(4):651–7.

Ness RB, Grisso JA, Klapper J, et al. Risk of ovarian cancer in relation to estrogen and progestin dose and use characteristics of oral contraceptives. Am J Epidemiol 2000;152(3):233–41.

Orr-Walker BJ, Evans MC, Ames RW, Clearwater JM, Cundy T, Reid IR. The effect of past use of the injectable contraceptive depot medroxyprogesterone acetate on bone mineral density in normal post-menopausal women. Clin Endocrinol 1998;49(5):615–18.

Schwartz SM, Petitti DB, Siscovick DS, et al. Stroke and use of low-dose oral contraceptives in young women: a pooled analysis of two US studies. Stroke 1998;29(11):2277–84.

Schwingl PJ, Ory HW, Visness CM. Estimates of the risk of cardiovascular death attributable to low-dose oral contraceptives in the United States. Am J Obstet Gynecol 1999;180:241–9.

Sidney S, Petitti DB, Soff GA, Cundiff DL, Tolan KK, Quesenberry CP Jr. Venous thromboembolic disease in users of low-estrogen combined estrogen-progestin oral contraceptives. Contraception 2004;70(1):3–10.

Sidney S, Siscovick DS, Petitti DB, et al. Myocardial infarction in users of low-dose oral contraceptives: a pooled analysis of 2 US studies. Circulation 1998;98(11):1058–63.

Vasilakis C, Jick H, del Mar Melero-Montes M. Risk of idiopathic venous thromboembolism in users of progestagens alone. Lancet 1999;354 (9190):1610.

WHO. Cardiovascular disease and use of oral and injectable progestogen-only contraceptives and combined injectable contraceptives. Results of an international, multicenter, case-control study. Contraception 1998;57: 315–24.

18

Perimenopausal Contraception

Susan A. Ballagh

Department of Obstetrics & Gynecology, Harbor-UCLA Medical Center, Torrance, CA, USA

The perimenopausal woman

The Stages of Reproductive Aging Workshop (STRAW) held in 2001 provided a framework for classifying the reproductive stage of a perimenopausal woman based on hormonal status (and ovarian aging) rather than age alone. Hormonal status is reflected by menstrual history, follicle stimulating hormone (FSH) level, and fecundity (Table 18.1). Studies in the 1970s showed that cycle length was most consistent for women aged 25–35, with 60% of cycles lasting 25–28 days. It is unclear how the increasing incidence of obesity, insulin resistance, and diabetes may have altered this pattern today.

As Table 18.1 shows, moving from the *reproductive stage* to the *first or early stage of the perimenopausal transition* is associated with reduced fecundity and elevations of early follicular-phase FSH. During this early stage, cycles usually remain regular and symptoms are uncommon. The beginning of a lowered risk of fertility is attributed to women 35–40 years of age, although this is variable.

The *middle stage of the perimenopausal transition* is a time of slightly reduced cycle length associated with elevated FSH and reduced inhibins. The current concept is that the ovary produces less inhibin with a resulting increase in early follicular FSH that accelerates follicular development and a resultant shortening of the follicular phase and elevated levels of estradiol by cycle days 1–3. This is most often noted in women aged 40–44 years.

The final or *late stage of the perimenopausal transition* is characterized by an extended lack of ovarian responsiveness—often with elevated FSH (>15–25 mIU/mL), resulting in skipped menses (spaced 60 or more days apart). On average, only 32% of the extended cycles are ovulatory, but 98% of regular cycles are ovulatory in women over 40. In 1985 Lindsay and Metcalf suggested that women with an early follicular FSH over 20 IU/L could discontinue contraception, but more recent data suggests that ovulation is common and women should be apprised of the risk of conception (The UK newpaper The Telegraph the oldest spontaneous pregnancy in a 59-year-old woman.)

During the delay of menstrual onset, women commonly experience a hypoestrogenic period associated with marked hot flashes that resolve once a follicle is coaxed to initiate a cycle. These cycles have higher luteal estradiol and lower luteal progesterone. The median age for these extended cycles is 47.5 years, but the age range that includes 95% of women is very wide (39–51 years).

The late stage of the perimenopausal transition includes the year following the last normal menstrual period.

As Table 18.1 implies, the perimenopausal changes in ovarian function occur in an orderly, linear fashion. The exceptions to this orderly pattern include those women who shift between early and late menopause based on stress, exercise and diet variation, medical conditions, surgery, or medication use.

Women, especially those under age 45, with typical menopause symptoms including fatigue, hypersomnia, or unexplained weight gain, may

Contraception, First Edition. Edited by Donna Shoupe.
© 2011 Blackwell Publishing Ltd. Published 2011 by Blackwell Publishing Ltd.

Table 18.1 Stages of reproductive aging in women. The reproductive stage starts at the time of the first menstrual period; the perimenopausal transition ends 1 year before the final menstrual period

Stages	Reproductive	Perimenopausal transition	Postmenopause
Typical age range	1st menses to age 35	Age 35–51	Age 51+
Typical pattern of menstrual cycles	Regular cycles begin 1–2 years after menarche, then cycles shorten over time (by a few days)	Variable patterns, further shortening of cycle length, skipped cycles until last year when there is no bleeding	Cessation of menses
Typical endocrine values	Day 3 normal FSH <10 mIU/ml	Day 3 FSH elevated, 10–25 mIU/ml, increasing to PM levels by late stage	FSH >35 mIU/ml
	Normal day 3 estradiol	Elevation of day 3 estradiol until late stage where estradiol levels are lower	Estradiol falls to <20–25 pg/ml by mid PM stage (~age 55)
	Declines in inhibin during middle to late stages		
Typical fertility	Peak fertility mid to late 20s, then declining over time	Faster declines in fertility, lower risk of pregnancy age 35–42, very low risk of pregnancy in middle and late states (after age 43–44)	None
Common symptoms	None	Hot flashes, headaches, sleep disturbances, mood problems, risk increases as progress through stages	Perimenopausal symptoms common in early PM; vaginal dryness, atrophy, bladder symptoms in mid PM; bone loss (physiologic loss in PM) eventually results in osteoporosis/fractures

FSH, follicle stimulating hormone; PM, postmenopause.
Adapted from The STRAW Menopause Stages (Stages of Reproductive Aging Workshop, Park City, Utah July 2001).

be suffering from hypothyroidism. Treatment of subacute hypothyroidism is controversial, in that the risks and benefits have not been well defined. In anecdotal reports, treatment is reported to provide relief of menopausal symptoms for some patients.

Contraceptive options

This chapter focuses on women 40 years old and older who begin to have a significant alteration in their ovarian function. The change in cyclicity often provides a false sense of security, resulting in low contraceptive compliance, and additionally make many forms of contraception more difficult to use.

Menstrual irregularity makes it difficult to practice natural fertility methods or periodic abstinence effectively. Many couples combine avoidance of mid cycle with other methods to improve efficacy. Similarly, withdrawal efficacy may be enhanced by mid-cycle avoidance of vaginal sex. Menstrual irregularities also make condom use more difficult, as women tend to use condoms during the mid cycle rather than near the menses. Older men may find condom use more difficult because of erectile problems.

Other barrier methods like the diaphragm and cervical cap may be more difficult to use and less effective, because of vaginal changes after childbirth.

Hormonal methods are highly effective for older women and additionally provide many contraceptive benefits, but health problems, especially cardiovascular disease, may limit the options (see Chapters 3, 4, 5, 6, 9 and 17). The progestin implant, progestin-only pills, and injectable progestin are good contraceptive options for a large percentage of perimenopausal women.

The increased use of sterilization of women in their fifth decade, and a recent increase in use of interauterine devices (IUDs) in women in all age groups, are positive trends. The two hysteroscopic tubal sterilization procedures now available (see Chapter 14) are cost-effective. The levonorgestrel (LNG)-releasing intrauterine system (LNG-IUS) is associated with significant decreases in blood loss that can be particularly valuable during the perimenopausal transition.

A high percentage of unintended and undesired pregnancies occur in women over 40, and except for a high rate of miscarriage (Figure 18.1), the use of elective termination among pregnant women in their forties would exceed that of teenagers. The increased risk of birth defects, particularly trisomies like Down syndrome, and greater use of prenatal diagnostic testing also contributes to a reduced rate of live birth per clinical pregnancy for older women.

Contraceptive needs

Seventy percent of women over 35 are married, but the number without children at home increases from 18% at age 35–39 to 49% in the 45–49 age group. Only 25% of women 50–54 have children at home. This provides increased opportunity for intimacy for most couples.

Most U.S. women over the age of 40 do not intend to conceive, as many have completed their families. However, a small but significant percentage of women in their forties still seek to conceive because they chose to delay childbearing or have experienced infertility.

Among sexually active women aged 40–49 who are able to become pregnant but do not want to become pregnant, 8% are not using any contraceptive method. This number is lower than the 19% in teenagers. By age 45, two thirds of women in the United States will report an unplanned pregnancy and one third will have had an abortion.

Fertility

Among infertile women who have not conceived by age 35 and seek in-vitro fertilization, egg quality is greatly reduced, resulting in a rapid decline of live birth rates beginning at age 37 (Figure 18.2).

It is important to note that these data from infertile women underestimate the fecundity of the population of women who have conceived without difficulty in the past. Among Hitterite women living in the Rockies who did not practice contraception, two thirds conceived after age 40. Similarly, natural fertility among rural Senegalese women fell after age 35, but more than half were still fertile at age 40. In short, while fertility declines, the decline is outpaced by the desire to prevent conception for all but a small fraction of women over 40.

For those who do desire pregnancy, prompt referral to fertility treatment is advisable to optimize the chances of conception. Those who regret their sterilization and seek pregnancy in this age group will achieve greater success with tubal reversal surgery than in-vitro fertilization.

Health issues

Recent surveys of perimenopausal women demonstrate a variety of common health issues.

- Data from the MMWR Surveillance indicates that two thirds of women 45–54 are overweight, with one quarter reaching obesity (BMI>30). Women continue to gain weight despite lower rates of gestation that are often correlated with overweight status in women 25–34 years old.
- Over half of perimenopausal women are sedentary.

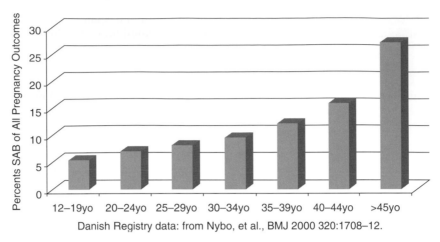

Figure 18.1 Miscarriage rate.

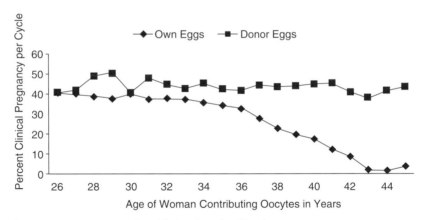

Figure 18.2 Pregnancy rate per cycle with in-vitro fertilization.

- One third are hypercholesterolemic and 28% have hypertension.
- One quarter smoke cigarettes and 11% report binge drinking with heavy drinking in 5% (Table 18.2).

Migraines are most frequent in women aged 30–59 years old, and 40% of sufferers have an associated aura. In women who experience an aura there is a doubling of the risk of cardiovascular disease, stroke and myocardial infarction. Use of estrogen-containing contraceptives confers an exponentially increased risk, similar to the increased risk to women over 35 years old who smoke. Women with common migraine without aura can safely use combination con-

traceptives provided they do not have other contraindications until age 35.

Women 35 years and older should be assessed for cardiovascular risk factors including *hypertension, nicotine use, diabetes, nephropathy,* and other *vascular diseases* as part of their primary care. Incidence of diabetes mellitus in women in their forties varies by ethnicity and body mass index. Women with prior gestational diabetes should be screened regularly for diabetes, since 3% develop the disease annually. There is no apparent effect of newer progestin-containing oral contraceptives (OCs) on glucose tolerance. In the BRFFS 2004 survey, a subset of women answered additional health questions about medical problems and identified similar rates

Table 18.2 Prevalences of health characteristics of perimenopausal women by age

Age (years)	25–34	35–39	40–44	45–49	50–54	55–59
BMI >25	47%	48%	50%	53%	58%	61%
BMI >30	22%	22%	23%	26%	27%	30%
Hypercholesterolemia	16%	21%	25%	31%	39%	46%
Hypertension	6.7%	11%	16%	22%	32%	41%
Diabetes	2.0%	2.9%	4.5%	6.0%	9.1%	13.2%
Current smoker	22%	20%	23%	22%	20%	18%
Heavy alcohol use	6.0%	4.8%	7.9%	7.9%	7.4%	7.2%

Source: 2005 BRFFS survey interactive database at http://apps.nccd.cdc.gov/s_broker/htmsql.exe/
weat/freq_analysis.hsql?survey_year=2005 (accessed April 18, 2010)

of hypercholesterolemia (25%), hypertension (11%), and diabetes (2%) as noted in the 2005 data (Table 18.2).

Of the 1% of women with a *prior myocardial infarction or stroke*, 40% and 53% respectively were not using contraceptives. Why would these women at highest risk of pregnancy complication not use contraceptives? This anomaly is explained in part by the fact that contraceptive provision to high-risk women is beyond the scope of many contraceptive providers, yet is often neglected by the specialists who care for their medical condition. A recent wave of unplanned conceptions at our institution was noted in women using sildenafil (Viagra) to treat pulmonary hypertension. Improved pulmonary function resulted in more physical stamina and likely increased sexual activity, if not libido. This is reminiscent of the wave of conceptions noted with the introduction of metformin (Glucophage) for glucose control that increased ovulation and unplanned conceptions in diabetic women.

It is imperative that women with medical contraindications to pregnancy, including those using teratogenic medications, receive thorough counseling that guides them to appropriate and effective methods to prevent conception.

Medical eligibility criteria

Chapter 19 provides information about specific choices of contraception for women with medical problems including diabetes, hypertension, and heart disease. In general, nonhormonal or progestin-only methods are safe to use. Equally effective as sterilization, yet reversible and underutilized, are the intrauterine and implant contraceptives. There are four progestin-only options including OCs, implants (Implanon in the United States), the LNG-IUS (Mirena), and depot medroxyprogesterone acetate (DPMA) injections (Depo-Provera).

Most women are unaware of the risks of pregnancy, especially in the fifth decade. These risks include increased pregnancy-associated hypertension, gestational diabetes, pulmonary embolism, anesthesia complications, and transfusions plus other rare but serious cardiovascular and pulmonary conditions (Figure 18.3).

> ☆ TIPS & TRICKS
>
> This is a time for good clinical judgment. When helping a patient select a method, always present the risk of pregnancy compared to the contraceptive risk to help her place the risks into proper perspective.

Actual perimenopausal contraceptive use

Age breakdown in contraceptive choices is possible from the 2002 National Survey of Family Growth, as outlined in Table 18.3. The most common method of contraception was sterilization, with female sterilization more prevalent than male. By the fifth decade, over half of women depend on sterilization as their contraceptive method. By age 40–44 years, nonuse was almost as common as abstinence, OCs, or condoms as a

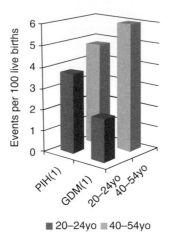

From Osterman MJK, et al.,
Natl Vital Stat Rep. 2009 Oct 28;58(5):1–24

■ 20–24yo ■ 40–54yo

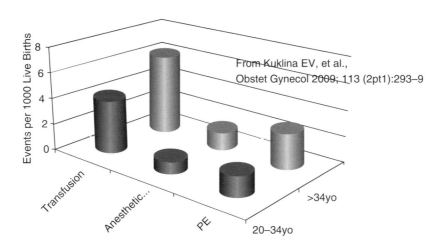

From Kuklina EV, et al.,
Obstet Gynecol 2009; 113 (2pt1):293–9

■ 20–34yo ■ >34yo

Figure 18.3 Selected pregnancy risks by age.

method. In women over 35 years old, less than 1% used an IUD or implants. OC use ranked fourth in popularity for 40–44 year olds, behind absti- nence (10.8%), condoms (8%), with 7.6% using the birth control pill. Nonuse of contraception among women exposed to intercourse was 6.8%—just a little behind OCs.

> ✋ CAUTION
>
> Dispel the myth that perimenopausal women are too old to conceive!

Contraceptive options for perimenopausal women

Sterilization considerations: interval, postpartum, and laparoscopic methods

Costs

Sterilization is an appealing method for women who have completed their families since it does not require additional effort and is highly effec- tive. Increased sterilization was noted after the early OCs (with significant side effects) were introduced. This increased sterilization rate was driven, at least in part, by the fact that at that

Table 18.3 Common methods of contraception by age for U.S. women in 2002

Method	Ages (years)			
	25–29	30–34	35–39	40–44
Sterilization				
Female	10.3	19.0	29.2	34.7
Male	2.8	6.4	10.0	12.7
Total	**13.1**	**25.4**	**39.2**	**47.4**
Reversible				
Oral contraceptives	25.6	21.8	13.2	7.6
Condoms	14.0	11.8	11.1	8.0
IUD	2.5	2.2	1.0	0.8
Injection (DMPA)	4.4	2.9	1.5	1.1
Other hormonal	1.7	0.9	0.5	0.2
Other barrier	0.3	0.1	—	0.4
Withdrawal	5.2	2.6	2.4	1.0
Periodic abstinence	0.7	1.1	1.4	1.6
Sponge, cap, female condom	0.4	0.4	0.5	1.1
Total	**54.8**	**43.8**	**32.1**	**21.2**
No method				
Pregnant,postpartum, or seeking pregnancy	13.9	13.9	8.9	4.1
No intercourse	8.9	7.6	9.1	10.8
Nonuse	8.0	7.0	7.8	6.8
Total	**30.7**	**28.5**	**25.9**	**21.6**

Advance Data from Vital and Health Statistics. Number 350, December 10, 2004.
Data from the 2002 National Survey of Family Growth. Download 4/18/10 from: http://www.cdc.gov/nchs/data/ad/ad350.pdf.

time, sterilization and not IUDs or OCs were paid for by insurance coverage.

Presently in California, Family Pact coverage for contraception rewards women for utilizing less expensive reversible methods by providing continued eligibility for annual examinations and cervical cancer screening with family planning services. Decisions about sterilization are based on parity rather than marital status. Five years after the last desired birth, 63% of black women, 60% of Hispanic women, and 55% of white women have been sterilized. The rate is only slightly lower among Catholic women.

Efficacy

Tubal ligation at the time of cesarean section or at postpartum minilaparotomy has the lowest failure rate. Since a segment of tube is resected and sent to pathology for evaluation, the provider is alerted to an incorrect technique. In addition, the increased separation between the tube and round ligament of the gravid uterus plus the dilated utero-ovarian veins simplify identification of the tubes.

The Filshie Clip or Falope Ring have a lower failure rate than bipolar cautery or the Hulka Clip (which is no longer marketed). Tubal ligation failures after the first 2 years usually implant outside the uterus. Although these failures lessen over time, there continues to be failures many years after a tubal ligation. Bipolar cautery has a tenfold increased risk of ectopic pregnancy at 10 years compared to partial salpingectomy. Ring and clip methods have an intermediate (fivefold) increase in ectopic pregnancy.

Complications

When tubal ligation is done at the time of cesarean section, there is no significant increased risk of complications. Since anesthesia contributes the greatest risk of the risk of postpartum tubal ligation, use of the laboring anesthetic also reduces the overall risk of the procedure. Interval sterilization is usually done via laparoscopy under general anesthesia in the United States. In other countries minilaparotomy with local anesthesia is more common. Unipolar cautery had a low failure rate but caused an unacceptably high incidence of bowel injury and is rarely used today. Failure is lessened with bipolar cautery when at least three sites of the tube are burned.

Laparoscopic sterilization has a reported laparotomy rate of 1.4/1000. Morbidity is rare and is almost entirely limited to anesthetic complications and large vessel injury.

Tubal ligation does not increase the risk of menstrual disorders but does replace hormonal contraceptives that would otherwise regulate perimenopausal bleeding. Women using hormonal methods should be advised at the time of the tubal ligation that latent cyclic irregularity may require continued use of hormones after surgery in some cases. Tubal ligation is not associated with earlier menopause and posttubal syndrome has not been well documented.

Regret

Sterilization becomes less cost-effective as a woman ages. Increasing age increases the risk of anesthetic complications at surgery. On the positive side, however, older women are less likely to regret their decision for sterilization: a significant consideration for women under 30 years of age.

Previously sterilized women aged 40–42 who desire to conceive should consider reversal of tubal sterilization since the cumulative intrauterine pregnancy rate is 50% over 2 years—equivalent to more than 5 cycles of in-vitro fertilization (IVF) for 40-year-old women (9.1 delivery rate per cycle) or over 70 cycles at 45 years old (0.7 delivery rate per cycle).

Hysterscopic methods

Hysteroscopic sterilization (Essure, Adiana) can be performed as an office procedure with local anesthetic with or without sedation. It has a lower risk of tubal failure than tubal ligation since tubal patency is rare with the inflammatory tissue ingrowth that obliterates the isthmic (intrauterine) portion of the tube.

There are a number of technical difficulties with device placement. Up to 14% of women who seek this method experience lack of placement of at least one side on the first attempt. At 3 months, displacement of one or both devices from the tubal ostia is noted in 4% and a failure of tissue ingrowth in 3.5%. Tissue ingrowth to block the tube is nearly always attained by 6 months but requires a second radiograph. Until a hysterosalpingogram confirms successful bilateral tubal blockage, women are not sterilized and must use another method to prevent pregnancy.

Use of DMPA a few weeks prior to hysteroscopy thins the endometrial lining to aid visualization and then provides highly effective contraception for the 3 month waiting period.

Vasectomy

Vasectomy is the least risky of the sterilization methods for a couple, but assumes a stable, faithful relationship to be effective for the woman. Little data documents that number of midlife women who have multiple partners, but divorce is common increasing by 3% per 5-year period and reaching 40% for women by age 50. Recent herpesvirus (HPV) testing of menopausal women suggests that recent exposure to multiple partners partly explains the 6% rate of HPV positivity. Interviews in Chicago suggest that 2% of married menopausal women had sex with another partner in the past year, while 15% of married women have ever had another partner outside their marriage.

For these women, vasectomy alone is a poor option. One third of women are unmarried at the time of tubal sterilization (from 20% of white women to 63% of black women). In contrast, only 7% of men are unmarried at the time of vasectomy.

Intrauterine contraception

The IUDs available in the United States are highly effective—as efficacious as sterilization—and yet they are vastly underutilized. Not surprisingly, a much larger percentage of physicians select these devices for themselves or their spouses compared to the general population. It is very unfortunate that so few women, especially women in their forties, take advantage of this form of contraception.

> ★ **TIPS & TRICKS**
>
> Women who use intrauterine contraception report the greatest method satisfaction and have the highest continuation rate of any reversible approach.

The LGS-IUD is ideally suited for women with anovulatory cycles because it protects the uterine lining from unopposed estrogen, reducing endometrial cancer risk by an estimated 40–60%. It also reduces total menstrual blood loss for women experiencing anemia due to heavy menses.

Either type of IUD can be used in most women with medical problems, since no estrogen is utilized by either device. Placement of the copper IUD (Cu-IUD) is the only contraceptive visit that a woman in her forties will need for the rest of her life. Standard clinical practice acknowledges 12 years' duration, but most devices still retain some copper and continue to work beyond that time.

Unless her menses are excessive and painful, the Cu-IUD is a great alternative for perimenopausal women. It is important to counsel women to expect altered bleeding patterns after IUD placement.

For the LGS-IUD, frequent spotting for the first 3–6 months is common. After that, most women will have lighter bleeding, and up to 20% will experience prolonged intervals without bleeding. For the Cu-IUD, menses are somewhat heavier and longer but menstrual timing is unaltered. See Chapter 9 for more specifics about intrauterine contraception.

Injectable contraceptive

Only one injectable contraceptive (available in two doses) is available in the United States, DMPA. It is highly effective, but requires quarterly visits to a provider to receive the shot. With perfect compliance it could be as effective as sterilization, but in typical use it has a 3% failure rate.

It is also may be associated with weight gain in sedentary women. Given the preponderance of weight issues in women in their 40s, it is rarely a "go to" method for a perimenopausal patient unless she is a long-standing satisfied user or bleeding problems are bothersome.

DMPA lowers circulating estradiol and is associated with temporary bone loss and may rarely be associated with vasomotor symptoms. Women generally will regain bone within 3 years of discontinuation For the perimenopausal woman who has long cycles after stopping the shot, use of hormone replacement for several years will help her regain lost bone. During use, adequate calcium intake is important to minimize bone loss.

Implant contraceptive

Another underutilized but highly effective reversible method, the implant is equivalent in efficacy to sterilization. The etonogestrel (or 3-keto-desogestrel) implant available in the United States comes packaged in a sterile inserter and is quickly placed subdermally in the nondominant arm. It provides 3 years of contraceptive protection with a single office visit.

The hormonal serum levels are equivalent to those of the minipill. During the first few months of use, hormone release is slightly higher, so women sensitive to hormone side effects can be counseled that hormone levels will drop by one third within the first 3 months.

Overall bleeding with the implant is lighter, with fewer bleeding days than would be expected during regular cycles. There is less predictability and women may experience occasional and seemingly random episodes of prolonged bleeding. The bleeding is rarely heavy enough to cause anemia, but counseling before insertion should include asking if she and her partner would be able to maintain their sexual relationship were she to experience a prolonged bleeding episode.

Removal of the single implant usually takes under 5 minutes and is well tolerated.

There is little or no weight gain with the method and it can be considered in almost all perimenopausal women, in contrast to estrogen-containing methods as discussed below.

Estrogen/progestin combined contraceptives

Combination products containing estrogen should only be offered to healthy women over 35 who do not smoke, do not have hypertension, and do not have migraine headaches (see Table 18.4).

Progestin-only pills

Progestin-only contraceptive pills, known as the minipill, are packaged in 28-day cycle packs containing only active pills that need to be taken at the same time every day. In typical use, progestin-

Table 18.4 Absolute contraindications to use of combination contraceptives

Prior or current DVT or stroke
Prior ischemic heart disease, MI or vascular disease
Complicated valvular heart disease with either: Pulmonary hypertension risk for subacute bacterial endocarditis atrial fibrillation
Systemic lupus erythematosus with antiphospholipid antibodies
Breast cancer within the previous 5 years
Diabetes complicated by vascular disease or diagnosed for 20+ years
Uncontrolled hypertension: systolic ≥160; diastolic ≥100 mmHg
Major surgery with prolonged immobilization
Women over 35 who smoke ≥15 cigarettes/day
Acute viral hepatitis or decompensated cirrhosis
Hepatocellular adenoma or hepatoma
Migraine with aura or migraine in women >35 years of age
Combination of age, diabetes, and/or hypertension

> **★ TIPS & TRICKS**
>
> **Think hormone free or progestin-only in perimenopausal women**
> Because of the increased prevalence of obesity, hypertension, diabetes, migraine with aura, and cigarette smoking it makes sense to avoid estrogen-containing but highly effective contraceptives and consider the following instead:
> - Minipills
> - Progestin—injectable or implant
> - IUDs: LGS-IUD and Cu-IUD

New products

New oral contraceptives

New agents have emerged in the past decade that contain a new progestin developed from modification of spironolactone. Three milligrams of drosperinone (DSP) has the equivalent diuretic action of 25 mg of spironolactone. DSP products are approved by the U.S. Food and Drug Authority (FDA) for premenstrual dysphoric disorder (PMDD) symptoms and moderate acne in addition to contraception. Pills with ethinyl estradiol (EE) and DSP have shown reduced weight gain compared to a LNG product, and reduced dysmenorrhea.

In May, 2010, a novel OC formulation containing estradiol valerate (instead of EE) and dienogest (an antiandrogenic progestin) was approved by the FDA. Natazia, the first contraceptive pill with four phases, contains only two placebo pills in a 28-day cycle. The same pill, named Qlaira, was released in Europe by Bayer in the fall of 2009. Natazia was highly efficacious in clinical trials. The substitution of estradiol valerate for EE reduced clotting factor changes and triglyceride elevation compared to a current EE formulation, but the clinical relevance of these biochemical changes is unclear. This dienogest formulation resulted in fewer withdrawal bleeds during the placebo pills, and less bleeding and spotting compared to a 20 μg EE/100 μg LNG pill (Alesse, Aviane).

only pills are less effective in preventing ovulation than combination OCs and have an overall typical failure rate around 8%. Failure rates in an older, perimenopausal population are lower due to lower underlying fertility. Once prescribed almost exclusively to breastfeeding women, the sales of progestin-only pills have increased for older women. The World Health Organization Medical Eligibility Criteria (WHO MEC) note that progestin-only contraceptives are less risky in women over 40.

Progestin-only pills are safer for women who are obese, smoke cigarettes, or have other risk factors for cardiovascular disease. Poor cycle control with irregular vaginal bleeding is the most common reason for method discontinuation.

There is only one formulation with norethindrone available in the United States at present, despite a successful European desogestrel product.

If larger population studies demonstrate less venous thromboembolism, an improved lipid profile, or less interaction with cigarette use, estradiol pills might become the preferred combination OC for the perimenopausal woman. Clinicians should keep alert for new data on these estradiol formulations.

New regimens

New regimens and packaging of combined OCs (COCs) include continuous regimens without any placebo pills, cycles with 84 active pills followed by 4 or 7 days of placebo, and a pill with a 28-day cycle with 24 active pills (24–4 regimen) (Figure 18.4) Compared to standard cycles with 21 active and 7 placebo pills, the newer 24–4 regimens are associated with lighter, shorter periods. All of the extended cycles (including the 24–4 cycles) have a potential advantage of reduced failure because of fewer pill-free days.

Extended or continuous regimens reduce menstrual migraine and headache symptoms, and decrease premenstrual complaints and dysmenorrhea when compared to standard OCs. Thyroid, androgen, and globulins do not appear to be altered significantly by reduced use of placebos. Extended and continuous regimens may have erratic, though typically lighter, bleeding episodes. Some women have complete absence of bleeding.

Several investigators have proposed a tailored regimen where women extend cycles to meet their individual needs based on convenience of menstrual avoidance and the inconvenience of unscheduled bleeding. Provided she has taken at least 21 active pills, the patient is encouraged to stop the pills (4 days) at a convenient time to cause a withdrawal bleed so she can reduce the risk of bleeding for 1–2 weeks and schedule bleeding around her activities or travel plans. Since many women over 40 experience vasomotor symptoms, these extended regimens have the added advantage of reducing perimenopausal hot flashes and other symptoms.

New delivery systems

New delivery systems have emerged that use *transdermal patch* or *vaginal ring* technology to deliver cyclic combination contraception with less frequent dosing. Both deliver EE and both provide the active agent of a progestin in standard OCs: 3-keto-desogestrel called etonogestrel (ring) and 17-Ac-norgestimate called norelgestromin (patch).The systemic delivery of EE does not change the metabolic effects on hepatic protein synthesis. Claims of "no first pass" liver metabolism are clinically irrelevant.

The advantage of these methods is the potential for improved compliance. This proved true for the weekly patch for teenagers, but has less effect in women over 40. While the 21-day ring dosing should afford better compliance, studies have not clearly documented improved efficacy in actual use situations.

The one study switching OC users to either the patch or ring found that more women who were randomized to the ring completed the 3 month study (95% versus 88%) with plans to continue the new method (71% vs 26%) compared to the patch. The bulk of patch users

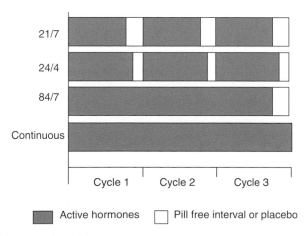

Figure 18.4 New pill dosing schedules.

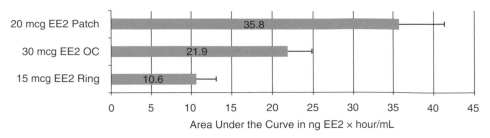

Figure 18.5 Ethinyl estradiol 21-day area under the curve. Reproduced from Van den Heuvel et al. Contraception 2005;72:169–74, with permission from Elsevier.

preferred the OC. The side effect that was more common with ring use was increased vaginal discharge, which may be advantageous for the subset of women in their 40s who report vaginal dryness.

The delivery of EE as measured by area under the curve is greater with the patch than with an OC containing 30 μg of EE (Figure 18.5). The EE area under the curve for the ring (labeled to release 15 μg daily) is less than half than that of the OC. Epidemiologic data has not correlated these variations in EE exposure with meaningful changes in thrombotic events, but this data does explain the difference in side effect profile of the two methods.

Rings and patches have also been used continuously, but few studies include women over 40. In general, continuous use has less vaginal bleeding than the 21–7 regimen.

Health concerns/side effects

Venous thromboembolism

Venous thromboembolism (VTE) is an adverse effect predominantly due to the estrogen component of the pill. There is little to no increased risk with progestin-only products. The WHO Collaborative Study of Cardiovascular Disease and Steroid Hormone Contraception from 1996 reported that the increased risk of idiopathic VTE associated with OC use among non-smokers constituted over 90% of all cardiovascular events for women aged 20–24 and more than 60% in those 40–44 years. The latest edition of the WHO MEC emphasizes that obese women (BMI ≥30) are at increased risk of VTE.

Hypertension/stroke

Combination contraception not an option for perimenopausal women with hypertension. A small proportion of women at any age starting a combination OC may experience an idiosyncratic reaction with increased blood pressure. The incidence is sufficiently frequent to recommend a blood pressure check before and during OC use. An earlier check within the first 2 months is preferred to assess this and other side effects. It affords interaction to reassure her about nuisance side effects, or switch her pill before she resorts to a less effective method. The current use of modern low-dose contraceptives does not appear to increase either ischemic or thrombotic stoke in women over 30 who do not have other risk factors.

Hyperlipidemia

All estrogen-containing contraceptives elevate triglycerides (in one study from 13% to 75%). They also alter enterohepatic circulation and production of bile acids that predisposes women to cholecystitis or cholelithiasis. Triglyceride levels over 500 mg/dL are associated with a significantly increased risk of acute pancreatitis. No meaningful or consistent changes in total cholesterol are noted with combination OCs. Desogestrel and lower dose norethindrone combination OCs reduce LDL cholesterol by 12–14% and increase HDL2 levels by 10–12%.

Lipids should be monitored in accordance with primary care screening guidelines. No special monitoring is required unless the patient has known hypertriglyceridemia that might be exacerbated with OCs.

Vascular disease

Whether due to long-standing diabetes, atherosclerosis, or other cause, vascular disease is a contraindication to combination contraceptive use. Conditions that predispose to arterial thrombosis or stroke are also contraindicated, such as antiphospholipid syndrome or migraine with and without aura.

Breast cancer

There is no evidence that breast cancer is more common in perimenopausal users of OCs than in nonusers. The Royal College study also verifies no change in risk of breast cancer in women who used the pill (RR 0.9; 95% CI 0.74–1.08). Some studies suggest that BRCA mutation carriers, as well as women with a significant family history of breast cancer are more vulnerable to the hormones in OCs.

Ovarian, uterine, and colon cancer

Based on a 2010 update from the Royal College of General Practitioners' Oral Contraceptive Study, the data suggest that ever users continue to enjoy a reduced incidence of ovarian cancer (RR 0.53; 95% CI 0.38–0.72) and endometrial cancer (RR 0.43; 95% CI 0.21–0.88). Both endometroid and clear cell endometrial cancers are reduced with OC use. There is also evidence of reduced colon cancer (RR 0.62; 95% CI 0.46–0.83) with a reduced risk of cancer overall (RR 0.88; 95% CI 0.82–0.93).

A new collaborative analysis of over 23,000 cases of ovarian cancer from over 40 countries confirms a significant, exposure-dependent ovarian cancer risk reduction for women whether they started OCs in the 1960s, 1970s, or 1980s. This large study found an attenuated but persistent benefit up to 30 years after the cessation of OC use. Mucinous ovarian cancers (12% of total cancers) were not reduced in OC users.

Cervical neoplasia and cancer

Estrogen enhances human papillomavirus (HPV) transcription and decreases HPV clearance, resulting in more persistence of HPV, an increase of cervical intraepithelial neoplasia, and an increased relative risk of cervical cancer. One group has demonstrated efficacy of applying a cream containing clomiphene citrate, a selective estrogen receptor modulator, for anogenital warts.

Fibroids

There is no significant change in fibroid size associated with OC use and no evidence that OCs promote the transformation of healthy cells into cells capable of creating fibroids.

Bone density

The WHO Consultation in 2005 reviewed the world literature and unpublished pharmaceutical data on the effect of combination contraceptives and DMPA on bone mineral density (BMD) with special consideration of perimenopausal women.

Combination contraceptives appear to have little influence on BMD overall. Bone loss was evident during DMPA use, but that loss was reversed by supplementing with estradiol during use. BMD was regained and exceeded nonuser values within 3 years of discontinuation if users initiated hormone replacement.

Women with type 1 diabetes have lower BMD than controls and are 6.4 times more likely to develop hip fracture after menopause. Women with type 2 diabetes are 2.2 times more likely to fracture, especially with longer disease or insulin use.

Barrier contraceptives

The most commonly used barrier, the *male condom*, has a 98% effectiveness if used correctly at every act of coitus. In the real world, efficacy is around 85–88%. Condom use increased markedly in the 1980s with the increase and publicity surrounding HIV infections. Condoms of sheep or other animal skin are porous and provide little protection. Latex or polyurethane condoms provide an effective barrier to sperm and to many sexually transmitted infections. Manufacturers are introducing new condom designs intended to enhance the sexual experience. These include textured or flavored models; some are even equipped with small vibrators.

Given the increase in divorce for women in the fifth decade noted above, a method with dual protection may be particularly appropriate.

A *female condom* is also marketed and can be applied before coitus. It is only 80% effective in actual use (see Chapter 11). Two cervical caps (FemCap, Lea Contraceptive) are also available.

All of these products are used with spermicide and are more effective for nulliparous (80%) than multiparous (75%) women.

Spermicide

Spermicide can also be used alone but is even less effective (65%). It is important to warn women that with frequent coitus (more than daily) the risk of transmission of infection may be increased with frequent use of spemicide.

Other

Other barriers now available include the *sponge* (of Seinfeld fame)

Compliance with barrier methods

Compliance with these methods is reduced because they are placed just before or during coitus. With the male condom, the penis must be erect for proper use. Female controlled methods can be positioned several hours ahead of coitus, but show less efficacy despite this theoretical advantage. For these methods to work, coitus must be planned and this implies that the female partner was prepared rather than "swept away" by the moment of passion.

Female barrier methods have been used most successfully in long-term stable relationships when their use becomes a comfortable part of sexually activity. They were popular in the 1950s, but the introduction of more convenient and effective choices has lead to a dramatic decline in use. Fewer than 2% of contraceptors now report use of these barrier methods, and for women in their 40s the figure is less than 1%.

For women with infrequent coitus, the barrier methods—especially male condoms—are good options. For infection prevention, male condom counseling should be provided to all women on any method, especially those with uncertain relationships.

Contraception use and compliance

The 2007 Pregnancy Risk Assessment System (PRAMS) identified that 39 58% of women who were not trying to get pregnant did not use any contraception in their conception cycle. This is similar to studies in the 1990s suggesting that many women still choose not to use contraception despite a dozen new contraceptive options that have been marketed in the interim.

> **EVIDENCE AT A GLANCE**
>
> Older women responding to contraceptive questions in the BRFSS 2004 survey were more likely to use no method, despite being exposed to pregnancy: 18.4% of women aged 35–39 and 23.2% of women aged 40–44.

Most women who did not use any contraception were married and were highly educated, with health insurance. It has been suggested that nonuse represents a latent unvoiced desire for pregnancy, or a desire to conceive that is not shared by the spouse. Similar dissonant behavior is noted in prevention sexually transmitted infections, where verbalized intentions often differ from actual practice.

Understanding the behavior associated with nonuse of contraception is likely to contribute more to preventing future pregnancy than refinement of current methods. Figure 18.6 outlines the reasons why women report that they do not use contraception. The biggest reason for short-term gaps in contraceptive use is *method inaccessibility*. Providers would be well advised to provide prescriptions for as many cycles of hormonal contraceptives as possible at each visit and to educate women about prescription plans and mechanisms that provide more contraception at one visit to reduce the need for refills. Many pharmacies and insurance plans now provide at least 3 months of drug at one time through certain mechanisms, often at a reduced rate of copayment.

Compliance in current users is also an important factor in the incidence of unplanned pregnancies. It is a fallacy to believe that older women practice contraception more effectively than younger women in their twenties. The actual rate of abortion and delivery to women in their forties is less than in younger women because of decreased fecundity, increased sterilization, and

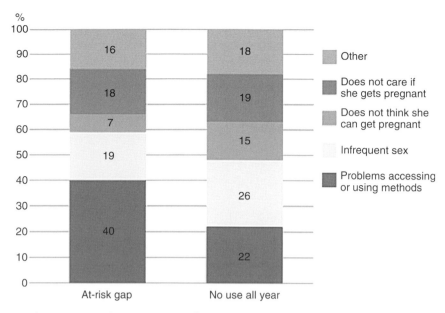

Figure 18.6 Why contraceptives are not used. Women commonly cite method problems or infrequent sex as reasons why they have gaps in use or do not use contraceptives at all. Source: Guttmacher Institute, 2007.

the very high rate of miscarriage, not because of improved compliance. In addition, Potter et al. showed that *practice does not make perfect!* Compliance deteriorates rapidly within the first few months of OC use.

> ★ TIPS & TRICKS
>
> The most important factor in compliance is making contraception effortless. IUDs and implants therefore show the most consistent use.

Another important positive factor for compliance is *user satisfaction* with a method. Women who like their method are more likely to practice it well, challenging clinicians and counselors to listen carefully to patient preferences. Although education and financial constraints contribute to compliance issues for some women, other factors such as autonomy and prior experience with specific methods are very important for women in their forties. Women who depend on withdrawal or rhythm methods were more, not less, educated and half reported incomes over $50,000.

Few contraceptive guidelines use age as a modifier of public policy. The approach to a woman in her forties must, however, be carefully individualized. She may desire to conceive, may have little motivation to prevent pregnancy, or may be very interested in avoiding future pregnancy. She may have a recently diagnosed medical problem or may face a new social situation that alters her ability to select and comply with contraceptive recommendations. In women over 40, the cost of an unintended pregnancy—in maternal and fetal health risks—is so high that special attention to her family planning needs is warranted.

> ★ TIPS & TRICKS
>
> The most important factor in compliance is making contraception effortless. The next most important is patient preference and method satisfaction.

Selected references

Guttmacher Institute publication and link previously sent. I cannot access it right now.

Hardman SM, Gebbie AE. Hormonal contraceptive regimens in the perimenopause. Maturitas 2009;63(3):204–12.

WHO. Medical eligibility criteria for contraceptive use, 4th ed. Geneva: World Health Organization; 2009. Available from: http://www.who.int/reproductivehealth/publications/family_planning/9789241563888/en/index.html

19

Medical Eligibility Requirements

Donna Shoupe

Division of Reproductive Endocrinology and Infertility, Keck School of Medicine,
University of Southern California, USA

Introduction

Ever since 1996, the World Health Organization (WHO) has published a series of evidence-based guidelines regarding the Medical Eligibility Criteria for Contraceptive Use (MEC). The fourth edition, published in 2010, includes 1870 recommendations for safe contraception covering more than 70 medical conditions. For each specific medical condition, the use of a particular contraceptive or sterilization method is assigned a category from 1 to 4.

- Category 1 is assigned when there are no restrictions for use of the method.
- Category 2 indicates that the advantages of using the method generally outweigh risks.
- Category 3 indicates that the health risks of use usually outweigh the contraceptive advantages.
- Category 4 is assigned if the use of the method presents an unacceptable health risk.

For example, the MEC recommends that for women with a history of gestational diabetes, oral contraceptives are a category 1 and for women with diabetes without vascular disease, oral contraceptives are a category 2. However, women with diabetes with vascular disease are assigned a category 3 or 4, depending on the severity of the disease.

Clinical judgment

The recommendation for use of the contraceptive method further takes into consideration the clinical judgment of the healthcare provider (Table 19.1).

The full version of the recommendations is available online. (See "Selected references" at the end of this chapter). The recommendations include updated medical eligibility criteria for provision of IUDs, all hormonal contraceptives, barrier methods, fertility awareness-based methods, coitus interruptus, lactational amenorrhea, emergency contraception, and male and female sterilization. The WHO MEC regarding specific contraceptive methods are also included in Chapters 3–14.

Consideration of conditions that expose a woman to increased risk as a result of unintended pregnancy

Clinical judgment is especially important when counseling women with conditions that may make pregnancy an unacceptable health risk. Because of their relatively higher typical-use failure rates, sole use of barrier methods or behavior-based methods may not be appropriate for some couples. These conditions are listed in Table 19.2

US Medical Eligibility Criteria for Contraceptive Use

In May, 2010, the U.S. Centers for Disease Control (CDC)'s Division of Reproductive Health released for the first time recommendations regarding contraceptive use entitled *U.S. Medical Eligibility Criteria for Contraceptive Use, 2010* (US MEC; see Chapter 1 and Tables 19.3 and 19.4). Because the

Table 19.1 Medical eligibility criteria and clinical judgment

	With clinical judgment	With limited clinical judgment
Category 1	Use the method under any circumstances	Use the method
Category 2	Generally use the method	Use the method
Category 3	Use of method not generally recommended unless other more appropriate methods are not acceptable	Do not use the method
Category 4	Method not to be used	Do not use the method

Table 19.2 Conditions associated with increased risk for adverse health events as a result of unintended pregnancy and where clinical judgment is very important

Breast cancer
Cirrhosis (severe, decompensated)
Diabetes (insulin-dependent; with nephropathy/retinopathy/neuropathy or other vascular disease; or of >20 years' duration)
Endometrial cancer
Epilepsy
Hypertension (systolic >160 mmHg or diastolic >100 mmHg)
History of bariatric surgery (within the past 2 years)
HIV/AIDS
Ischemic heart disease
Malignant gestational trophoblastic disease
Malignant liver tumors and hepatocellular carcinoma of the liver
Ovarian cancer
Peripartum cardiomyopathy
Schistosomiasis with fibrosis of the liver
Sickle cell disease
Solid organ transplantation within the past 2 years
Stroke
Systemic lupus erythematosus
Thrombogenic mutations
Tuberculosis
Valvular heart disease (complicated)

Adapted from WHO Medical Eligibility Criteria for Contraceptive Use, 4th ed., 2010.

scientific evidence regarding contraceptive use is the same globally, and because the CDC worked with the WHO to develop their guidelines, the CDC accepted most of the WHO guidelines. Some of the WHO recommendations, however, were modified for use in the United States. The changes in classification are shown in Table 19.3 and a summary of the changes is listed in Table 19.4.

★ TIPS & TRICKS

The US MEC guidelines are designed to "assist healthcare providers when they

Table 19.3 US MEC: Changes in classifications from WHO MEC. WHO recommendations are in {brackets}. Consult the clarification column when available. Consult the website for further clarification (as listed in references)

Condition	COC/P/R	POP	DMPA	Implants	LNG-IUD	Cu-IUD	Clarification
Breast-feeding							
<1 mo postpartum {WHO: <6 wks postpartum}	3 {4}	2 {3}	2 {3}	2 {3}	—	—	The US Department of Health and Human Services recommend that infants be exclusively breast-fed during the first 4–6 months of life, preferably for a full 6 months and ideally, continue through the first year of life
1 mo to <6 mos {WHO: ≥6 wks to <6 mos postpartum}	2 {3}	—	—	—	—	—	
Postpartum (in breast-feeding or non-breast-feeding women)							
<10 min after delivery of the placenta {WHO: <48h, including insertion immediately after delivery of the placenta}	—	—	—	—	2 {1 if not breast-feeding and 3 if breast-feeding}	—	—
b. 10 min after delivery of the placenta to <4 wks {WHO: ≥48h to <4 wks}	—	—	—	—	2 {3}	2 {3}	—
DVT/PE							
History of DVT/PE, not on anticoagulant therapy							
Lower risk for recurrent DVT/PE (no risk factors)	3 {4}	—	—	—	—	—	—
Acute DVT/PE	—	2 {3}	2 {3}	2 {3}	2 {3}	2 {1}	—
Higher risk for recurrent DVT/PE (≥1 risk factors)	—	—	—	—	—	2 {1}	—

(Continued)

Table 19.3 *Continued*

Condition	COC/P/R	POP	DMPA	Implants	LNG-IUD	Cu-IUD	Clarification
Active cancer (metastatic, on therapy, or within 6 mos after clinical remission)							
Lower risk for recurrent DVT/PE (no risk factors)	3 {4}	—	—	—	—	2 {1}	Women on anticoagulant therapy are at risk for gynecologic complications: hemorrhagic ovarian cysts and severe menorrhagia. Hormonal contraceptive methods can be of benefit in preventing or treating these complications.
Valvular heart disease							
Complicated (pulmonary hypertension, risk for atrial fibrillation)	—	—	—	—	1 {2}	1 {2}	—
Ovarian cancer	—	—	—	—	1 {Initiation 3; Continuation 2}	1 {Initiation 3; Continuation 2}	—
Uterine fibroids	—	—	—	—	2 {1 if no uterine distortion and 4 if uterine distortion is present}	2 {1 if no uterine distortion and 4 if uterine distortion is present}	—

							Comments
History of bariatric surgery							
Restrictive procedures: (vertical banded gastroplasty, laparoscopic adjustable gastric band, laparoscopic sleeve gastrectomy)	1	1	1	1	1	1	—
Malabsorptive procedures: shortening the functional length of the small intestine	COCs: 3 P/R: 1	3	1	1	1	1	—
Peripartum cardiomyopathy							
Normal or mildly impaired cardiac function (NYHA functional class I/II)							
<6 mos	4	1	1	2	2	2	
≥6 mos	3	1	1	2	2	2	
Moderately or severely impaired cardiac function (NYHA functional class III/IV)	4	2	2	2	2	2	
Rheumatoid arthritis							
On immunosuppressive therapy	2	1	2/3	1	Initiation 2; Continuation 1	Initiation 2; Continuation 1	DMPA in women on long-term corticosteroid therapy with history of, or risk factors for, nontraumatic fractures is category 3. DMPA for women with rheumatoid arthritis is category 2.

(Continued)

Table 19.3 *Continued*

Condition	COC/P/R	POP	DMPA	Implants	LNG-IUD	Cu-IUD	Clarification
Not on immunosuppressive therapy	2	1	2	1	1	1	—
Endometrial hyperplasia	1	1	1	1	1	1	
IBD (ulcerative colitis, Crohn disease)	2/3	2	2	1	1	1	For women with mild IBD, with no other risk factors for VTE, COC/P/R use category 2. women with IBD with active or extensive disease, surgery, immobilization, corticosteroid use, vitamin deficiencies, fluid depletion), COC/P/R use is category 3.
Solid organ transplantation							
Complicated: graft failure (acute or chronic), rejection, cardiac allograft vasculopathy	4	2	2	2	Initiation 3; Continuation 2	Initiation 3; Continuation 2	
Uncomplicated	2	2	2	2	2	2	Women with Budd–Chiari syndrome should not use COC/P/R because of the increased risk for thrombosis.

COC, combined oral contraceptive; Cu-IUD, copper intrauterine device; DMPA, depot medroxyprogesterone acetate; DVT, deep venous thrombosis; IBD, inflammatory bowel disease; LNG-IUD, levonorgestrel-releasing intrauterine device; NYHA, New York Heart Association; P, combined hormonal contraceptive patch; PE, pulmonary embolism; POP, progestin-only pill; R, combined hormonal vaginal ring; VTE, venous thromboembolism.
Note: When a contraceptive method is used as a therapy, rather than solely to prevent pregnancy, the risk/benefit ratio may be different and should be considered on a case-by-case basis.

Table 19.4 Summary of changes to the US MEC

Condition/contraceptive method	US MEC change
Emergency contraceptive pills	History of bariatric surgery, rheumatoid arthritis, inflammatory bowel disease, and solid organ transplantation added and given a category 1
Barrier methods	History of bariatric surgery, peripartum cardiomyopathy, rheumatoid arthritis, endometrial hyperplasia, inflammatory bowel disease, and solid organ transplantation—barrier methods classified as category 1
Sterilization	In general, no medical conditions would absolutely restrict a person's eligibility for sterilization. Recommendations from the WHO MEC about specific settings and surgical procedures for sterilization are not included. The guidance has been replaced with general text on sterilization
Other deleted items	Guidance for combined injectables, levonorgestrel implants, and norethisterone enanthate removed because these methods are not currently available in the United States. Guidance for "blood pressure measurement unavailable" and "history of hypertension, where blood pressure CANNOT be evaluated (including hypertension in pregnancy)" is removed
Unintended pregnancy and increased health risk	The following conditions are added to the WHO list of conditions that expose a woman to increased risk as a result of unintended pregnancy: history of bariatric surgery within the past 2 years, peripartum cardiomyopathy, and receiving a solid organ transplant within 2 years

counsel women, men and couples about contraceptive methods. Although they should serve as a source of clinical guidance, healthcare providers should always consider the individual clinical circumstances of each person seeking family planning services."

Selected references

Criteria Committee of the New York Heart Association. Nomenclature and criteria for diagnosis of diseases of the heart and great vessels. 9th ed. Boston, MA: Little, Brown & Co; 1994.

Office on Women's Health, US Department of Health and Human Services. HHS blueprint for action on breastfeeding. Washington, DC: US Department of Health and Human Services, Office on Women's Health; 2000.

U.S. Medical Eligibility Criteria for Contraceptive Use (US MEC), 2010. Available from: http://www.cdc.gov/mmwr/preview/mmwrhtml/rr59e0528a1.htm

WHO. Medical eligibility criteria for contraceptive use, 4th ed. Geneva: World Health Organization; 2009. Available from: http://www.who.int/reproductivehealth/publications/family_planning/9789241563888/en/index.html

20

Hormonal Contraception and Mood

Andrea Rapkin[1] and Sarita Sonalkar[2]

[1]Department of Obstetrics and Gynecology, David Geffen School of Medicine at UCLA, Los Angeles, CA, USA
[2]Department of Obstetrics and Gynecology, Boston University School of Medicine, Boston, MA, USA

Introduction

Forty percent of reproductive-age women use some form of hormonal contraception, composed of ethinyl estradiol (EE) in combination with a synthetic progestin or containing a progestin alone, including the pill, patch, vaginal ring, injectable, implant, or intrauterine device. These hormonal treatments not only provide excellent fertility control, but also have noncontraceptive benefits including menstrual cycle regulation, treatment of dysmenorrhea, endometriosis, menorrhagia, acne, and severe premenstrual syndrome; they also lower the risk of developing endometrial and ovarian cancers. One of the major reasons cited for hormonal contraceptive discontinuation is the development of undesirable affective symptoms such as depression, irritability and anxiety. Although many women report adverse mood changes while using hormonal contraceptives, establishing causation between the exposure to the sex steroids in the contraceptives and negative mood is challenging.

Randomized controlled trials studying their effect on mood are limited, and outcomes are often conflicting.

This chapter summarizes the relevant evidence-based studies of the effects of hormonal contraceptives on mood and will discuss recommendations for women with and without affective disorders.

> ⋆ TIPS & TRICKS
>
> It is important to counsel patients regarding the potential psychological effects of hormonal contraception and to be aware of what the studies to date demonstrate in this regard.

Background

Mood disorders are common among reproductive-age women. Approximately 10–12% of women of reproductive age in the United States suffer from depression. The almost twofold higher incidence of depression in women as compared to men begins to emerge with puberty. Women are particularly vulnerable during times of hormonal fluctuation such as during the premenstrual phase of the menstrual cycle, the postpartum period, and during the climacteric. In contrast, after menopause, women tend to enjoy mood stabilization.

> EVIDENCE AT A GLANCE
>
> Notably, between 5% and 20% of ovulating women report significant interference with their daily activities because of mood symptoms associated with premenstrual dysphoric disorder (PMDD) or premenstrual syndrome (PMS).

Contraception, First Edition. Edited by Donna Shoupe.
© 2011 Blackwell Publishing Ltd. Published 2011 by Blackwell Publishing Ltd.

Given this association between mood disorders and times of hormonal variability, sex steroids provide a plausible explanation. Sex steroids modulate many of the relevant neurotransmitter systems in the brain. Progesterone and A-ring-reduced pregnane steroid metabolites of progesterone, also called neuroactive steroids, are vital for central nervous system (CNS) functioning, modulating the major inhibitory neurotransmitter system in the brain, γ-aminobutyric acid (GABA). Estrogen and progesterone also influence the opioid, serotonergic, and cholinergic neurotransmitter systems.

The neuroactive metabolites of progesterone, specifically allopregnanolone and pregnanolone, are synthesized in the ovary, adrenal gland, and brain. They have potent sedative and anxiolytic properties, similar to other GABA-active agents such as benzodiazepines, barbiturates, and ethanol. In women, concentrations of allopregnanolone increase after ovulation in the luteal phase of the menstrual cycle and with pregnancy, and decrease after menopause. CNS neuroactive steroid levels are decreased postpartum, and in rodent chronic stress models, such as social isolation and in depression.

Peripheral and brain allopregnanolone levels are clearly affected by the administration of exogenous sex steroids. In one study, the hormonal constituents of combined oral contraceptives (COCs) suppressed neurosteroids in the periphery and brain in rats and in the plasma of reproductive aged women. Synthetic progestins with or without estrogen have the ability to increase neurosteroids when administered to postmenopausal women. Similar to ethanol, the neuroactive steroids can have variable effects on mood, manifesting a U-shaped dose–response curve with the lower and higher concentrations of the GABA-active steroids having a sedative effect, and the moderate levels (approximating those seen in the luteal phase) increasing irritability and dysphoria. Exogenous progestins in hormonal contraceptives may alter mood and behavior by similar mechanisms.

The progestins used in hormonal contraceptives are a chemically diverse group of steroids. They can be divided into those related to progesterone: pregnanes and norpregnanes (medroxy-progesterone acetate, megesterol acetate, chlormadinone acetate, cyproterone acetate) and those related to testosterone: estranes and 13-ethyl gonanes. Estranes include norethindrone, norethindrone acetate, ethynodiol diacetate, norethinodrel, lynesterol, and tibilone; gonanes include levonorgestrel (LNG), desogestrel, norgestimate, dienogest, and gestodene. A separate class of progestin derived from spirolactone includes drospirenone (DRSP). DRSP is an analog of spirolactone that has both antimineralocorticoid and antiandrogenic properties, unlike the earlier generations of COCs formulated with the 19-nortestosterone-derived progestins that potentially have a range of androgen-like effects.

The COCs available in the United States contain estranes, gonanes or the spirolactone-derived progestagen; outside the United States, some COCs have pregnane constituents. As a class, progestins vary substantially in their biological effects, and the CNS effects of the different synthetic progestins and of progesterone are dependent on their individual chemical structure, binding capabilities, and metabolism.

Although endogenous estrogen and progesterone are at their lowest levels in the cycle during menses in normally cycling women, even lower serum levels of endogenous estrogen and progesterone are seen during the COC cycle and in the beginning of the pill-free week. This may have some effect on mood. Other proposed biochemical theories of hormone-mediated mood changes include progestin-mediated increase in monoamine oxidase (MAO) activity with resultant lowering of serotonin levels, estrogen-mediated inhibition of the MAO pathway, and estrogen-induced pyridoxine deficiency.

Effect of hormonal contraceptives on mood in women without mood disorders

Combined oral contraceptives

Oral contraceptives are the most widely used method of contraception in the United States. Approximately 30% of women using any method of contraception are using the COC pill. Despite this widespread use, only 68% continue to use the pill after 1 year. In a prospective study of 293 patients initiating or switching to a new COC,

28% discontinued use after 6 months. Of these patients, 5% cited mood changes as a reason for discontinuation.

Data from randomized controlled trials fail to support the assertion that COCs commonly cause adverse psychological symptoms. One randomized double-blind study of 462 women looked at the percentage of traditionally "hormone-related" side effects in a 6-month comparison of COC versus placebo pill users. Symptoms of emotional lability and physical symptoms of headache, nausea, breast pain, abdominal bloating, back pain, weight gain, and decreased libido were studied, and there were no differences in the incidence of these symptoms between the COC and placebo groups. Emotional lability was common in the COC group, and approached but did not reach statistical significance.

Depressive symptoms

EVIDENCE AT A GLANCE

- In a review of oral contraceptives and depression written by Gail Slap in 1981 9 of the 12 major studies reported an association between COCs and depressed mood, but only two studies showed that COC use clearly preceded depression.
- Common to all the studies of the psychological effects of COCs was a beneficial outcome: there was less variability in negative affect and less negative affect during menstruation in patients taking COCs.
- Many of these studies were retrospective cohort studies of never-users, past-users, and current users of oral contraceptives that assessed mood symptoms one to three times over the course of several months. In addition, these studies were all done before the major reduction of estrogen dosage in 1985.

More recent studies focusing on specific COC regimens have used a prospective design and have incorporated daily self-rating of symptoms. This methodology permits assessment of mood variability and identification of affective changes related to the menstrual cycle.

In a 2002 review of prospective, controlled studies of the effect of COCs on mood, four studies found no significant group differences in negative affect across the entire menstrual cycle, one study found that COC users reported less negative affect across the cycle, one study found higher negative affect throughout the cycle of a monophasic but not a triphasic COC, and two studies found that COC users experienced higher positive affect.

Affect variability refers to affective fluctuations on a moment-to-moment or day-to-day basis. Some studies have suggested that COC use is associated with less variability across the menstrual cycle. *Affect reactivity* refers to the magnitude of affective change in response to a specific experience. In a study of 107 students, COC users experienced a blunted affect response to a series of mood-induction procedures that elicited feelings of positive affect, jealousy, social ostracism, and parental feelings. In another large review, eight studies showed either no difference or improvement in mood, and three studies showed worsening of mood with COCs.

It is difficult to generalize across these studies on COCs and mood, as mood disturbance is not characterized in a standard way, and measurements used to assess mood vary. In addition, the formulations studied differed significantly.

A recent randomized controlled trial in adolescents treated with placebo pills reported types and quantities of side effects similar to those adolescents treated with COCs, with no difference in depressive symptoms between those treated with COCs and those treated with placebo; in fact there was a modest decrease in depression scores in both groups.

Progesterone as a contributor to mood symptoms

Many studies have focused on the role of the progestin as a contributor to dysphoric mood. Two studies showed worsening of mood with a higher progestin/estrogen ratio. One of these, by Akerlund *et al.* in 1993, compared two formulations of COCs, and found that a higher percentage (28%) of women taking 150 µg desogestrel/20 µg EE dropped out of the study due to mood changes, as compared to those in 150 µg desogestrel/30 µg

EE group. Another study by Graham in 2005 compared a COC containing 0.15 mg LNG with a progestin-only pill containing 0.03 µg LNG and found that the lower-dose progestin-only pill group had a reduction in depression.

Estrogen is less likely to be a contributing factor to these depressive symptoms, as clinical and preclinical studies have shown that estrogen alone has serotonin and mood enhancing effects. Given the potent effects of neuroactive steroids on mood, it was hypothesized that neurosteroid suppression could contribute to adverse mood in women.

In a prospective observational study of 35 women who were naive to COCs, Rapkin *et al* in 2006 measured levels of serum neuroactive steroids allopregnanolone, allotetrahydrodeoxycorticosterone, and dihydroepiandrosterone (DHEA) before and after a 3-month period of low-dose COC use. Mood and anxiety were assessed before and after the period of contraceptive use with validated assessment tools. Although a significant reduction in neuroactive steroids was seen over the 3-month period, no adverse psychological symptoms related to the COCs were noted.

Recommendations

EVIDENCE AT A GLANCE

On the basis of the limited work that has been done, it seems that COCs do not cause significant mood disturbances. Of course, any new mood symptoms that develop during the use of COCs should be fully evaluated. If there is any concern about an underlying mood disorder, evaluation by a mental health professional and judicious treatment is necessary. Patients with severe mood or behavioral changes, or suicidal ideation should have immediate mental health assessment in an emergency room, if necessary.

A lower progestin/estrogen ratio may improve mood in women who have negative mood symptoms with COCs. In addition, COCs may result in stabilization of affect variability over the pill cycle. It remains difficult to formulate evidence-based conclusions as there are few placebo-controlled trials, the doses and chemical compositions of the formulations of COCs differ, and the tools used to assess mood vary significantly.

Contraceptive patch and vaginal ring

There is no data specifically addressing the effects on mood of the nonoral combined contraceptive methods such as the transdermal patch or vaginal ring. However, given the similar mechanism of these methods to COCs, similar recommendations apply until further studies have been done.

Depot medroxyprogesterone acetate

The U.S. Food and Drug Administration (FDA) approved depot medroxyprogesterone acetate (DMPA) for contraceptive use in 1992. This injectable method provides excellent contraceptive efficacy for 3 months, and acts by altering the endometrial lining, thickening cervical mucus, and blocking the luteinizing hormone surge to prevent ovulation. Serum estradiol levels in DMPA users range from 10 to 92 pg/mL, and for one third of users, remain unchanged from early to mid follicular levels of 40–50 pg/mL. For most users, however, estradiol levels may vary, and may reach postmenopausal levels of <20 pg/mL. The progestin likely suppresses any vasomotor symptoms that may result from lower levels of estrogen. Serum concentrations of medroxyprogesterone acetate (MPA) vary among women but range from 1.5 to 3 ng/mL for the first few days after injection, gradually decline, and plateau at about 1.0 ng/mL for about 3 months and then decline further.

Since ovulation is inhibited, serum endogenous progesterone levels remain low (<0.4 ng/mL) for several months following an injection of DMPA, as published by Mishell in 1996. The current product labeling cautions against use in women with a history of "psychic depression," based on clinical data submitted to the FDA showing that 1.5% of 4200 users reported depression, and 0.5% discontinued use of DMPA for this reason. However studies supporting this advice are limited and conflicting.

In a study of 180 DMPA users (who had used DMPA from anywhere from 1 to 132 months) and 257 nonusers, DMPA users were more likely than nonusers to report depressive symptoms. In addition, discontinuers of DMPA were more likely to report depressive symptoms, with the highest proportion reporting these symptoms at their visit before discontinuation, and at their first discontinuation visit. The proportion of women with depressive symptoms decreased with each visit after discontinuation. *A causal relationship could not be evaluated from this data*. Proposed causes of this association include a pharmacologic effect of DMPA itself, or other factors that were associated with both an increased likelihood to use DMPA and an increase in depressive symptoms. Although the study controlled for age, ethnicity, education level, and history of depression, other variables that may be related to an increase risk of depression (such as stress, relationship conflict, and poverty) were not measured. Women with higher stress levels may be more likely to choose a more reliable and long-acting contraceptive such as DMPA.

Other studies did not show an association between DMPA and depressive symptoms. In a study of 393 women who chose to use DMPA for the first time, depressive symptoms were evaluated with a questionnaire and a "depressive symptom score" before initial administration of DMPA and 1 year later. Fifty-six percent of these women had discontinued the DMPA at the end of a year. However, in both continuers and discontinuers, there was no increase in depressive symptom scores over 12 months.

A 1995 study identified 80 DMPA users and interviewed them at two time periods: once during an interval of relatively high DMPA exposure (1 month after an injection) and once in an interval of low exposure (either immediately before a first injection, or before a scheduled reinjection). No association was found between depression and presumed DMPA exposure.

Finally, in a study comparing adolescents using DMPA and those using no hormonal contraception (controls), the well-validated Beck Depression Inventory was administered at baseline prior to DMPA administration, and at 3, 6, and 12 months after exposure. Although the adolescents who chose DMPA had higher depression scores at baseline, the mean Beck Depression Inventory score 12 months later did not differ significantly

from controls. In fact, users of DMPA showed an improvement in depression scores over the year.

Recommendations

> **EVIDENCE AT A GLANCE**
>
> - Most research has shown that DMPA does not increase depressive symptoms.
> - Studies earlier than those discussed above were limited by smaller sample sizes, lack of pretreatment information about depression, and lack of standardized measurement scales.

A history of depression is not a contraindication to DMPA use, but caution should be used when prescribing DMPA for a woman with current depression based on FDA labeling. Consultation with mental health personnel is prudent at the offset for these women, to ensure adequate mental health follow-up after DMPA administration.

Levonorgestrel intrauterine system

No research has been done specifically studying the effect on mood of the LNG intrauterine system (LNG-IUS). The package insert reports a clinical trial of the IUS in which 6.4% of 2339 women reported altered or depressed mood. Extrapolations of mood effects can be made by comparing serum levels with the LNG-IUS with other modes of delivery of LNG.

A 1986 study by Nilson *et al* of an intrauterine device (IUD) designed to release 20 μg/day of LNG showed that serum levels of LNG were 150–200 pg/mL within the first few weeks of use, with a gradual decline over time. The currently marketed LNG-IUS, as stated in the package insert, releases 20 μg of LNG per day and a stable serum concentration of 150–200 pg/mL occurs after the first week following insertion with concentrations after long-term use of 12, 24, and 60 months being 180 ± 66 pg/mL, 192 ± 140 pg/mL, and 159 ± 59 pg/mL, respectively.

Serum levels of LNG are higher with oral contraceptive pill use or with transdermal progestin implants. Studies of the six-rod LNG implant (now discontinued in the United States) have shown that mean serum concentrations can be as high as 900 pg/mL. Five case reports have described onset of major depression after insertion of the six-rod levonorgestel implant but prospective trials have not substantiated this association. A prospective trial of 910 women using these implants showed no increase in depression scores at 6 months after insertion.

Oral administration of a 150 µg LNG/30 µg EE COC yields serum concentrations of LNG of 2900 pg/mL after 1 hour and 500 pg/mL after 24 hours, according to Goebelsmann in a 1986 study, and most research has shown that this higher level of LNG does not cause mood symptoms.

Recommendations

Given that serum levels of LNG are low with the currently marketed LNG-IUS, it is unlikely that significant mood symptoms would occur with this method. However, additional studies need to be done to specifically address this issue.

★ TIPS & TRICKS

At this time, the IUS appears to be an excellent choice for women with mood symptoms using the COC, and it can be removed easily if such symptoms ensue.

Effect of hormonal contraceptives on mood in women with mood symptoms or disorders

PMDD and PMS

EVIDENCE AT A GLANCE

Premenstrual symptoms are common; most surveys have found that as many as 85% of menstruating women report one or more premenstrual symptoms. However, severe symptoms that meet the American Congress of Obstetricians and Gynecologists (ACOG) criteria for PMS are much less common, occurring in 13–20% of women. PMDD is even less prevalent, affecting approximately 3–8% of reproductive-age women.

The criteria for PMDD are much more specific and stringent than for PMS. A diagnosis of PMDD requires the presence of five or more severe premenstrual symptoms present during the last week of the luteal phase and at least one of the symptoms must be a core mood symptom (anxiety, irritability, mood swings, or depression). For the American Psychiatric Association DSM-IV diagnosis of PMDD, the symptoms must markedly interfere with work, school, social activities, and relationships with others. The degree of social and role impairment and lowered quality of life in women with PMDD is similar to that of dysthymia and only slightly lower than major depressive disorder.

The premenstrual symptoms are triggered by ovulation and may be related to fluctuations in gonadal hormones, particularly progesterone, during the luteal phase of the menstrual cycle. Since COCs replace the fluctuating levels of endogenous ovarian steroids with more stable levels of exogenous hormones, they have been used in an attempt to reduce premenstrual symptoms.

However, in two randomized controlled trials studying this treatment for PMS, no significant improvement in symptoms was noted in the COC group compared with placebo. Formulations used included 35 µg EE with 0.5 mg, 1.0 mg, and 0.5 mg norethindrone in a 1992 trial by Graham et al., and 30 µg EE with 3 mg drosperinone in a 21–7 formulation in a 2001 trial by Freeman et al.

The mechanism underlying these residual symptoms remains unclear but it has been suggested that PMS-like symptoms may accrue from the following mechanisms:

- Adverse central and/or peripheral effects of the hormonal constituents of the COCs.
- Exposure to and/or withdrawal from endogenous sex steroids in predisposed women.
- Exposure to and/or withdrawal from the exogenous steroids comprising the COCs.

A 1987 publication by Bancroft et al. showed that among women with PMS symptoms before taking COCs, triphasic preparations had more negative mood changes as compared with monophasic preparations, both of which contained L-norgestrel. Another study found that a monophasic pill containing EE and desogestrel and both monophasic and triphasic pills containing EE and LNG had beneficial effects on PMS symptoms, but these effects only lasted for three of the four cycles studied by Backstrom *et al* (1992).

In a 2003 case-control study, previous depression was shown to be a predictor of premenstrual mood deterioration in women taking COCs. Of 658 women who had previously used COCs, 16.3% reported premenstrual mood improvement, and 12.3% reported mood deterioration with COC use. However, of the 71 women with a history of depression, premenstrual mood deteriorated in 25.4%.

In a 2005 open-label, head-to-head 6-cycle study by Sangthawan et al., women receiving DRSP 3 mg/EE 30 µg in a 21–7 formulation showed an approximately 50% decrease from their baseline level of premenstrual symptoms including water retention, weight gain, irritability, anxiety, and feeling blue, whereas the comparison group receiving LNG/EE experienced no changes in their premenstrual symptoms. DRSP 3 mg/EE 30 µg was more effective in a regimen extended for 42–126 days compared in another open-label study, with a standard cyclic 21–7 regimen, by Sillem et al. in 2003.

Trials studying a newer formulation of EE 20 µg and DRSP 3 mg in a 24–4 (24 active pills followed by 4 placebo pills) formulation have shown great promise in the treatment of PMDD. In a double-blinded, randomized, placebo-controlled study comparing Yaz to placebo in women with PMDD, the Daily Record of Severity of Problems scale was used to assess women's symptoms. A 50% decrease in daily symptom scores occurred in 48% of the active treatment group, and 36% of the placebo group. A crossover trial had similar findings, with the response corresponding to a number-needed-to-treat of eight patients.

Recommendations

In general, most COC formulations do not influence premenstrual mood, although a history of depression may predispose to worsening premenstrual symptoms, and monophasic preparations are preferred.

A 24–4 regimen of 3 mg DRSP/20 µg EE is recommended for the treatment of PMDD in women desiring hormonal contraception. The 24–4 regimen with 3 mg DRSP/20 µg EE has been approved by the U.S. FDA for this purpose.

It is unclear which PMDD symptoms respond better to this COC compared with the other FDA approved treatment for PMDD—the selective serotonin reuptake inhibitors (SSRIs). Whether the combination of this COC and an SSRI will improve treatment outcome, either increasing number of responders or the magnitude of response, is unknown, but there are no significant metabolic interactions between the two classes of drug.

This COC will likely be prescribed off label for women with the whole range of PMS symptoms, mild to severe, and studies should be completed in this group of women. Additional possibilities for the treatment of resistant symptoms of PMS or PMDD could include other more extended regimens for DRSP/EE with brief respite of 3–4 days every 3 months, or with no break at all.

Major depressive disorder

EVIDENCE AT A GLANCE

The lifetime rate of major depression is 7.4 in 100 women, and the annual rate for depressive symptoms (both men and women) is 3/100 persons. As the underlying basis of the relationship between depression and sex steroids has not been elucidated, it is unclear whether the various exogenous estrogen and progestins in COCs have a differential effect on women with underlying mood disorders.

A major depressive syndrome or episode by DSM-IV definition manifests with five or more of the following symptoms, present most of the day nearly every day for a minimum of two consecutive weeks, with at least one symptom being either depressed mood or loss of interest or pleasure. Symptoms include depressed mood, loss of interest or pleasure in most or all activities, insomnia or hypersomnia, change in appetite or weight, psychomotor retardation or agitation, low energy, poor concentration, thoughts of worthlessness or guilt, or recurrent thoughts about death or suicide.

One study of the effects of hormonal contraception on women with major depressive disorder (MDD) was done through a subanalysis of a larger study, the Sequenced Treatment Alternatives to Relieve Depression (STAR*D). The study population comprised women younger than 40 years of age on COC, progestin-only contraception, or no contraception. Women in the COC group manifested a decline in the severity of depression and better physical functioning, as well as less obsessive-compulsive behavior. Women in both hormone groups were more likely to show hypersomnia compared to the nonhormone group. Women in the progestin-only group were significantly more likely to show weight gain and gastrointestinal symptoms but not mood symptoms. Although the study was limited by its exploratory design, there was no evidence that any of the hormone treatments worsened depressive symptoms.

Another study, by Joffe et al. in 2007, evaluated a group of 25 women with depression who were successfully treated with antidepressants except during the luteal phase of the menstrual cycle. Women were given EE 30 mg/day plus DRSP 3 mg/day for 21 days and then randomly assigned to double-blinded treatment with EE 30 µg/day or placebo for days 22–28 of two study cycles. Statistically significant improvement in depression scores was seen in both groups and there were no differences between the two groups.

Recommendations

> ⭒ TIPS & TRICKS
>
> Oral contraceptives can be used safely in women with major depressive disorder (MDD). Some women with MDD may have additional premenstrual symptom control from use of a DRSP-containing oral contraceptive.

Postpartum depression

> ⭒ TIPS & TRICKS
>
> Women have an increased frequency of all types of psychiatric illness in the postpartum period. Three types of puerperal disorders have been described: postpartum blues, postpartum depression, and postpartum psychosis.

- Most women experience *postpartum blues* in the early postpartum period, with symptoms peaking at approximately the fifth postpartum day, and rapidly diminishing afterward. This syndrome may represent normal variation of emotional changes after delivery and may be caused by fluctuation in hormone levels. Supportive care is all that is usually needed for treatment.
- *Postpartum depression* affects approximately 13% of women. Criteria for postpartum depression are the same as for major depression but occur in the postpartum period. Although the DSM-IV requires that symptoms of major depression with postpartum onset begin within 4 weeks of childbirth, research suggests that episodes of depression are common up to 1 year after delivery. The etiology of postpartum depression is not fully understood, although biochemical, sociocultural, and biopsychosocial causes have been proposed. A hormonal basis has been hypothesized as well, given the sudden and substantial fluctuation in progesterone, estrogen, cortisol, and β-endorphin levels in the postpartum period.
- *Postpartum psychosis* is a severe psychotic syndrome, occurring after 1–4 of every 1000 deliveries. The cause of psychosis is unknown but has been proposed to be related to low estrogen levels precipitating supersensitization of dopamine receptors.

Two randomized controlled trials have been conducted investigating the effect of contraceptive doses of hormones in postpartum depression. In one trial by Lawrie in 1998, 180 women received a single 200 mg dose of the synthetic progestogen norethistrone enanthate (also known as norethindrone enanthate, a bimonthly progestin-only contraceptive not available in the United States) or placebo within 48 hours of delivery. Participants were not selected based on increased risk of having or developing postpartum depression. Women receiving the norethisterone enanthate injection were more likely to report minor/major depressive symptoms at 6 weeks postpartum compared to those receiving placebo, although mean depression scores remained below the criteria for major or minor depression. At 12 weeks postpartum, no significant differences were seen.

In a noncontraceptive hormone treatment study by Gregoire et al. in 1996, 61 women with postpartum depression were randomized to 12 weeks of 200 μg of daily transdermal 17-β-estradiol followed by 12 weeks of added cyclical dydrogesterone 10 mg 12 days/month or placebo. Women in the estrogen group had a significant decrease in mean depression scores as compared to placebo at 4 and 12 weeks postpartum Although these findings were encouraging, there were some methodological limitations with the study, including significant attrition rate (27%), increased number of women in the estrogen group using concurrent SSRIs, and increased length of time of depression in women in the placebo group.

Recommendations

Results of these studies should be interpreted carefully within each clinical situation. The one study evaluating the relationship between hormonal contraception and postpartum depression showed that the 2-month norethindrone enanthate injection may have a negative effect on mood in the postpartum period. It is unclear if the 3-month DMPA formulation has the same effect as norethisterone enanthate on mood in the postpartum period.

☆ TIPS & TRICKS

- Given the convenience, efficacy, and safety profile of DMPA, it is still an excellent option for postpartum women, as long as appropriate counseling and precautions are given.
- There is no current evidence recommending for or against other hormonal methods with regard to postpartum depression.

Regarding estrogen in the prevention of postpartum depression, additional studies are needed before recommendation can be made for this therapy. In addition, the prothrombotic effects of estrogen should be kept in mind, and estrogen should be used with caution in the postpartum period.

Other psychiatric disorders

Data regarding hormonal contraception in women with other mood disorders including anxiety, bipolar disorder, and schizophrenia are sparse, but some extrapolations and recommendations can be made.

Schizophrenia

Schizophrenia and other psychoses have been hypothesized to be related to estrogen deficiency in some women from as early as 1909, and estrogens may exert a protective effect in the development of schizophrenia. In a study of 125 schizophrenic women with regular menses, significant improvements in psychotic scores, but not depressive scores, were seen with the higher estrogen levels in the luteal phase in a study by Bergemann et al. in 2007.

Life cycle studies have shown that women are more likely to have either a first episode or a relapse of existing illness during the postpartum period and during menopause, during times of decreased estrogen. In contrast, chronic psychoses and psychotic relapse rates tend to improve during pregnancy, when estrogen plasma levels are high.

In a randomized controlled double-blinded trial by Kulkarni et al. in 2001, 102 women with schizophrenia, schizoaffective disorder, or schizoform disorder were given transdermal estrogen or placebo for 28 days. Women in the estrogen group had statistically significantly improved psychosis scores over time.

☆ TIPS & TRICKS

Given these findings, we can extrapolate that estrogen-containing contraceptives do not adversely affect symptoms in schizophrenia and may even improve them. However, women with schizophrenia are more likely to have problems with compliance with a daily oral contraceptive regimen, so COCs are not ideal as compared with long-acting methods, for which there is no data.

Bipolar disorder

Minimal research has been undertaken on hormonal contraception for women with bipolar disorder. Bipolar disorder briefly is defined as a clinical course characterized by the occurrence of one or more manic or hypomanic episodes, as well as one or more major depressive episodes.

A 2009 cross-sectional study by Vieira et al. looked at the prevalence of women using contraception in a group of 139 patients with bipolar disorder. Forty percent of women in this group were not using any contraceptive method, and this proportion was similar in those women using lithium, a known teratogen. No associations were found with hormonal contraception and symptom or illness severity.

These findings underscore the need for effective contraception in this group, and the limited research shows no contraindication to hormonal methods.

Anxiety and panic disorder

No studies addressing these populations could be found.

Conclusions

> ### ☆ TIPS & TRICKS
>
> Contemporary studies of hormonal contraception show a favorable profile with regard to affective side effects in asymptomatic women and those with mood and other psychiatric disorders. All reversible contraceptive methods carry a World Health Organization category 1 classification for medical eligibility for depressive disorders, meaning that there is no restriction for the use of the contraceptive method.

Further studies are certainly necessary, but at this time, there are no contraindications to combined or progestin-only hormonal contraceptives in women with mood disorders. However, if there is any concern about exacerbation of underlying mood disorder or emergence of significant depression, anxiety or irritability during the course of treatment, explicit evaluation and management is necessary. In most settings, the hormonal contraceptive will be changed or discontinued. The risks of unplanned pregnancy must be balanced against the benefits of hormonal contraceptive continuation combined with pharmacologic or psychological treatment of the mood symptoms or disorder.

Selected references

Andreen L, Nyberg S, Turkmen S, van Wingen G, Fernandez G, Backstrom T. Sex steroid induced negative mood may be explained by the paradoxical effect mediated by GABA-A modulators. Psychoneuroendocrinology 2009;34(8): 1121–32.

Birzniece V, Backstrom T, Johoansson IM, et al. Neuroactive steroid effects on cognitive functions with a focus on the serotonin and GABA systems. Brain Res Rev 2006;51(2): 212–39.

Civic D, Scholes D, Ichikawa L, et al. Depressive symptoms in users and non-users of depot medroxyprogesterone acetate. Contraception 2000;61(6):385–90.

Gupta N, O'Brien R, Jacobsen LB, et al. Mood changes in adolescents using depot-medroxyprogesterone acetate for contraception: a prospective study. J Pediatr Adolesc Gynecol 2001; 14(2):71–6.

Jarva JA, Oinonen KA. Do oral contraceptives act as mood stabilizers? Evidence of positive affect stabilization. Arch Womens Ment Health 2007;10(5):225–34.

Joffe H, Cohen LS, Harlow BL. Impact of oral contraceptive pill use on premenstrual mood: Predictors of improvement and deterioration. Am J Obstet Gynecol 2003;189(6):1523–30.

Kahn L, Halbreich U. Oral contraceptives and mood. Expert Opin Pharmacother 2001;2(9): 1367–82.

Magalhaes PV, Kapczinski F, Kauer-Sant'Anna M. Use of contraceptive methods among women treated for bipolar disorder. Arch Womens Ment Health 2009;12(3):183–5.

O'Connell K, Davis AR, Kerns J. Oral contraceptives: side effects and depression in adolescent girls. Contraception 2007;75(4):299–304.

Oinonen, KA, Mazmanian D. To what extent do oral contraceptives influence mood and affect? J Affect Disord 2002;70:229–40.

Pearlstein TB, Bachmann GA, Zacur HA, Yonkers KA. Treatment of premenstrual dysphoric disorder with a new drospirenone-containing oral contraceptive formulation. Contraception 2005;72(6):414–21.

Rapkin AJ, Biggio G, Concas A. Oral contraceptives and neuroactive steroids. Pharmacol Biochem Behav 2006;84(4):628–34.

Redmond G, Godwin AJ, Olson W, Lippman JS. Use of placebo controls in an oral contraceptive trial: methodological issues and adverse event incidence. Contraception 1999;60:81–5.

Rosenberg M, Waugh M. Oral contraceptive discontinuation: a prospective evaluation of frequency and reasons. Am J Obstet Gynecol 1998;179(3):577–82.

Stanczyk FK. All progestins are not created equal. Steroids 2003;68:879–90.

Westhoff C, Truman C, Kalmuss D, et al. Depressive symptoms and Depo-Provera. Contraception 1998;57(4):237–40.

Westhoff C, Wieland D, Tiezzi L. Depression in users of depo-medroxyprogesterone acetate. Contraception 1995;51(6):351–4.

Westhoff C, Truman C, Kalmuss D, et al. Depressive symptoms and Norplant contraceptive implants. Contraception 1998;57(4):241–5.

Yonkers KA, Brown C, Pearlstein TB, Foegh M, Sampson-Landers C, Rapkin A. Efficacy of a new low-dose oral contraceptive with drospirenone in premenstrual dysphoric disorder. Obstet Gynecol 2005;106(3):492–501.

Young EA, Kornstein SG, Harvey AT, et al. Influences of hormone-based contraception on depressive symptoms in premenopausal women with major depression. Psychoneuroendocrinology 2007;32(7):843–53.

21

Contraception in Women with Abnormal Uterine Bleeding

Ian S. Fraser

Department of Obstetrics, Gynaecology and Neonatology, Queen Elizabeth II Research Institute for Mothers and Infants, University of Sydney, NSW, Australia

Introduction

Abnormal uterine bleeding (AUB) is one of the commonest gynecological symptoms presenting both to family practitioners and to specialists. For women in the reproductive age who are seeking treatment for AUB, many healthcare providers will look to one of the contraceptive options in order both to treat the bleeding problem and to supply contraceptive protection.

The approach to management in this situation requires attention to some basic principles and necessitates several steps. The first and most important step is close attention to the description of the bleeding problems, followed by assessment and diagnosis of the cause underlying abnormal bleeding (see algorithm in Fig. 21.1).

The timing and nature of each abnormal bleeding symptom and the range of underlying causes may have significant influence on the choice of suitable contraception. Malignancy or premalignancy should be ruled out in women with long-standing or persistent AUB. Many contraceptive methods can be expected to have a beneficial impact on pre-existing AUB, but this direct beneficial effect needs to be balanced against the tendency of some methods to cause other types of bleeding problems.

Combined oral contraceptive pills (OCs) and the levonorgestrel-releasing intrauterine system (LGN-IUS) will provide a substantial beneficial effect in reducing menstrual blood loss in most women with heavy menstrual bleeding (HMB).

Bleeding patterns are predictable with both of these methods, although on occasion abnormal bleeding may continue or worsen.

The other progestogen-only methods (e.g., "minipills," injectables, and subdermal implants) may reduce menstrual blood loss in women with HMB but frequently convert the bleeding patterns into unpredictable episodes of light bleeding or spotting, or more rarely prolonged or frequent bleeding. Continued use of the injectable progestin is associated with improved bleeding control.

The potential impact of transdermal and intravaginal delivery of hormonal estrogen–progestogen combinations on AUB have not been formally tested, although they could be expected to have beneficial effects.

Need for uniform terminology

It has become clear that there is considerable international confusion in the definitions and usage of many terminologies relating to AUB, and an international group has made initial recommendations on simplification and tightening of these terminologies. In particular, the group has recommended that the most confusing terms (menorrhagia, metrorrhagia, and dysfunctional uterine bleeding) be discarded and replaced with simpler terms describing volume, duration, regularity, and frequency, which professionals and patients alike can understand (Table 21.1).

Presentation of patient

AUB 'complaint' with contraceptive need

Assessment of the symptom of AUB

Investigation, diagnosis and precise assessment of underlying cause

Blood count, including platelets, ferritin, transvaginal ultrasound scan

± sonohysterogram (± hysteroscopy, biopsy, curettage)

Others if indicated – e.g. coagulation screen

Consideration of structural or non-structural underlying

reproductive tract causes

Presentation of contraceptive options to patient

And/or surgical options

Figure 21.1 Algorithm for the initial assessment and management of the patient with abnormal uterine bleeding.

Table 21.1 Currently recommended terminology for description of menstrual bleeding

Clinical dimensions of menstruation and menstrual cycle	Recommended terminology	Normal limits (5th to 95th percentiles)[a]
Volume of monthly blood loss (mL)		
Heavy	Heavy menstrual bleeding (HMB)	>80
Normal		5–80
Light		<5
Duration of flow (days)		
Prolonged	Prolonged menstrual bleeding	>8.0
Normal		4.5–8.0
Shortened		<4.5
Regularity of menses, cycle to cycle variation over 12 months (days)		
Absent variations		1–2
Regular variations	Regular menstrual bleeding	Variation ±2–20
Irregular variations		Variation >20
Frequency of cycles (days)		
Frequent		<24
Normal		24–38
Infrequent	Infrequent menstrual cycles	>38

[a] It is recommended that definitions of normality or abnormality for all these parameters be based on published population data (of general populations) and the limits be related to the median and 5th–95th centiles (see Fraser et al., 2007 for detailed discussion).

Abnormal uterine bleeding (AUB) is nowadays regarded as the overarching symptom to describe any significant departure from normal menstrual bleeding or from the normal menstrual cycle.

- Terms like "menorrhagia", "metrorrhagia," and "dysfunctional uterine bleeding" are defined so differently in different parts of the world (and often not defined at all!), that it is recommended, in the interests of accurate international communication, at both clinical and scientific levels, that these terms be abandoned. They should be replaced by simple terms, as shown in Table 21.1. Further thorough discussion of the background of these recommendations is provided in Fraser et al. (2007) and Woolcock et al. (2009).
- "Dysfunctional uterine bleeding" (DUB) has previously been used to describe a range of conditions where there is no evidence of a structural lesion of the reproductive tract, and the cause is presumed to be "molecular." There is much evidence to confirm that disturbances of such molecular systems do occur within the endometrium, within the hypothalamic-pituitary–ovarian (HPO), system and as systemic coagulopathies. The means now exist to separate these at a research level, although this is not usually clinically required.
- In clinical situations the assessment of heavy menstrual bleeding (HMB) has to be made on the basis of carefully elicited clinical "complaint." HMB is therefore defined as excessive menstrual blood loss, which interferes with a woman's physical, social, emotional, and/or material quality of life. It can occur alone or in combination with other symptoms; see the U.K. National Institute for Health and Clinical Excellence (NICE) guidelines, 2007.

- Intermenstrual bleeding (IMB) is regarded as bleeding between otherwise reasonably normal menstrual periods.
- Amenorrhea and oligomenorrhea are terms which should remain because their definitions of absent or very infrequent cycles (longer than 6 weeks) are uniformly accepted.
- The terms 'menstruation/ menses/cycles' are almost universally agreed.

Adapted from Fraser et al., (2007).

There is a very limited published literature on intermenstrual bleeding (IMB) and postcoital bleeding (PCB), except with regard to techniques used to accurately exclude underlying malignancy. Additionally, the existing literature on IMB and PCB overlaps in a confusing manner with the literature on unscheduled (or "breakthrough") bleeding in women using hormonal contraception or other hormonal therapies. By contrast, there is a much more comprehensive and focused literature on HMB, even though the confusion of terminologies persists.

Types of abnormal uterine bleeding symptoms

- *HMB* is one of the most common complaints (Table 21.2).
- *Prolonged bleeding* presents at a rate of about 1 in 10 cases of HMB, and many cases of prolonged bleeding are also heavy (HPMB).
- *Excessively frequent menstruation* is rare (<1% of all cases of AUB).
- *Irregular bleeding* (sometimes variably frequent) is common, especially in adolescence and the menopause transition.
- *IMB* is a specific and common type of irregular bleeding; it is usually defined as erratic bleeding, often light in volume, occurring between otherwise fairly normal periods.
- IMB may occur in women experiencing PCB.
- Occasionally, bleeding may be completely *erratic or acyclic.*

All these different bleeding symptoms need individual attention for diagnosis prior to start-

Table 21.2 Different types of abnormal uterine bleeding and their symptoms

		Causes	
	Comment	Structural[a]	Nonstructural[b]
AUB	Overarching term		
HMB	Commonest symptom	Leiomyomas	Endometrial causes
Prolonged ± HMB	10–20% of HMB	(Adenomyosis (moderate to severe) Endometrial polyps, submucous myoma, or enlarged cavity from intramural myomas	HPO causes (ovulatory DUB) Disorders of hemostasis
Frequent menses	Rare	None known	Presumed primary HPO disturbance
IMB ± PCB	Fairly common	Surface lesions: endometrial polyps, intramural submucous myomas Cervical ectropion or polyps, cervicitis Cervical or endometrial cancer	–
Irregular menses	Common in adolescence; perimenopause; PCOS		Primary HPO disturbance

AUB, abnormal uterine bleeding; DUB, dysfunctional uterine bleeding; HMB, heavy menstrual bleeding; HPO, hypothalamic–pituitary–ovarian; IMB, intermenstrual bleeding; PCB, postcoital bleeding; PCOS, polycystic ovary syndrome.
[a] Structural causes are those causes where there is a recognizable structural lesion within the reproductive tract.
[b] Nonstructural causes are those causes where there is a presumed disturbance of the molecular systems responsible for controlling endometrial, HPO, or coagulatory function.

ing specific contraception. Condoms may need to be recommended for contraceptive protection while diagnosis of the underlying cause is being pursued.

Underlying causes of HMB and HPMB

Structural pelvic causes

As a group, structural pelvic anomalies are a common cause of HMB, and sometimes several structural causes may coexist. Typically, structural pelvic lesions will result in IMB, PCB, or heavy cyclic bleeding.

Uterine leiomyomas (fibroids)

Fibroids are the commonest structural pelvic cause of HMB. Submucous myomas cause the heaviest bleeding and surgical removal before starting specific contraceptive methods is often considered. Intramural and subserous myomas rarely require removal before initiating hormonal methods, but may in individual cases, especially if there has been persistent bleeding despite previous contraceptive use.

Adenomyosis

Adenomyosis is a poorly understood, benign gynecological condition that may not be associated with symptoms in mild forms. Moderate to severe cases often result in HMB and menstrual pain. Adenomyosis may coincide with other potentially symptomatic conditions such as fibroids, endometrial polyps, or endometriosis.

Endometriosis

Endometriosis is often associated with HMB and is typically associated with pre- and postmenstrual spotting. No current noninvasive test yet exists for definite diagnosis of this condition, although biomarkers are being pursued.

Endometrial polyps

Endometrial polyps are also mysterious, but are they are very common benign intrauterine or intracervical lesions, whose pathophysiology is currently unexplained. They typically cause erratic and variably heavy IMB or spotting, and may cause HMB.

Endometrial hyperplasia

Endometrial hyperplasia is typically the end result of excessive anovulatory endometrial proliferation. Establishing the degree of severity of the lesion prior to initiating a specific contraceptive method is advised. Endometrial hyperplasia with atypia is managed as a premalignant lesion.

Nonstructural causes

- endometrial molecular disturbances (submicroscopic aspects of disease)
- hypothalamic–pituitary–ovarian causes (H-P-O; pathophysiologic disturbances around menarche and the menopause transition; polycystic ovaries, chronic anovulation)
- disorders of hemostasis ("coagulopathies").

The endometrial and H-P-O causes of abnormal uterine bleeding are not well understood but there continues to be extensive investigation into a range of molecular causes (submicroscopic aspects of disease) underlying these symptoms. The molecular causes so far described are many and complex, but they are not amenable to routine assessment in clinical practice. Fortunately, many of these women will respond well to hormonal therapies geared to suppressing the endometrium, no matter which of the underlying molecular systems is primarily involved.

Investigations prior to starting contraception

These investigations need to be individualized, depending on symptoms and prior investigations, and may include the following:

- Menstrual history and characteristics of current bleeding describing volume, duration, regularity, and frequency
- Accompanying symptoms or problems
- Health history and medications
- Physical examination, vital signs, pelvic examination, Pap smear, and/or endometrial biopsy (if indicated)
- Transvaginal ultrasound ± sonohysterogram
- Laboratory tests: full blood count including platelets, pregnancy test, serum ferritin or iron studies, metabolic panel, clotting panel
- Hysteroscopy, D&C; and colposcopy ± biopsy (if there is evidence of cervical anomaly).

> ☆ **TIPS & TRICKS**
>
> General principle of all investigations:
> 1. General health assessment
> 2. Transvaginal ultrasound imaging
> 3. Direct visualization /palpation of any lesion
> 4. Tissue diagnosis, if required

These investigations will usually be negative in women with one of the nonstructural causes of HMB or other AUB. If bleeding appears to be truly excessive or long-standing, a coagulation screen may be warranted. Rarely, other investigations may be indicated to rule out unusual causes or a specialist consultation may be indicated.

Contraceptive choices for women with AUB

There is now a large body of good quality evidence to assist physicians in making recommendations to women with AUB who require contraception (Table 21.3). This evidence is comprehensively presented in the publications of the U.K. National Institute for Health and Clinical Excellence and the excellent systematic reviews of the Cochrane Collaboration. An excellent systematic review by Kaunitz et al.

Table 21.3 Use of different contraceptive methods in women with HMB

Cause of HMB	Surgery 1st line	LNG-IUS	COC	DMPA	Oral P minipill
Structural					
Uterine leiomyomas (fibroids)					
subserous	–	+++	+++	++	–
intramural	+	+++	++	++	–
submucous	+++	+	+	+	–
Adenomyosis	+	+++	+	+	–
Endometriosis	++	++	++	++	–
Endometrial polyps	+++	++	+	+	–
Endometrial hyperplasia: (only with endometrial biopsy monitoring)					
simple benign	Diagnosis only	+++	++	+	+
adenomatous/complex		+++	+		–
with nuclear atypia		++	–		–
arteriovenous malformation		+	+++	+	–
Nonstructural					
Endometrial molecular causes	–	+++	+++	+	+
HPO causes	–	+++	++	+	+
Disorders of hemostasis	–	+++	++	+	–

+++, recommended strongly; ++, a reasonable alternative, "worth a try"; +, may be considered, but may be ineffective or cause side effect (usually unscheduled or breakthrough bleeding), works well in some; -, not first line, little or no evidence, anecdotal evidence.

(2009) also provides sound advice (see "Selected references").

Contraceptive options for women with HMB/HPMB

Fortunately most women with nonstructural causes of AUB, and many with structural change (where malignancies are excluded and surgical options are declined), will respond well to hormonal therapies geared at suppressing the endometrium.

The primary options for these women are the hormonal contraceptives. The most extensive evidence is available on the use of the LNG-IUS for HMB and HPMB.

LNG-IUS (Mirena, Bayer Schering Pharma)

This is widely recommended as the first choice therapy for medical management of HMB in those women for whom it is deemed suitable (see Chapter 9).

★ **TIPS & TRICKS**

The average patient with HMB can expect an 80–90% reduction in menstrual blood loss after placement of a LNG-IUS.

There is now considerable published evidence to support LNG-IUS use in many situations where HMB is a complaint. This therapy seems able to effectively reduce measured menstrual blood loss in most women with HMB no matter what the underlying cause. This includes adenomyosis, coagulopathies, benign endometrial hyperplasias and intramural and subserous myomas. It may also prevent endometrial polyp recurrence.

Combined oral contraceptives

One of the well-known noncontraceptive benefits of combined oral contraceptives (COCs) is control of bleeding and a reduction in menstrual cramps (see Chapter 3). COCs reduce the overall incidence of bleeding problems by about 50% from what occurs in non-pill-users. Bleeding days, amount of blood loss, IMB and breakthrough bleeding is decreased in COC users in general.

There is increasing evidence to support use of monophasic ethinyl estradiol-based COCs or the new estradiol-based COC for management of HMB.

- Objective measurements of menstrual blood loss during treatment are currently limited, but users of a monophasic 30μg COC can expect a 35 to 40% reduction in blood loss.
- Preliminary data indicate that the new estradiol-based COC will reduce measured loss by over 70%.

The package insert of the 20-μg COC with 24 active pills (ethinyl estradiol plus norethindrone acetate) followed by 4 days (iron only) pill is associated with a 1–1.5 day menses blood/month. It is marketed as "an effective low-dose birth control pill that can give you shorter, lighter periods"

Intramuscular injections of depot medroxyprogesterone acetate (DMPA)

DMPA will often initially cause infrequent, light bleeding in most women whether or not they initially experienced HMB. With continued use, 50% of women have amenorrhea at 1 year of use and by 2 years of use, 80% of women will have amenorrhea (see Chapter 8). Many women with HMB do not take favorably to the occurrence of erratic and sometimes prolonged light bleeding, which many women starting DMPA initially experience or to the requirement of periodic visits for injections.

Progestogen-releasing subdermal implants

Implants also reduce menstrual bleeding in most women with HMB (according to very limited data), but again, these women may experience episodes of prolonged or frequent light bleeding, especially during the initial 'settling in' period. Since the pattern of bleeding that these women will experience cannot be predicted, this method

is regarded as second line contraceptives for women with HMB or IMB.

Oral high-dose progestogens

Oral progestogens may be very suitable therapies for HMB and HPMB, but are particularly suitable for those women with anovulatory or disturbed ovulatory cycles, however they should always be treated with 'long-cycle' therapy, where the progestogen is given for at least three weeks out of four. These long-cycle regimens will also work well for ovulatory women. Shorter cycles of therapy (eg. ten days per month) are no better than placebo. The contraceptive efficacy of these regimens has not been formally tested. Extensive data clearly indicate that the LNG-IUS is a preferable means of delivering contraceptive progestogen for HMB.

Other methods

Two other effective methods of HMB treatment exist: the antifibrinolytic agent, tranexamic acid, and nonsteroidal anti-inflammatory agents (NSAIDs) such as mefenamic acid, naproxen, and ibuprofen. These methods are not contraceptives, but they are effective at reducing menstrual blood loss in most women. Hence, they may be considered as an adjunct for contraceptive methods which do not have the intrinsic capacity to reduce HMB on their own (see below).

Transdermal and intravaginal combined estrogen–progestogen methods

These combined methods may also be effective in reducing menstrual bleeding, but substantive data do not yet exist.

Contraceptive options for women with IMB and PCB

Very limited data exist for guiding the selection of contraceptives for women with these symptoms, however, the basic principle is to identify a structural defect prior to selecting a contraceptive option. If the problem can be correctly identified, treatment options may result in resolution of the problem. Following this, most women will be able to choose from the full range of available contraceptive methods.

Table 21.4 Potential adverse menstrual effects of steroidal contraceptives used for AUB

LNG-IUS
Unpredictable "spotting" or light bleeding is common in the first 3–6 months after insertion of the LNG-IUS. Thereafter, infrequent light bleeding or amenorrhea is expected
Unpredictable spotting and light bleeding are much commoner when the LNG-IUS is used for HMB, particularly in the presence of uterine leiomyomas (intramural or small submucous), but steadily improve over 6–12 months is common
Women in whom the LNG-IUS is inserted for HMB may experience recurrence of symptoms before the nominal 5-year contraceptive lifespan of the device, requiring early insertion of a replacement device

COCs
Unscheduled "IMB" (usually light) may occur in any user of a combined oral contraceptive, but anecdotally may be more frequent or heavier in the woman presenting with HPMB. This usually improves with time
Any COC may reduce HPMB, but anecdotally the 30-µg ethinyl estradiol pills, 24/4 regimen OC, or the new multiphasic estradiol valerate/dienogest pill (Natazia, Qlaira, Bayer Schering Pharma, for which there is good recent evidence) are effective therapies

COC, combined oral contraceptive; HMB, heavy menstrual bleeding; HPMB; heavy/prolonged menstrual bleeding; IMB, intermenstrual bleeding.

Adverse effects of hormonal contraceptives on bleeding patterns

It is well recognized that hormonal contraceptives may have some undesired effects on menstrual bleeding patterns, and these may also occur in women being treated for HMB or other types of AUB (Table 21.4). These tend to settle with time for most methods, but may require empirical manipulations of hormonal dosage to try and improve the patterns.

Roles of other nonpreferred methods of contraception in women with HMB or other types of AUB

Condoms

The male condom is a good temporary contraceptive option (with oral iron supplements!), but specific additional HMB therapy, such as tranexamic acid, a NSAID, or progestin therapy options is needed to control the bleeding problems.

Diaphragms

The diaphragm is not a good option as it has a relatively high failure rate and needs the addition of specific HMB therapies (as for condoms and other barrier methods above).

Tubal sterilization

Sterilization may be a good, permanent contraception option in women with HMB, if combined with a combination of diagnostic hysteroscopy, diagnostic curettage, endometrial polypectomy, myomectomy, or endometrial ablation.

Essure or Adiana

These hysteroscopic implant techniques may have a role if the cause of HMB is removed (i.e., polypectomy or myomectomy) at the same time of insertion, or if combined with endometrial ablation (see Chapter 14).

Copper-containing intrauterine device

Copper IUDs generally will increase menstrual blood loss and may also cause unpredictable IMB in some women. Although they are a very cost-effective method of contraception (see Chapter 2), they need to be combined with specific HMB therapy.

Acute and severe HMB

Women with a history of acute, severe HMB requiring hospital or emergency room admission need urgent investigations for cause and control of bleeding, then prevention of future episodes. The options for long-term management and contraception will be dependent on the cause.

Role of surgery for HMB or IMB before contraception

Minor surgical procedures (hysteroscopy, endometrial biopsy, curettage and/or endometrial polypectomy) are commonly required to make a clear diagnosis prior to the initiation of contraception. In some cases, other lesions may require specific surgical procedures such as hysteroscopic or abdominal myomectomy, or endometriosis excision prior to the initiation of hormonal or other contraception. These will need consideration on a case by case basis.

Benefits associated with long-term contraceptive use

- There is evidence that medium to long-term use of both LNG-IUS and some COCs will help to prevent or delay the development of new leiomyomas, endometriosis, endometrial hyperplasia and endometrial polyps.
- There is long-standing and extensive evidence that the COC protects against endometrial and ovarian carcinoma.
- The LNG-IUS is now used to prevent and treat endometrial hyperplasia and cancer (see Chapter 9) but further evidence is needed to firmly establish the guidelines.
- The effectiveness of transdermal and intravaginal ring estrogen-progestogen contraceptives for these purposes is less well studied.

Switching contraception in women with persistent HMB or IMB

Since few good quality published data exist to support particular courses of action, there is a need for sensible extrapolation from the data that does exist and individualization.

Further investigations may include:

- CBC with platelets to confirm there is no persisting anemia
- TV/US or MRI to exclude overlooked, or new, structural myometrial and endometrial lesions, or rare ovarian pathology

- If TV/US or MRI is normal, check full coagulation screen
- Serum TSH—hypothyroidism is a rare cause of HMB

Persistent unscheduled bleeding of the "intermenstrual" type is most likely to be a side effect of the hormonal contraceptive used, but should not be ignored if there is a possibility of an overlooked surface lesion within the reproductive tract.

> ### ⚕ SCIENCE REVISITED
>
> The endometrium is the organ that usually bleeds, and hormonal therapies with an 'endometrial focus' are most likely to be effective for AUB (provided lesions requiring surgical excision have been treated).
>
> Disturbances of the complex molecular mechanisms responsible for the control of the volume of blood lost at menstruation are common causes of HMB (especially: excessive endometrial plasminogen activator and local fibrinolysis; disturbances of local platelet function; disturbances of prostaglandin synthesis and metabolism; probable disturbances of local release of matrix metalloproteinases, endothelins and other endometrial vasoactive substances
>
> Hormonal therapies usually effectively suppress some of these disturbed mechanisms, but noncontraceptive drugs like the fibrinolytic inhibitor, tranexamic acid, or one of the nonsteroidal anti-inflammatory, anti-prostaglandin agents, may be combined with a contraceptive barrier method or copper intrauterine contraceptive device.

Selected references

Fraser IS. The promise and reality of the intrauterine route for hormone delivery for prevention and therapy of gynaecological disease. Contraception 2007;75(suppl):S112–17.

Fraser IS, Critchley HOD, Munro MG, Broder M. A process designed to lead to international agreement on terminologies and definitions used to describe abnormalities of uterine bleeding. Fertil Steril 2007;87:466–76.

Kaunitz AM, Meredith S, Inki P, Kubba A, Sanchez-Ramos L. Levonorgestrel-releasing intrauterine system and endometrial ablation in heavy menstrual bleeding: a systematic review and meta-analysis. Obstet Gynecol 2009;113: 1104–16.

Livingstone M, Fraser IS. Mechanisms of abnormal uterine bleeding. Hum Reprod Update 2002;8:60–7.

Munro MG. Abnormal uterine bleeding. Cambridge Clinical Guide. Cambridge, UK: Cambridge University Press, 2010.

Woolcock J, Critchley HOD, Munro MG, Broder M, Fraser IS. Review of the confusion in current and historical terminology and definitions for disturbances of menstrual bleeding. Fertil Steril 2008;90:2269–80.

Guidelines

National Institute of Health and Clinical Excellence (NICE). Available from: www.nice.org.uk

Long acting reversible contraception—full guideline; CG30; 2005.

Heavy menstrual bleeding—full guideline; CG44; 2007.

Systematic reviews

Cochrane Collaboration. Available from: www.thecochranelibrary.com

Farquhar C, Brown J. Oral contraceptive pill for heavy menstrual bleeding. Cochrane Menstrual Disorders and Subfertility Group, Cochrane Database Syst Rev 2010;2.

Lethaby A, Cooke I, Rees MC. Progesterone or progestogen-releasing intrauterine systems for heavy menstrual bleeding. Cochrane Menstrual Disorders and Subfertility Group, Cochrane Database Syst Rev 2009;1.

Lethaby A, Augood C, Duckitt K, Farquhar C. Non-steroidal anti-inflammatory drugs for heavy menstrual bleeding. Cochrane Menstrual Disorders and Subfertility Group, Cochrane Database Syst Rev 2009;1.

Grimes DA, Hubacher D, Lopez LM, Schulz KF. Non-steroidal anti-inflammatory drugs for heavy bleeding or pain associated with intrauterine-device use. Cochrane Menstrual Disorders and Subfertility Group, Cochrane Database Syst Rev 2009;1.

Lethaby A, Irvine GA, Cameron IT. Cyclical progestogens for heavy menstrual bleeding. Cochrane Menstrual Disorders and Subfertility Group, Cochrane Database of Syst Rev 2009;1.

Lethaby A, Farquhar C, Cooke I. Antifibrinolytics for heavy menstrual bleeding. Cochrane Menstrual Disorders and Subfertility Group, Cochrane Database Syst Rev 2009;1.

22

Hirsutism and Acne

Jennefer A. Russo[1] and Anita L. Nelson[1,2]

[1]Department of Obstetrics, Gynecology, and Reproductive Sciences, University of Pittsburgh Medical Center, Magee-Womens Hospital, Pittsburgh, PA, USA
[2]Department of Obstetrics and Gynecology, David Geffen School of Medicine at University of California, Los Angeles, CA, USA

Introduction

In the age of direct-to-consumer marketing, the average clinician will encounter many patients presenting for birth control consultations who are seeking more than just contraception from their birth control method. A patient will want the pill that is "better for acne," or she may have heard that taking a certain oral contraceptive pill (OCP) will decrease her need for hair removal with waxing or shaving. Are these claims true? What other issues should be explored with patients who seek birth control for these reasons? At the conclusion of this chapter, you will understand how to approach the patient with hirsutism or acne who presents seeking an optimal birth control method.

Causes of hirsutism and acne in women

> **SCIENCE REVISITED**
>
> - Acne results from excess androgen activity causing increased production of sebum in the skin. The excess sebum, presence of bacteria on the skin, and abnormal shedding of follicular skin cells (hyperkeratinization) may result in blockage of the follicles and development of an inflammatory process.

> - Hirsutism, or excessively heavy hair growth in hormonally sensitive areas in women, results from hair follicles being stimulated by androgens to convert vellus hair, which is fine and unpigmented, to terminal hair, which is thicker and darker.

Located in the skin are microscopic glands that secrete an oily/waxy material called sebum that is designed to lubricate the skin and hair. These glandular structures that consist of a hair follicle, hair, sebaceous gland and an arrector pili muscle are known as a pilosebaceous unit. At the local level, testosterone is converted to dihydrotestosterone (DHT) by 5α-reductase, an enzyme found in the hair follicle. DHT is very potent androgen that stimulates the sebaceous gland to produce extra sebum and the growth of the hair follicle. Testosterone and other androgens stimulate 5α-reductase activity, while estrogens and a long list of commercially available products reduce its activity.

Most commonly, hirsutism and acne are associated with polycystic ovarian syndrome (PCOS). Although the cause of PCOS is unknown, it is associated with hyperinsulinemia, anovulation, and androgen excess. A patient with PCOS might present with complaints of irregular menses or infertility, or she may simply present complaining of the symptoms of androgen excess—excessive hair growth and acne.

Hirsutism may be due to ethnic or family trait, or androgen excess. Up to 10% of U.S. women report some degree of hirsutism. Women of Mediterranean, Middle Eastern and South Asian ancestry are the most likely to develop idiopathic hirsutism. *These women will often have normal menses and normal androgen levels. An inherited increased 5α-reductase activity in the pilosebaceous unit is thought to be the underlying cause.*

Hirsutism commonly appears on the face, chest, and back.

Patient evaluation

The first step in evaluation of a patient complaining of acne and hair growth is to examine the patient and determine the severity of the condition. In terms of hair growth, the Ferriman-Gallwey Score may be consulted (http://www.gfmer.ch/Cours/Hirsutism_ferriman_gallwey_score.htm). This describes the extent of male pattern hair growth on the face, arms, legs, chest, pubic area, and intergluteal area. However, the patient's level of distress due to excess hair growth may not coincide with the score she is given on this scale.

Acne can also occur in different levels of severity, from closed or open comedones to nodulocystic acne, the most severe form. Circulating levels of androgens do not always correlate with amount of acne, although androgen's action at the hair follicle is thought to be the mitigating factor.

It is important to treat "patient-important" hair growth and acne. Although a woman may have what appears to be mild hirsutism and acne, she may have already been using products to remove hair and treat acne. This is usually a chronic problem that plagues a patient over the course of her life, at great financial and psychological expense.

Which conditions should be ruled out before treating hirsutism and acne?

Rapid onset or extensive hair growth and acne should prompt evaluation for more serious and life-threatening conditions than PCOS. In the differential diagnosis, one must consider:

- Cushing syndrome
- Nonclassical (or adult onset) congenital adrenal hyperplasia
- Androgen-secreting tumor of ovary or adrenal gland
- Exogenous androgens (anabolic steroid exposure).

Less likely, and more commonly associated with oligomenorrhea or amenorrhea along with other symptoms characteristic of the diagnosis:

- Acromegaly
- Genetic defects in insulin action
- Primary hypothalamic amenorrhea
- Thyroid disease
- Prolactinoma
- Primary ovarian failure.

Cushing syndrome

This extremely rare condition is found in only 1 in 1,000,000 people. Patients should be screened for Cushing syndrome only if there is suspicion based on symptoms other than hirsutism and oligomenorrhea. Symptoms that should arouse suspicion are presence of muscle wasting, moon facies, abdominal striae, buffalo hump, centripetal fat distribution, or hypertension. Cushing syndrome involves oversecretion of cortisol either from the pituitary, adrenal tumor, or an ectopic source of adrenal corticotropic hormone. The standard test for cortisol excess is either a 24-hour urinary cortisol or a dexamethasone suppression test.

Adult-onset congenital adrenal hyperplasia

Approximately 1–5% of hirsute women have adult-onset congenital adrenal hyperplasia, which can be ruled out by a normal 17-hydroxy-progesterone level less than 4 ng/mL (random) or 2 ng/mL (fasting).

Androgen-secreting tumors

These tumors are extremely uncommon. A testosterone level above 150–200 ng/dL is suspicious. These levels are not very sensitive or specific, and it is important to be familiar with the normal reference range of your local laboratory.

Clinical signs of masculinization/virilization include temporal (frontal) baldness, clitoral enlargement, increased muscle mass, or deeping of the voice. Any patient with a palpable ovarian mass, masculinization, and/or elevated testosterone should undergo a pelvic and/or abdominal ultrasound. *Keep in mind that approximately 50% of women with hirsutism have normal total and free testosterone levels.*

Laboratory studies

- Androgen studies: total testosterone, free testosterone, dehydroepiandrosterone sulfate (DHEAS).
- Anouvulatory patients: LH, prolactin. Select anovulatory patients should be evaluated for insulin resistance with a two hour glucose tolerance test or hemoglobin A1c, thyroid stimulating hormone level, and fasting lipids.
- Those with a prolonged periods irregular menses or menorrhagia may require an endometrial biopsy or pelvic ultrasound to evaluate the endometrial stripe and ovaries.
- 17-hyroxyprogesterone if hirsutism/acne is long-standing or severe.

✋ CAUTION

Patient with rapid onset of symptoms, a pelvic mass, temporal balding, clitoromegaly, or stigmata of Cushing syndrome should have a more extensive workup. However, the majority of PCOS patients seen in a clinical practice will have had a gradual onset of symptoms since puberty and the extent of hair growth and acne will be less marked than those of a patient with a tumor, congenital adrenal hyperplasia, or other more serious condition.

Diagnosis

Approximately 7% of reproductive-aged women have the diagnosis of PCOS. Its diagnosis is generally based on the findings of hyperandrogenism, oligomenorrhea or amenorrhea, and polycystic ovaries by ultrasound. Diagnosing the condition will enable women with PCOS to be treated for the associated metabolic syndrome which may include hypercholesterolemia, diabetes, and hypertension.

Treatment

Hirsutism

- A patient may be assigned a Ferriman–Gallwey score, or she may simply be treated for hirsutism based on her own discomfort with her amount of hair growth.
- The treatment for existing hirsutism includes laser, electrolysis, or topical depilatories plus OCPs and/or other antiandrogenic medications. OCPs are a good option for women with hirsutism who desire birth control.

✋ CAUTION

- When a patient presents with hirsutism and acne, always think about polycystic ovarian syndrome (PCOS). PCOS may be associated with diabetes, hypercholesterolemia, hypertension, and endometrial cancer, and has important preventive health ramifications.
- No combined hormonal contraceptive has been approved by the U.S. Food and Drug Administration (FDA) for the treatment of hirsutism.

Treatment options

OCPs

Although pharmaceutical companies would prefer us to believe their claims that their own OCP is "better" than another company's, in regard to hirsutism, there are no studies demonstrating that one pill has a benefit over any other pill. Most OCPs offer some improvement in the extent of hair growth, and the pills that are approved for acne are popular options. The most effective form of therapy involves treatment with a OCP in combination with a hair removal

★ TIPS & TRICKS

In general, treatment effects should be monitored by the patient noting if she is requiring less treatment with waxing, shaving, or other hair removal methods. She should be advised that it may take 6 months to notice a difference in hair growth or regrowth (6 months is the half-life of a hair follicle).

method and possibly another antiandrogenic medication.

OCPs are the first line of pharmaceutical treatment for patients who do not desire fertility. Some literature quotes effectiveness in the range of 60–100% of patients seeing results, but studies are small and the effect of birth control may take place over a prolonged period of time. Patients may need to be treated for months to years before noting an effect. For patients with anovulation, OCPs add cycle control and endometrial protection.

The mechanisms of action of the OCP in controlling androgen effects seem to be multifactorial.

- Oral contraceptives inhibit secretion of luteinizing hormone (LH) and thereby decrease ovarian androgen production.
- Estrogen in oral contraceptives stimulates hepatic production of sex hormone binding globulin (SHBG). The increase in SHBG causes a decrease in circulating free testosterone, binding up and preventing the end tissue effects of testosterone.
- Oral contraceptives may also decrease adrenal androgen production.
- Oral contraceptives inhibit 5α-reductase and androgen receptor activity.

Few studies examine OCPs for hirsutism side-by-side with other treatment modalities. A recent meta-analysis showed that there was little difference between insulin-sensitizing drugs and OCPs for the treatment of hirsutism and acne in PCOS. Another meta-analysis demonstrated little benefit from insulin sensitizers.

Most of the beneficial effect of combined oral contraceptives is derived from estrogen, with progestin-only birth control methods not having the same beneficial effect on hirsutism and acne. The progestin may, however, have a synergistic effect, especially if it is a less androgenic progestin. Estrogen found in OCPs is ethinyl estradiol in varying doses or estradiol valerate, and progesterone may be present in the form of norethindrone, norethindrone acetate, norethisterone, norethynodrel, ethynodiol diacetate, norgestrel, levonorgestrel, desogestrel, gestodene, norgestimate, dienogest, cyproterone acetate, drospirenone, and dienogest. The latter seven are the most recently developed "third-generation" progestins, selected for their low androgenic to progestogenic activity.

- Drospirenone has antiandrogenic characteristics, but at the dose of 3 mg in oral contraceptives it has minimal impact on androgenic symptoms such as acne and hirsutism. Although the more recent progestins are thought to be less androgenic, and they have been shown to decrease free testosterone and increase SHBG, there has been no appreciable difference in clinical hirsutism across studies.
- Cyproterone acetate is an androgen receptor blocker that is derived from 17-hydroxyprogesterone and is found in oral contraceptives outside the United States. It has been found to be effective for hirsutism when used alone or as a component of OCPs.
- Dienogest is now available in the United States in a recently approved OCP also containing estradiol valerate. It has antiandrogenic activity and is reported to improve androgenic symptoms when combined with ethinyl estradiol in a combination OCP.

Other treatment options

Weight loss

First, for patients with PCOS, weight loss may result in a decrease in circulating androgens and provide some improvement in hirsutism. Any patient who has anovulation and hirsutism should be suspected of having PCOS. Up to 80% of women with hirsutism have the diagnosis.

Antiandrogens

Antiandrogens appear to have a more pronounced effect on hirsutism. Specifically, the medication *spironolactone* (Aldactone) has been more extensively studied and found to have a lower side effect profile and toxicity than other antiandrogens. Its mechanism of action is to compete with dihydrotestosterone for androgen receptors in the skin. It increases liver clearance of testosterone and decreases 5α-reductase activity. Sex hormone binding globulin levels are also increased in patients taking spironolactone.

A recent meta-analysis demonstrated an improvement in patients who were treated with 100 mg/day of spironolactone versus placebo, but only in patients' self-reported outcomes, and not Ferriman–Gallwey scores. There may be added benefit when oral contraceptives are prescribed in combination with spironolactone.

Other antiandrogens used for hirsutism include *flutamide*, an androgen-receptor antagonist, and *finasteride*, a 5α-reductase inhibitor. Both are highly teratogenic in male fetuses and seem to offer little benefit over spironolactone, which does not appear to have as many risks. Flutamide may also be hepatotoxic in some patients.

Topical treatments

Topical treatments such as *eflornithine* (Vaniqa), which is an inhibitor of the enzyme ornithine decarboxylase, are showing promise in the treatment of facial hair. However, this treatment is only effective during the time it is applied. If there is a continued androgen stimulus, vellus hairs will continue to be converted to terminal hairs.

Laser treatments

Laser hair removal/electrolysis shows promise, but hair regrowth may occur after stopping treatment when the androgenic stimulus remains. Therefore, continued therapy with antiandrogens or OCPs while using a topical treatment, or a combination of topical treatments, may be advisable for those patients not desiring fertility.

Other methods
- Chemical depilatories, waxing, shaving, plucking, or bleaching are generally effective but temporary methods

- Topical 5α-reductase inhibitors are indicated for benign prostatic hyperplasia and androgenic alopecia.

Acne

Acne, like hirsutism, can have a huge impact on a patient's self-esteem and self-concept. Prevalence is high, with approximately 50% of people between 20 to 29 years reporting acne, and 20–35% of those between 30 and 39 years reporting it. Postadolescent acne is more common among women. Women may also have a component of acne associated with premenstrual flares.

Acne is a result of a toxic mix of excess sebum, abnormal shedding of follicular skin cells (keratinization), and bacterial overgrowth at the level of the hair follicle. Depending on the degree of each problem, the pimple, or "microcomedo," develops into a closed comedo (whitehead), open comedo (blackhead), or inflammatory lesion. Inflammatory lesions, or nodulocystic acne, are associated with severe acne. Most patients with acne have normal androgen levels, although elevated androgen levels have been found to be pathogenic for acne in certain conditions such as PCOS.

Acne and hirsutism therapies, because they are geared toward altering the effects of androgens, have a great deal of overlap. The effectiveness of different antiandrogens for acne vulgaris differs significantly.

Treatment options

Combined oral contraceptives

A combined oral contraceptive is effective for women with acne as primary therapy (especially if acne is mild), or as an adjunct to therapy with topical antibiotics or topical retinoid treatment. In women who are using isotretinoin for severe acne, it is imperative that birth control be used to prevent pregnancies as birth defects may result from this medication.

Every clinician has likely heard the request for "the pill that gets rid of acne." Although Ortho Tri-Cyclen was the first OCP to be marketed as an adjunct treatment for acne because of the positive profile of its progestin, norgestimate, most second- and third-generation pills have been shown to improve acne.

Meta-analyses performed between 2004 and 2009 have shown little benefit of one OCP over another across randomized controlled trials. Trials have shown conflicting results, failing to yield one OCP as superior. In addition, OCPs have not been compared head-to-head with other acne treatments. Finally, progestin-only contraceptives seem to have little effect on hirsutism and acne, although they do provide a protective effect on the endometrium in patients with PCOS.

Spironolactone
Although it has a favorable profile when used for the treatment of hirsutism, spironolactone seems to have less of an effect when used for acne.

Most commonly, the recommendation of dermatologists is to use topical therapy such as a *retinoid, benzoyl peroxide,* or a topical antibiotic to treat mild acne. Combination topical products *with both an antibiotic and tretinoin* are available with prescription.

- For more severe acne, topical therapy may be combined with OCPs.
- Patients with nodular acne (the most severe form of acne) may consider using *oral isotretinoin and oral antibiotics.* In women of reproductive age, it is critical to offer OCPs with isotretinoin because of its teratogenic effects.

Are there other contraceptive methods that work for hirsutism and acne?

Again, the beneficial effect of contraception appears to derive from the estrogen component more than the progestin. Therefore, only combined methods should have the antiandrogenic results of decreasing hirsutism and acne. Minimal research exists on the contraceptive vaginal ring (NuvaRing) and contraceptive patch (Ortho Evra) with regard to hirsutism and acne. NuvaRing contains the progestin etonorgestrel and Ortho Evra contains norelgestromin. A few studies looking at androgen levels and self-reported improvement in acne and hirsutism have demonstrated positive outcomes for patients, but these studies have again been small. No meta-analyses yet exist to compare these birth control methods to placebo, OCPs, each other, or other acne and hirsutism treatment modalities.

Conclusions

When a patient presents with acne or hirsutism that is bothersome to her, a clinician should be aware that her treatment options include combined oral contraceptives. Furthermore, the patient who presents specifically for birth control while also seeking benefits for acne or hair growth should be counseled on the positive profile of combined oral contraception in comparison to other birth control methods.

Any patient with a rapid onset of hirsutism or acne should be evaluated for conditions such as Cushing syndrome, adult-onset congenital adrenal hyperplasia, or an androgen-producing tumor. If the onset has been gradual or consistent since puberty, PCOS should be suspected. As a diagnosis alone, the significance of PCOS may mean irregular ovulation and infertility, but in association with diabetes, hypertension, obesity, endometrial hyperplasia, and cancer, among other conditions, PCOS can be a life-threatening condition as it associated with long-term medical problems. It is imperative that the diagnosis be made, that patients undergo screening tests for the above conditions, and counseling is done concerning the diagnosis and potential associated conditions.

⚙ SCIENCE REVISITED

The use of **OCPs** in these patients is extremely valuable for a number of reasons, especially for protection of the endometrium and for decreasing circulating androgens, which may affect insulin metabolism and weight. With the decrease in androgens will also come the improvement in hirsutism and acne, which may sometimes be even more important to the patient.

Any patient who is choosing a birth control method should be counseled about the beneficial side effects of combined hormonal contraceptives as a part of her process in choosing a method. For those patients who have what appears to be clinically mild acne or hirsutism but are bothered by the conditions and also desire birth control, combined oral contraceptives are an excellent choice. *The vaginal ring and contraceptive patch likely also offer these advantages.*

Selected references

ACOG Practice Bulletin No. 108. Polycystic ovary syndrome. Obstet Gynecol 2009;114(4):936.

Arowojolu A, Gallo M, Lopez L, Grimes D, Garner S. Combined oral contraceptive pills for treatment of acne. Cochrane Database Syst Rev 2009;3: CD004425.

Azziz R. Use of combination estrogen-progestin contraceptives in the treatment of hyperandrogenism and hirsutism. Up to Date, Sept 30, 2009. Available from: http://www.uptodate.com/

Breitkopf D, Rosen M, Young S, Nagamani M. Efficacy of second versus third generation oral contraceptives in the treatment of hirsutism. Contraception 2003;67;349.

Brown J, Farquhar C, Lee O, Toomath R, Jepson R. Spironolactone versus placebo or in combination with steroids for hirsutism and acne. Cochrane Database Syst Rev 2009;4: CD000194.

Cosma M, Swiglo B, Flynn D, et al. Insulin sensitizers for the treatment of hirsutism: a systematic review and metaanalyses of randomized controlled trials. J Clin Endocrinol Metab 2008;93(4):1135.

Costello M, Shrestha B, Eden J, Sjoblom P, Johnson N, Moran L. Insulin-sensitizing drugs versus the combined oral contraceptive pill for hirsutism, acne and risk of diabetes, cardiovascular disease, and endometrial cancer in polycystic ovary syndrome. Cochrane Database Syst Rev 2007;1: CD005552.

Martin K, Chang J, Ehrmann D, et al. Evaluation and treatment of hirsutism in premenopausal women: an Endocrine Society clinical practice guideline. J Clin Endocrinol Metab 2008;93(4): 1105.

Ofori, A. Hormonal therapy for acne vulgaris. Up to Date, Sept 30, 2009. Available from: http://www.uptodate.com/

Ofori, A. Pathogenesis, clinical manifestations, and diagnosis of acne vulgaris. Up to Date, Sept 30, 2009. Available from: http://www.uptodate.com/

Speroff L, Glass RH, Kase NG (eds) Clinical gynecologic endocrinology and infertility, 6th ed. Baltimore, MD: Lippincott Williams & Wilkins; 1999.

Swiglo B, Cosma M, Flynn D, et al. Antiandrogens for the treatment of hirsutism: a systematic review and metaanalyses of randomized controlled trials. J Clin Endocrinol Metab 2008;93 (4):1153.

23

HIV and Other Sexually Transmitted Infections

Alice Stek

Department of Obstetrics and Gynecology, Keck School of Medicine, University of Southern California, Los Angeles, CA, USA

Contraception in HIV-infected women

As of the end of 2009, approximately 33 million people were living with HIV/AIDS worldwide. Half of the adults are women; the great majority of these 16 million women are of reproductive age. An estimated 430,000 HIV-infected children are born annually.

> **SCIENCE REVISITED**
>
> Prevention of unwanted pregnancy is the most effective way to reduce mother-to-child transmission of HIV (MTCT). Women with HIV need effective, reversible contraceptive options.

Especially in resource-poor settings, effective contraception protects maternal health and quality of life, prevents maternal mortality and prevents children from becoming orphans. In settings with adequate resources, the outcomes of pregnancies in women receiving optimal care are very good, with mother-to-child transmission (MTCT) rates of <1%; pregnancy has no effect on maternal HIV disease progression; and the long-term maternal prognosis keeps improving.

With advances in maternal and infant prognosis, fewer HIV-infected women are choosing sterilization and the ability to plan pregnancies has become more important. For women with HIV infection, as for all women, efficacy of the contraceptive method is of great importance. Additional considerations unique to HIV-infected women are:

- safety of the various methods in the setting of immunocompromise
- impact on sexual transmission to a partner
- possible pharmacologic interactions with medications for treating HIV.

Barrier methods

Control of viral load by use of highly active antiretroviral therapy (HAART) is also very effective in preventing sexual HIV transmission. Although the viral load in the genital tract is strongly correlated with viral load in the blood, the genital pool of HIV is not identical to the systemic one, and occasionally genital tract shedding of the virus can occur even with undetectable blood viral load. All HIV-infected women should therefore use condoms, unless attempting to conceive.

The female condom and the diaphragm have not been studied as extensively as the male condom in HIV-discordant couples, and there are no conclusive data on the efficacy of these barrier methods in preventing HIV transmission.

The contraceptive efficacy of any barrier method is unlikely to be altered by HIV.

Contraception, First Edition. Edited by Donna Shoupe.

- Male condoms are proven to reduce the risk of heterosexual HIV transmission by at least 80%. Because of this, condom use is often emphasized to the exclusion of more effective contraceptive methods. It is recommended that condoms be used even if both partners are HIV-infected.
- Ideally, women should use dual methods.
- HIV-infected women should not be denied access to more effective contraceptive methods.

Spermicides

The spermicide nonoxynol-9 has anti-HIV activity in vitro. However, in a trial among HIV-negative commercial sex workers in Africa, use of nonoxynol-9 several times daily resulted in increased HIV acquisition, probably as a result of epithelial irritation. It is not known if spermicides increase the risk of HIV transmission from an HIV-infected woman to her HIV-negative male partner.

Hormonal contraception

Hormonal contraception may be appropriate for HIV-infected women. However, there are concerns regarding safety, efficacy, and drug interactions. Adherence by women who may be taking a number of other medications should also be considered.

DMPA

In several large prospective studies of hormonal contraception (combined oral contraceptives [COCs] and depot medroxyprogesterone acetate [Depo-Provera, DMPA]) among HIV-infected women in Africa and the United States, no adverse impact of hormonal contraception on women's health was found. No significant effect on HIV viral load, CD4 count, or progression of HIV disease to AIDS or death was demonstrated.

- One study (Stringer et al. 2007) randomized 600 postpartum HIV-infected women in Zambia to a copper-containing intrauterine device (Cu-IUD versus hormonal contraception (DMPA or COCs). The women were not using antiretrovirals and had at least 2 years of follow-up. The women randomized to hormonal contraception were 2.4 times as likely to become pregnant again. Among the women randomized to hormonal contraception, the risk of HIV disease progression or death was increased 1.5-fold.
- In a larger retrospective study among HIV-infected postpartum women in 7 African countries and Thailand, Stringer et al. compared 1,045 women using hormonal contraception—most using DMPA or injectable norethisterone enantate, some on COCs—to 3,064 women not using hormonal contraception. Reassuringly, they found no significant difference in HIV disease progression.
- A more recent prospective study in Uganda among 625 recently infected HIV-positive women also found no difference in HIV progression to AIDS or death with use of hormonal contraception versus nonhormonal contraception.

Although it appears that hormonal contraception does not accelerate HIV disease progression, drug interactions with antiretroviral medications present another potential safety concern.

DMPA slightly increases the activity of CYP3A4, as does nevirapine, while some other antiretrovirals, particularly ritonavir, inhibit CYP3A4.

Hormonal contraception may alter the metabolism of antiretroviral drugs and the antiretroviral drugs may increase or inhibit the metabolism of contraceptive hormones. Contemporary medical management of HIV infection usually includes combination antiretroviral therapy with at least two categories of antiretrovirals. Of particular concern are drugs that induce or inhibit the cytochrome P450 3A4 (CYP3A4) pathway.

The available data on DMPA are generally reassuring. Serum levels of medroxyprogesterone acetate were no different in women using nelfi-navir, efavirenz, or nevirapine than in women not on these antiretrovirals, and ovulation was effectively suppressed. Nelfinavir exposure was slightly decreased and nevirapine levels were slightly increased with DMPA use; these changes were considered clinically insignificant. In the same study HIV viral load and CD4 count were unaltered. Similarly, blood levels of levonorgestrel (LNG) in women using the LNG-IUD were similar in women using and not using antiretroviral therapy.

Few data are available regarding interaction between progestins and newer antiretrovirals. The most up-to-date drug interaction data can be found at http://hivinsite.ucsf.edu and www.hiv-druginteractions.org.

EVIDENCE AT A GLANCE

Current data support the use of DMPA and probably other parenterally administered progestins in women with HIV, whether on antiretrovirals or not. WHO currently classifies DMPA as category 1 (no restrictions for use of the contraceptive method) and norethisterone enantate as category 2 (advantages generally outweigh risks) for women on antiretrovirals.

(http://www.who.int/reproductivehealth/publications/family_planning/9789241563888/en/index.html)

Drug interactions are of greater concern with combined hormonal contraception:

- There is a variable effect of antiretrovirals on hormonal contraceptive levels, even within the same antiretroviral class.
- Some antiretrovirals increase ethinyl estradiol levels: the protease inhibitors amprenavir, atazanavir, and indinavir and the non-nucleoside reverse transcriptase inhibitors efavirenz and etravirine.
- Often, antiretrovirals decrease ethinyl estradiol levels: the protease inhibitors darunavir, lopinavir/ritonavir, nelfinavir, ritonavir and tipranavir, and the non-nucleoside reverse transcriptase inhibitor nevirapine.

- The nucleoside reverse transcriptase inhibitors such as zidovudine, lamivudine, abacavir, emtricitabine and tenofovir have no clinically significant effect on contraceptive steroid levels.

Combined hormonal contraceptives and progestin-only pills

☆ TIPS & TRICKS

WHO regards combined hormonal contraceptives and progestin-only pills category 1 for women on nucleoside reverse transcriptase inhibitors only, category 2 for women on non-nucleoside reverse transcriptase inhibitors, and category 3 for women using ritonavir-boosted protease inhibitors.

- Norethindrone levels can be increased with amprenavir, atazanavir, indinavir, and tipranavir, and decreased with lopinavir, nelfinavir, nevirapine, and etravirine. It is also important to ensure the antiretroviral levels remain in the therapeutic range.
- Ethinyl estradiol can decrease amprenavir, tipranavir, and ritonavir levels. If there is a significant drug interaction, an alternative contraceptive method or a dose adjustment is recommended.
- Current recommendations for amprenavir, lopinavir/ritonavir, nelfinavir, nevirapine, ritonavir, and tipranavir are shown in Table 23.1.

✋ CAUTION

- Be aware of drug interactions. Data are evolving; refer to these websites for the most recent data:
- http://hivinsite.ucsf.edu
- www.hiv-druginteractions.org
- Avoid using combined hormonal contraceptives with amprenavir, darunavir, lopinavir/ritonavir, nelfinavir, nevirapine, ritonavir, tipranavir
- Avoid efavirenz with norgestimate or levonorgestrel.

Table 23.1 Antiretroviral interactions with combined hormonal contraceptives and recommendations for use

Antiretroviral	Effect on antiretroviral levels	Effect on contraceptive steroid levels	Recommendations
(fos)Amprenavir	↓Amprenavir	↑EE ↑Norethindrone ↑Norgestimate	Consider alternate contraception
Atazanavir	Not studied	↑EE ↑Norethindrone	No change
Darunavir	No change	↓EE ↓Norethindrone	Use alternate contraception
Indinavir	Not studied	↑EE ↑Norethindrone	No change
Lopinavir/ritonavir	Not studied	↓EE ↓Norethindrone	Use alternate contraception
Nelfinavir	Not studied	↓EE ↓Norethindrone	Use alternate contraception
Ritonavir	↓ Ritonavir	↓EE	Use alternate contraception
Tipranavir	↓ Tipranavir ↓Ritonavir	↓EE ↑Norethindrone	Use alternate contraception
Efavirenz	No change	↑EE ↓Norgestimate ↓Levonorgestrel	Avoid use with norgestimate or levonorgestrel
Etravirine	Not studied	↑EE ↓Norethindrone	No change
Nevirapine	No change	↓EE ↓Norethindrone	Avoid coadministration

EE, ethinyl estradiol.

The literature is not conclusive regarding whether the risk of HIV shedding from the female genital tract is increased with the use of hormonal contraception. Viral shedding could increase the risk of transmission to an HIV-negative partner. There is a developing consensus that neither hormonal contraception nor IUDs increase genital tract HIV shedding.

Intrauterine devices

The copper IUD has been evaluated in several African studies. Overall, complications and infectious morbidity were not increased in HIV-infected women. In the previously mentioned randomized Zambian study by Stringer et al. (2007), pregnancy rates were much lower in the IUD group than in the hormonal contraception group. IUD use was safe, with only 1 case of pelvic inflammatory disease (PID), for a rate of 0.2/100 woman–years.

There is much less data on the use of the levonorgestrel intrauterine system (LNG-IUS) in HIV-infected women:

- Reports of 2 small studies in Finland found no adverse outcomes in women receiving LNG-IUS. They were able to demonstrate an increase in hemoglobin after LNG-IUS insertion.

- In a recent abstract, investigators from Kenya followed 30 HIV-infected women after LNG-IUS insertion. The LNG-IUS was tolerated well, there was no increase in genital tract HIV shedding, and fewer women had anemia 6 months after insertion compared to baseline.

> **EVIDENCE AT A GLANCE**
>
> None of these studies found an increase in genital tract HIV shedding in women using an IUD.

Sterilization

> **☆ TIPS & TRICKS**
>
> Sterilization is an ideal contraceptive method for HIV-infected women who are certain they want no more children.

Careful counseling is essential to ensure the woman has an accurate understanding both of the very low risk of vertical transmission in most cases and of her own prognosis. Tubal ligation is particularly appropriate for women who undergo a cesarean delivery. Some women are poor surgical candidates for a postpartum or interval surgical sterilization. For these women and for others, hysteroscopically placed tubal inserts may be good alternatives, although this has not yet been studied.

Other sexually transmitted infections

> **✋ CAUTION**
>
> **Except for the restrictions regarding IUD placement (Chapter 9),** the presence of sexually transmitted infections (STIs) does not usually influence the choice of contraceptive method.

Hormonal methods

Among women at high risk for STIs, there may be an increased risk of chlamydial cervicitis with the use of combined hormonal contraception or DMPA; for other STIs there is no association. All women at high risk should be encouraged to use condoms, which are proven to provide some protection against STIs.

According to WHO guidelines (Table 23.2) there is no restriction in the initiation or continuation of hormonal contraception in women with STIs other than hepatitis or HIV, or PID.

Combined hormonal contraception should not be in initiated in women with acute viral hepatitis, but the advantages of continuation of combined hormonal contraception in these women generally outweigh the theoretical or proven risks.

There are no restrictions for hormonal contraception in women who are carriers or who have chronic viral hepatitis. Progestin-only contraception is appropriate in women with acute or chronic viral hepatitis and in carriers.

IUDs

The WHO guidelines (Table 23.2) state that in women with PID in the past, the benefits of IUD insertion or continuation generally outweigh the risks.

- Women with current PID need treatment with appropriate antibiotics, but do not need removal of their IUDs.
- IUDs should not be inserted in women with current PID, current purulent cervicitis, gonorrhea, or chlamydia.
- Among women having an IUD inserted, the risk of subsequent PID is higher among women with an STI at the time of insertion.
- In women with very high risk of exposure to gonorrhea or chlamydia, the risks of IUD insertion may outweigh the benefits. There is no need to remove the IUD in a woman who acquires an STI.

> **☆ TIPS & TRICKS**
>
> IUDs can be used without restriction in women with viral hepatitis or using antibiotics.

Spermicides

There are no contraindications to use of spermicides except in women with HIV or at high risk for acquiring HIV. Although typical use of

Table 23.2 WHO MEC for women with STIs

Condition	Cu-IUD	LNG-IUD	CHC	POC	Sterilization
HIV	2	2	1	1	Accept
AIDS	2/3[a]	2/3[a]	1	1	AIDS-related illness may require delay
Hepatitis					
Acute	1	1	2/3/4[b]	2/3/4[b]	Delay
Chronic/carrier	1	1	1	1	Accept
PID					
Past	1/2[c]	1/2[c]	1	1	Accept
Current	2/4[d]	2/4[d]	1	1	Delay
STIs					
Current purulent cervicitis, gonorrhea, chlamydia	2/4[d]	2/4[d]	1	1	Delay
Vaginitis, other STIs	2	2	1	1	Accept

CHC, combined hormonal contraceptives; Cu-IUD, copper-containing IUD; LNG-IUD, levonorgestrel intrauterine system; PID, pelvic inflammatory disease; POC, progestin-only contraceptives; STI, sexually transmitted infection.
[a] Category 3 for insertion unless clinically well on antiretroviral therapy.
[b] Category 2 for continuation, category 3 or 4 for initiation of method.
[c] Category 1 if PID in past with subsequent pregnancy; category 2 without subsequent pregnancy.
[d] Category 2 for continuation; category 4 for insertion.
Key:
Category 1: Condition for which there is no restriction for use of the contraceptive method.
Category 2: Condition where the advantages of using the method generally outweigh the theoretical or proven risks.
Category 3: Condition where the theoretical or proven risks usually outweigh the advantages of using the method.
Category 4: Condition which represents an unacceptable health risk if the contraceptive method is used.
From WHO medical eligibility criteria for contraceptive use, 4th edition, 2009.

spermicides is probably safe, repeated and high-dose use of nonoxynol-9 was associated with genital lesions and increased acquisition of HIV among commercial sex workers in one study. Therefore, WHO recommends against its use by women with HIV or at high risk of acquiring HIV.

Surgical sterilization

Surgical sterilization should be postponed in women with acute viral hepatitis, current PID, purulent cervicitis, chlamydia, or gonorrhea.

Antibiotics for STIs and other indications

There have been anecdotal reports of oral contraceptive failure with use of antibiotics. Pharmacokinetic studies have not shown any significant interaction with COCs and tetracycline, doxycycline, ampicillin, metronidazole, quinolones, or fluconazole.

> ✋ CAUTION
>
> - Use of rifampin or rifabutin decreases steroid levels in women taking COCs; alternate contraceptive methods should be used.
> - The effectiveness of DMPA is not decreased with rifampin or rifabutin, but the effectiveness of other progestin-only methods may be reduced.

Selected references

Cohn SE, Park J-G, Watts DH, et al. Depo-medroxyprogesterone in women on antiretroviral therapy: Effective contraception and lack of clinically significant interactions. Clin Pharmacol Therapeut 2007;81(2):222–7.

Curtis KM, Nanda K, Kapp N. Safety of hormonal and intrauterine methods of Curtis contraception for women with HIV/AIDS: a systematic review. AIDS 2009;23 (suppl 1):S55–67.

Database of Antiretroviral Drug Interactions. UCSF Center for HIV Information, University of California San Francisco. http://hivinsite.ucsf.edu.

Heikinheimo O, Lehtovirta P, Suni J, Paavonen J. The levonorgestrel-releasing intrauterine system (LNG-IUS) in HIV-infected women—effects on bleeding patterns, ovarian function and genital shedding of HIV. Hum Reprod 2006;21(11):2857–61.

Lehtovirta P, Paavonen J, Heikinheimo O. Experience with the levonorgestrel-releasing intrauterine system among HIV-infected women. Contraception 2007;75:37–9.

Liverpool HIV Pharmacology Group and Department of Pharmacology and Therapeutics, University of Liverpool, Liverpool, UK. http://www.hiv-druginteractions.org.

Stringer EM, Kaseba C, Levy J, et al. A randomized trial of the intrauterine contraceptive device vs hormonal contraception in women who are infected with the human immunodeficiency virus. Am J Obstet Gynecol 2007;197:144.e1–144.e8.

Stringer EM, Gigantia M, Carter RJ, El-Sadr W, Abrams EJ, Stringer JSA, for the MTCT-Plus Initiative. Hormonal contraception and HIV disease progression: a multicountry cohort analysis of the MTCT-Plus Initiative. AIDS 2009;23 (suppl 1):S69–77.

Stringer EM, Levy J, Sinkala M, et al. HIV disease progression by hormonal contraceptive method: secondary analysis of a randomized trial. AIDS 2009;23:1377–82.

Watts DH, Park J-G, Cohn SE, et al. Safety and tolerability of depo-medroxyprogesterone acetate among HIV-infected women on antiretroviral therapy: ACTG A5093. Contraception 2008;77(2):84–90.

WHO. Medical eligibility criteria for contraceptive use, 4th ed. Geneva: World Health Organization; 2009. Available from: http://www.who.int/reproductivehealth/publications/family_planning/9789241563888/en/index.html.

24

Contraception Following Ectopic Pregnancy, and Induced or Spontaneous Abortion

Paula H. Bednarek and Alison B. Edelman

Department of Obstetrics and Gynecology, Oregon Health & Science University, Portland, OR, USA

Introduction

Contraceptive counseling and provision are important components of care for women after pregnancy. Ovulation can occur as early 10 days following the end of a pregnancy. Many women want to delay or avoid getting pregnant again; therefore it is important to initiate contraception as early as possible. Assuming no immediate complications, nearly all methods are considered safe and feasible to begin right away, including the intrauterine device (IUD), the subdermal implant, or sterilization.

This chapter focuses on contraceptive issues following pregnancies that have ended in the first- or second-trimester induced or spontaneous abortion, or following treatment for ectopic pregnancy. The chapter will first address the clinical presentation of each of these clinical situations and then the associated advantages and concerns for various contraceptive options.

Induced abortion

Each year, almost half of all pregnancies among American women are unintended, and about half of these unplanned pregnancies end in abortion. Planned and wanted pregnancies may also end in induced abortion for indications such as fetal anomaly, maternal health concerns, or other unexpected circumstances that may arise during the prenatal course. In 2005, approximately 1.2 million abortions were performed in the United States, with nearly 90% performed in the first trimester (before 12 weeks).

> ★ TIPS & TRICKS
>
> Contraceptive counseling and the option of immediate initiation of effective contraception are critical components of abortion care.

First-trimester surgical abortion

Over 90% of first-trimester surgical abortions are performed in outpatient settings, using either electric or manual (handheld syringe) vacuum aspiration. Perioperative antibiotics are routinely provided to patients, which has been proven to decrease postoperative infection rates. Women typically experience cramping and bleeding similar to a menstrual period for a few days to several weeks following the procedure, with regular menses usually returning within 4–6 weeks after the procedure.

First-trimester medical abortion

In the United States, medical abortion with mifepristone and misoprostol is offered at 9 weeks gestation or less. Prophylactic antibiotic provision is becoming more routine and may reduce the rates of serious postabortion infection. The duration of bleeding after medical abortion varies significantly between patients and is usually slightly longer than after surgical abortion. Other symptoms of recovery following medical abortion are similar to those with surgical abortion.

Women are asked to return within 2 weeks of their medical abortion, to confirm pregnancy expulsion. If an ultrasound is utilized at this visit, the main goal is to determine the presence or absence of the gestational sac.The thickness of the endometrial lining on ultrasound does not predict abortion success or diagnose complications.

Second-trimester abortion

Beyond the first trimester, abortion can be performed surgically or medically. Surgical second-trimester abortion can be performed in an outpatient setting using specialized forceps and vacuum aspiration, while medical abortion is generally performed in a hospital setting similar to the delivery of a term pregnancy. Recovery following second-trimester abortion is generally similar to first-trimester abortion. However, it may take 1–2 weeks longer for the uterus to return to its nonpregnancy size and position.

Spontaneous abortion

Approximately 15% of clinically recognized pregnancies end spontaneously. Women usually present with bleeding and/or cramping. However, miscarriage can also be asymptomatic. Risk factors for spontaneous abortion are listed in Table 24.1. Depending on a patient's gestational age, symptoms, and personal preference, miscarriage can be managed medically, surgically, or expectantly.

Surgical management of a miscarriage utilizes the same technique as for an induced abortion and thus recovery is similar. As compared to expectant management, medical management with misoprostol provides greater predictability of time to expulsion, higher rates of successful expulsion, and lower rates of surgical intervention. The recovery process following medical or expectant management of spontaneous abortion is similar to the recovery following induced medical abortion. Spontaneous abortion beyond the first trimester is managed like a second-trimester induced abortion and thus recovery is no different.

Table 24.1 Risk factors for spontaneous abortion

Advancing maternal age
Maternal smoking
Maternal diabetes
Uncontrolled maternal thyroid disease
Maternal infection
Polycystic ovarian syndrome
Previous spontaneous abortion
Parental structural chromosome abnormality
Short interpregnancy interval (generally less than 3–6 months following term pregnancy)
Thrombophilias (more associated with second trimester loss)
Fetal genetic syndrome (more associate with second-trimester loss)

There is theoretical concern that getting pregnant too soon after spontaneous or induced abortion may lead to a higher risk of repeat miscarriage or other pregnancy complications such as preterm labor or fetal growth restriction. *Contraceptive counseling and provision is therefore an integral part of care for women experiencing pregnancy loss.*

Ectopic pregnancy

In the United States, ectopic pregnancy accounts for 2% of all first-trimester pregnancies and 6% of all pregnancy-related deaths, making it the leading cause of maternal death in the first trimester. Risk factors for ectopic pregnancy are listed in Table 24.2. Ectopic pregnancy can be managed medically or surgically.

Medical management of ectopic pregnancy

Methotrexate is used to treat early, nonruptured ectopic pregnancies using single-dose, two-dose, or multidose protocols. Success depends on the treatment regimen used, gestational age, and human chorionic gonadotrpin (hCG) level—the overall success rate with methotrexate ranges from 71% to 94%.

Table 24.2 Risk factors for ectopic pregnancy

Pelvic inflammatory disease
History of prior ectopic
History of tubal surgery
Use of fertility drugs or assisted reproductive technology
Current use of IUD
Advancing maternal age
Maternal smoking

Surgical management of ectopic pregnancy

An ectopic pregnancy can be treated surgically via laparoscopy or laparotomy, with either salpingectomy (removal of the fallopian tube) or more conservatively with salpingostomy (incision into the fallopian tube). Surgical treatment is recommended if a woman is not a candidate for methotrexate, is hemodynamically unstable, or would be unable to comply with the follow-up requirements of methotrexate treatment. Another reason to consider surgical management is in a patient with an ectopic pregnancy following a previous sterilization procedure. While surgically treating the ectopic pregnancy, a bilateral *salpingectomy* can be concurrently performed to provide effective sterilization for the future.

In comparing methrotrexate to salpingostomy, randomized trials have shown no difference in overall tubal preservation, tubal patency, repeat ectopic pregnancy, or future pregnancies.

Contraceptive considerations

> ✭ TIPS & TRICKS
>
> Following treatment for ectopic pregnancy, or induced or spontaneous abortion, women should be informed about their ability to get pregnant quickly, less than 2 weeks after the procedure. **A woman's short- and long-term reproductive plans should be discussed to help guide her choice of contraceptive method.**

Specific counseling considerations include:

- If the recent pregnancy was unplanned and was the result of a contraceptive failure, it is important to identify the factors that may have contributed to the failure.
- Following a desired pregnancy that ended prematurely, future desires for pregnancy are likely to vary for each patient. Some women hope to get pregnant again as soon as is medically safe. Others may prefer more time to ensure emotional wellbeing before trying to get pregnant again. Still others may not desire another pregnancy in the foreseeable future, and would prefer long-term effective contraception immediately.
- Women with certain medical issues before or during pregnancy may need to delay or avoid pregnancy. Some medical conditions may preclude the use of certain contraceptive methods: refer to the chapter about each specific contraceptive for detailed discussion of cautions and contraindications.
- In general, contraceptive counseling should also include information on method safety, effectiveness, mechanism of action, side effects, protection from sexually transmitted infections, and other method-specific characteristics such as noncontraceptive benefits (e.g. beneficial impact on menstrual bleeding).

Most contraceptive methods can be initiated immediately following treatment or management of ectopic pregnancy and induced or spontaneous abortion. All women should be informed about emergency contraception, especially women who choose not to start a contraceptive method immediately.

> ✭ TIPS & TRICKS
>
> Assuming no immediate complications, nearly all forms of contraception are safe and feasible to begin on the day of a first- or second-trimester abortion or following surgical treatment for ectopic pregnancy, including IUD insertion, placement of subdermal implant, or sterilization.

Contraceptive options for immediate initiation

For most women, it is safe to start any *combined (estrogen-progestin)* or *progestin-only* method of contraception immediately (same day) after treatment of an ectopic pregnancy or at the end of a first- or second-trimester pregnancy. This includes immediate placement of a progestin-only *subdermal implant* at the time of surgery.

Concerns have been raised over early initiation of the vaginal ring; however, no adverse events have been reported when the ring was initiated as early as 5 days following first trimester abortion. Although there is limited data, no adverse reports have been reported with the common clinical practice of immediate initiation of the ring on the day of surgical abortion at Planned Parenthood.

Barrier methods (i.e. condoms) may be used immediately, except for diaphragms and cervical caps (see below).

Immediate IUD insertion

An IUD can safely be inserted at the conclusion of a surgical first- or second-trimester (induced or spontaneous) abortion and after surgical treatment of ectopic pregnancy. There is a higher expulsion rate if an IUD is placed immediately following a second-trimester procedure (approximately 10–15%) compared to the expulsion rate following immediate insertion with first-trimester procedures (approximately 4–6% or interval insertion (approximately 2–5%)). However, the provision of this highly effective contraceptive outweighs the increased risk of expulsion for most women who request this option.

Medical treatment for an induced or spontaneous abortion or an ectopic pregnancy does not always have a clearly defined day of completion to know when to "immediately" initiate an IUD. With medical abortion, it has been shown to be safe to place an IUD at the same visit as ultrasound confirmation of pregnancy expulsion (as early as 1 week following mifepristone).

Following medical treatment of ectopic pregnancy, the serum hCG level is usually followed to zero. However, the patient's ovulatory function often returns before this. Contraception, including IUD insertion, should be initiated as soon as it is apparent that further methrotrexate doses or surgical management will not be necessary—usually within 1 week.

Immediate sterilization

Tubal ligation via laparoscopy or minilaparotomy can also be safely performed at the same time as a first- or second-trimester abortion. However, special attention should be given to counseling patients who request sterilization, to ensure that their choice is not influenced by the stress of their immediate situation and to avoid regret in the future.

If an ectopic pregnancy was the result of a failed female sterilization, greater consideration may be given to surgical management of the ectopic pregnancy if the patient wants to continue to rely on female sterilization for contraception. A concurrent bilateral *salpingectomy* can be performed to ensure effective contraception.

Contraceptive options for delayed initiation

The *diaphragm* or *cervical cap* should not be started for at least 2 weeks following first-trimester abortion, because it is generally recommended to avoid putting anything in the vagina for 2 weeks following the procedure to minimize the risk of infection. Although there is no specific data, the World Health Organization (WHO) recommends waiting 6 weeks after a second-trimester abortion to initiate a diaphragm or cervical cap due to possible changes in anatomy that would affect the fit, similar to following term delivery.

Fertility awareness methods should not be initiated immediately. A woman's menses may take several months to return following an abortion. WHO recommends waiting for three postprocedure menses before utilizing fertility awareness methods.

If a patient wants to use contraception but is unable to choose a method at the time of the abortion, she should be scheduled for a follow-up visit within 1–2 weeks to readdress this. At the very least she should be recommended to use a method such as condoms and/or emergency contraception during the interim.

Contraceptive effects on post-treatment recovery

Multiple studies have evaluated the use of combined oral contraceptives and progestin-only methods immediately following abortion, and there have been no reports of serious adverse events with this practice, including thromboembolic events. No differences in infection rates or patient reported pain have been found.

> **⚗ SCIENCE REVISITED**
>
> - Interestingly, bleeding patterns (amount or duration) are not affected by the immediate initiation of **hormonal contraception**.
> - Patients who have an **IUD** in place following their abortion may experience the same complications as other abortion patients, but pain, irregular or heavy bleeding, or infection are unlikely to be specifically caused by the IUD.

Use of contraception following surgical complications

Complications following induced or spontaneous abortion and treatment for ectopic pregnancy are rare but may impact the initial contraceptive choice, especially the immediate insertion of an IUD. It is generally recommended that an IUD *not* be placed immediately in the setting of hemorrhage, uterine perforation, infection, or hematometra. The patient should be offered an interim contraceptive method, and can return after the complication has resolved for IUD insertion.

Most other complications do not preclude the use of any of the contraceptive methods, except if a woman has experienced a thrombotic event (such as deep vein thrombosis or pulmonary embolus). Patients with these complications should not use estrogen-containing contraceptives.

IUDs and ectopic pregnancy

IUDs are highly effective at preventing pregnancy. However, if there is a contraceptive failure and a pregnancy does occur with IUD use, it is more likely to be ectopic. It is important to note that since the overall pregnancy rate in IUD users is lower compared to noncontraceptors, the absolute number of ectopic pregnancies is lower among IUD users.

> **EVIDENCE AT A GLANCE**
>
> - Past use of an IUD does not lead to an increased risk of ectopic pregnancy
> - Current use of an IUD decreases the risk of ectopic pregnancy as compared to a woman that uses no contraception (0.5 versus 3.25–5.25/1,000 women years, US data).
> - Women with a prior history of ectopic pregnancy can safely use an IUD.

In addition to the changes in FDA labeling, the WHO also supports the routine use of IUDs (both copper T380A and LNG-IUS) in women with a past history of ectopic pregnancy.

Conclusion

Effective contraceptive services are integral to the care of patients undergoing treatment for ectopic pregnancy, and induced or spontaneous abortion. After pregnancy, many women want to delay or avoid getting pregnant again. Therefore, women should be counseled about all available contraceptive options in order to help them choose the method that is safe, effective, convenient, and best meets their short- and/or long-term family planning needs.

Selected references

ACOG Practice Bulletin No. 59. Intrauterine device. Obstet Gynecol 2005;105:223–32.

ACOG Practice Bulletin No. 94. Medical management of ectopic pregnancy. Obstet Gynecol. 2008;111:1479–85.

Davis A, Westhoff C, DeNonno L. Bleeding patterns after early abortion with mifepristone and misoprostol or manual vacuum aspiration. J Am Med Womens Assoc 2000;55:141–4.

Fine PM, Tryggestad J, Meyers NJ, Sangi-Haghpeykar H. Safety and acceptability with the use of a contraceptive vaginal ring after surgical or medical abortion. Contraception 2007;75:367–71.

Finer LB, Henshaw SK. Disparities in rates of unintended pregnancy in the United States, 1994 and 2001. Perspect Sex Reprod Health 2006;38:90–6.

Hajenius PJ, Mol F, Mol BWJ, Bossuyt PMM, Ankum WM, Van der Veen F. Interventions for tubal pregnancy. Cochrane Database Syst Rev 2007;1:CD000324.

Nanda K, Peloggia A, Grimes D, Lopez L, Nanda G. Expectant care versus surgical treatment for miscarriage. Cochrane Database Syst Rev 2006;2:CD003518.

Reeves MF, Lohr PA, Harwood BJ, Creinin MD. Ultrasonographic endometrial thickness after medical and surgical management of early pregnancy failure. Obstet Gynecol 2008;111:106–12.

Sivin I. Dose- and age-dependent ectopic pregnancy risks with intrauterine contraception. Obstet Gynecol 1991;78:291–8.

Sivin I, Stern J. Health during prolonged use of levonorgestrel 20 micrograms/d and the copper TCu 380Ag intrauterine contraceptive devise: a multicenter study. International Committee for Contraception Research (ICCR). Fertil Steril 1994;61:70–7.

Stanwood NL, Grimes DA and Schulz KF. Insertion of an intrauterine contraceptive device after induced or spontaneous abortion: a review of the evidence. Br J Obstet Gynaecol 2001;108:1168–73.

Vonher H. Contraception after abortion and post-partum. Am J Obstet Gynecol 1973;117:1002.

WHO. Medical eligibility criteria for contraceptive use, 4th ed. Geneva: World Health Organization; 2009. Available from: http://www.who.int/reproductivehealth/publications/family_planning/9789241563888/en/index.html.

WHO. Safe abortion: Technical and policy guidance for health systems. Geneva: World Health Organization; 2003.

Xiong X, Buekens P, Wollast E. IUD use and the risk of ectopic pregnancy: a meta-analysis of case-control studies. Contraception 1995;52:23–34.

Zhang J, Gilles JM, Barnhart K, et al. A comparison of medical management with misoprostol and surgical management for early pregnancy failure. N Engl J Med 2005;353:761–9.

Index